# The Medical Interview

## The Three Function Approach

# The Medical Interview

## The Three Function Approach

**STEVEN A. COLE, MD, MA, FAPA**
Professor of Psychiatry, Emeritus
Stony Brook University School of Medicine
Stony Brook, NY

**JULIAN BIRD, MA (CANTAB), FRCP, FRCPSYCH**
Lately Senior Lecturer in Psychiatry
Guy's Kings and St. Thomas's School of Medicine
University of London
London, United Kingdom

SAUNDERS

ELSEVIER

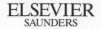

SAUNDERS

1600 John F. Kennedy Blvd.
Ste 1800
Philadelphia, PA 19103-2899

THE MEDICAL INTERVIEW: THE THREE FUNCTION APPROACH        ISBN: 978-0-323-05221-4

---

**Notices**

---

**Library of Congress Cataloging-in-Publication Data**

Cole, Steven A., author, editor of compilation.
 The medical interview: the three function approach / Steven A. Cole, Julian Bird.—Third edition.
     p. ; cm.
 Includes bibliographical references and index.
 ISBN 978-0-323-05221-4 (pbk.)
 I. Bird, Julian, author, editor of compilation. II. Title.
 [DNLM: 1. Medical History Taking. 2. Communication. 3. Physician-Patient Relations. WB 290]
 RC65
 616.07′51–dc23

                                                                                2013037383

*Senior Content Strategist:* James Merritt
*Content Development Specialist:* Jacob Harte
*Publishing Services Manager:* Hemamalini Rajendrababu
*Project Manager:* Saravanan Thavamani
*Design Manager:* Ellen Zanolle
*Marketing Manager:* Debashis Das

Printed in United States of America
Last digit is the print number:   9  8  7  6  5  4  3  2  1

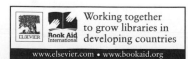

TO

my parents

John and Clara Cole

*I wish you could have lived to see and enjoy this book*


My children and grandchildren

Jamie, Eugenia, Ethan, Monika, Anna, Doug,

Kristen, MaryBeth, Michael,

Siena, Aria, Elliot, Kyra, and Naomi

*You broaden and brighten my life.*


AND

my wife

Mary

*You bring peace and joy.*

*I cherish and treasure our life and love.*

**Thomas L. Campbell, MD**
William Rocktaschel Professor and Chair
Department of Family Medicine
University of Rochester School of Medicine
  and Dentistry
Rochester, NY

**Cecile A. Carson, MD**
Integrated Health Institute
Honeoye, NY

**William Clark, MD, FAACH**
Fellow, Past President, American Academy
  on Communication in Healthcare
Lecturer in Medicine, Harvard Medical
  School
Woolwich, ME

**Mary DeGenaro Cole, MS, FNP-BC**
Faculty, Stony Brook University School of
  Nursing, Stony Brook, NY

**Kathy Cole-Kelly, MS, MSW**
Professor of Family Medicine
Director, Communication in Medicine
Case Western Reserve University School of
  Medicine
Cleveland, OH

**Connie Davis, MN, RN, ARNP, GNP-BC**
Program Director
Centre for Comprehensive Motivational
  Interventions
Hope, BC Canada
Adjunct Clinical Faculty
University of British Columbia
Vancouver, BC Canada

**Roxane Gardner, MD, MPH, DSc**
Assistant Professor Obstetrics & Gynecology
Harvard Medical School
Brigham and Women's Hospital, Boston
Division of Adolescent Gynecology, Boston
  Children's Hospital
Simulation Faculty—Center for Medical
  Simulation
Associate Medical Director, Obstetrics,
  CRICO Patient Safety
Boston, MA

**Geoffrey H. Gordon, MD, FACP**
Staff Physician, Department of Pain
  Management
Northwest Permanente Medical Group
Portland, OR

**Damara Gutnick, MD**
Clinical Assistant Professor of Medicine and
  Psychiatry
New York University Langone School of
  Medicine
New York, NY
Centre for Comprehensive Motivational
  Interventions
Hope, BC Canada

**Khati Hendry, MD, CCFP, FAAFP**
Department Head of Family Practice,
Penticton Regional Hospital and
Managing Partner
Rosedale Medical Associates,
Summerland, BC Canada

**Susan Lane, MD, FACP**
Associate Professor of Clinical Medicine and
Residency Program Director and Vice-Chair
  for Education
Department of Medicine
Stony Brook University School of Medicine
Stony Brook, NY

**Steven Locke, MD**
Associate Psychiatrist
Massachusetts General Hospital
Associate Clinical Professor of Psychiatry
Consultant, The Center for Medical
  Simulation
Boston, MA

**Catherine Nicastri, MD**
Associate Professor of Clinical Medicine
Program Director, Geriatric Fellowship
  Program
Department of Medicine
Stony Brook University School of Medicine
Stony Brook, NY

**Dennis H. Novack, MD**
Professor of Medicine
Associate Dean of Medical Education
Drexel University College of Medicine
Philadelphia, PA

**David J. Steele, PhD**
Senior Associate Dean for Medical
  Education
Professor, Family and Community Medicine
Paul L. Foster School of Medicine
Texas Tech University Health Sciences
  Center at El Paso
El Paso, TX

**Guy Undrill, MB, ChB, MRCPsych**
Consultant Psychiatrist, 2gether NHS Trust
Clinical Lecturer, University of Bristol
Gloucester, UK

**Toni B. Walzer, MD**
Assistant Clinical Professor of Obstetrics,
  Gynecology, and Reproductive Biology
Harvard Medical School
Brigham and Women's Hospital, Boston,
  MA and
Co-Director, Labor & Delivery Program,
  Center for Medical Simulation
Boston, MA

**Joseph Weiner, MD, PhD**
Associate Professor of Clinical Psychiatry and
  Medicine
Hofstra North Shore-LIJ School of Medicine
Hempstead, NY

The publication of the third edition of *The Medical Interview: The Three-Function Approach* is a milestone in the field it introduces: communication between practitioner and patient. Foremost, it is a classic educational book in the field, a leader in use for teaching student doctors, nurse practitioners, and others. In writing a new edition, Dr. Cole and colleagues have updated the book's evidence base, advanced it conceptually, enhanced its practicality, and improved its likely teaching effectiveness. The third is the best edition yet.

When the first edition came out, the field of doctor-patient communications, as it was then called iatrocentrically, had emerged from its charismatic era into first rounds of theoretical and empirical research. This volume moves well beyond that to include an interdisciplinary perspective, a cogent crystallization of what learners need to know and understand, and inclusion of a behaviorally sophisticated yet brief method called Brief Action Planning to help activate patients to commit positively in their own care (i.e., to support patients' self-management of their own health and illnesses). The addition as well of new chapters on specific situations such as health literacy challenges, dealing with bad news, managing chronic care, alcoholism, dealing with errors, and the like, further strengthen the potential curriculum based on this book. The book is now sufficiently strengthened to warrant its adoption for higher levels of learners and to be of interest to practitioners seeking new insight and clarity about their most important clinical tool.

The medical interview is the most important clinical tool available to health practitioners, for both personal and professional reasons. On the personal level, the interview is the task in medicine a practitioner will do the most often and spend the most time on from now until he or she retires. An average primary care practitioner may do between as many as 250,000 interviews in a professional lifetime of 40 years; therefore it is worth doing expertly, cogently, and efficiently.

Professionally the interview is the major medium of care. It determines the problems addressed and helped. It forms the doctor-patient relationship central to the satisfaction of both practitioner and patient. It determines knowledge of the life context of the illness, which may hold the secrets of etiology and healing. It is the medium of patient education about the illness, the diagnostic process, and the therapy. For all these reasons, the interview is well worth the attention of practitioners at every level, throughout a professional lifetime.

In the 1970s, the interview was the subject of charisma and speculation. Teaching was based on the precept that students should do as the teachers do. Teachers were chosen on the basis of self-assertion or charismatic appeal. That all changed with the advent of fast, economical taping of interviews combined with analytic reliability, pioneered by Barbara Korsch and Deborah Roter. Since then, thousands of articles have looked at the content, process, outcomes, and correlates of interviews and interviewers. A pending meta-analysis of communication's impact on cardiovascular outcomes found more than 3500 articles! The medical interview is a subject about which specific, empirical knowledge is expanding rapidly. It is the responsibility of each diligent clinician or future clinician to know at least the main points of this literature, and this book represents one useful starting point.

The bottom line of the literature is that these skills matter every day in each encounter. If one has 10% inefficiency in one's interviewing, one will lose more than 2 years of practice time as a result. If one fails to identify one of the three problems the average patient has in mind during a typical visit, one will overlook more than 200,000 problems over a professional lifetime, many of them critically important!

Some deans and program directors believe skill in the interview just requires talent. It is true that each trainee has a unique complex of interactive strengths and weaknesses, some beginning stronger than others. But virtually everyone can get better through deliberative skills practice with cogent feedback based on sound core concepts and outcomes research. A variety of authors, in the United States, the Netherlands, and the United Kingdom have shown that simple efforts to improve interviewing skills will succeed in changing behavior and improving clinical care. In one such experiment, a single interview practice course of six sessions led to durable improvements still measurable after 6 years. Although there is always room for improvement, the reading of a text such as this accompanied by appropriate exercises can be expected to lead to significantly enhanced mastery of the basics of effective interviewing.

The opposite is equally true. Those interviewing without adequate training and supervision are likely to make one or more serious errors regularly. This will damage diagnostic ability, practitioner satisfaction, and patient satisfaction and adherence.

Both research and practical clinical learning about the interview have been enhanced by recent conceptual advances. The first of these is the recognition that the interview has anatomy and physiology, structure and functions. The structure may be viewed simply as beginning, middle, and end, or more complexly with up to 10 structural elements. Each of these encompasses a series of specific behaviors that if mastered leads to better results. In our own work, around 63 discrete skills were found to be important to teach and learn.

The interview also has functions. Julian Bird and Steven Cole led in the definition of the three function model of the interview, which has enormous heuristic utility in learning about interviewing. The three functions get expressed variously, but the formulation in this book is both authoritative and clear. The three functions, like the structural elements, have specific skills underlying their execution that can and must be learned, practiced, and mastered.

One way in which every level practitioner can uniquely benefit from this volume, as I did, relates to a major revision and evidenced-based evolution of Function Three, "Collaborate for Management."

This development of Function Three parallels an important shift in our understanding of optimal patient care: from clinician-centric "management" to the more powerful, relationship-centered focus on "collaborative management." Function Three now addresses collaboration for patient education and collaborative management to motivate and plan patient self-management of their own health and illnesses. Dr. Cole and colleagues have developed an eight-step, self management support technique, called Brief Action Planning. Chapter 5 describes Brief Action Planning and Chapter 18 adds "Stepped Care Advanced Skills for Action Planning," more advanced applications of Function Three skills for more complex patient care.

To complement the text and classroom, Dr. Cole and colleagues have also developed a web-based training program for Brief Action Planning, an abridged version of which purchasers of the text can use at no cost.

Several approaches enhance the learning of the material taught here. The first is to attempt to practice often and with focused awareness of specific behaviorally defined learning goals. One's chances of accomplishing something are increased if one knows what that something is. Second, expert performance in most fields derives from what Ericsson has called deliberative practice—practice with feedback followed by improved practice. The total amount of practice an individual does correlates in many fields, from playing the violin to chess to surgery, with improved performance, but only a few practice enough to approach mastery. And do your patients not deserve mastery from you? Direct feedback about one's performance through self-review and review with a skilled tutor increases the breadth and depth of possible learning because solo practice is handicapped by one's own blind spots. A sense of scientific curiosity and humanistic wonder will make the work more effective and more fun. The human drama is heightened by illness and we practitioners have the privilege of front row seats. Our patients share with us most of the wisdom and understanding to be obtained in life and we are in a wonderful position to learn from them and their experience.

Dr. Cole and colleagues have created a brief, conceptually clear, clinically relevant text initially focused on beginning students of the practitioner's arts. The book is organized along the lines of the three function model, making the steps to mastery explicit, understandable, and discrete. But there is much here also for the experienced clinician who seeks an introduction to the study of the interview. I would have loved to have a book like this when I started to learn to talk with patients. Despite 40 or so years of scholarship and research in this field, I learned new things and I was genuinely stimulated by this third edition. Students who embark with this book on a lifetime of practice and learning about their core clinical skill will be well and truly launched.

*Mack Lipkin, Jr., MD*
Professor of Medicine, New York University School of Medicine
Founding President, American Academy on Communication in Healthcare
Past President, Society of General Internal Medicine
New York, NY
August, 2013

## What's New?

The second edition of *The Medical Interview: The Three-Function Approach* (2000) has been the assigned or required text in many US medical schools and physician assistant programs, translated into Japanese, and widely adopted internationally. That it may have had even modest educational impact or touched some patients' lives feels both gratifying and humbling. I feel honored and privileged to have this opportunity to develop a third edition.

But it's taken eight years to complete because I had ambitious goals, the most important of which involved a conceptual and operational reformulation of Function Three. Now called, "Collaborate for Management," Function Three focuses on developing partnerships with patients to better support their own self-care for health and illness. With contributions of colleagues, (Mary Cole, Damara Gutnick, and Connie Davis) Chapter Five presents a cornerstone of Function Three, "Brief Action Planning (BAP),"[1] a stepped-care self-management support technique consistent with the principles and practice of Motivational Interviewing (MI) and behavioral change research. A learner-directed web-based training program is available to assist in mastering the knowledge and skills of BAP. Chapter 18, written with Damara Gutnick and Joe Weiner, advances the core skills of BAP into more complex applications of action planning for patients with persistent unhealthy behaviors.[2]

The third edition has many other advances worth noting. Elements of Functions One and Two have matured and also been enriched with evidence-based developments in medical care and communication.

A new chapter on "Presentation and Documentation" will help students learn how to organize the information they collect for oral or written purposes.

Six new topics have been added on important subjects like interviewing about risky drinking and alcohol use, disclosure of medical errors and apology, health literacy, chronic illness, communicating with the psychotic patient, and giving bad news with a new nine-step structured roadmap on sharing "difficult" news. Four chapters have been substantially updated or re-written: interviewing the elderly patient, sexual issues in the interview, culturally competent medical interviewing, and troubling personality styles and somatization.

The last chapter of the book, on integrating structure and function, has also been substantially revised. This chapter delves into other domains of higher-order interviewing in an attempt to provide guidance for experienced clinicians moving toward mastery. Six types of clinical flexibility and six "rules" of interviewing, observed and developed from nearly 40 years of practice, may prove of interest to experienced clinicians and educators for consideration in their own work in patient care or training. The information and ideas presented in Chapter 33 are mostly my own, somewhat speculative, all grounded in my own clinical experience, and based on what Michael Polanyi would call "personal knowledge."[3]

## Who is the Audience?

The book began as a textbook for medical students and retains this focus. However, the core concepts themselves as well as the entire second half of the text has been enriched and expanded to meet the needs of medical residents as well as practicing physicians.

Students and practitioners in allied medical fields, such as nurse practitioners and physician's assistants, as well as dieticians, physical therapists, dentists, health coaches, social workers, psychologists, occupational therapists, etc, will also find the concepts and skills of the Three Function Model useful in their own training and clinical practice. So, although the third edition continues to address the needs of medical students, it has also been consciously enriched to meet the needs of a broad spectrum of other clinicians as well.

## A Note on Language

Because the text will be used by medical students, physicians, allied health practitioners, social workers, psychologists, and others, I often use the generic word "clinician" to describe the person who is reading and learning from the text and speaking to the patient in the dialogues quoted in the text. In many cases, however, I revert back to the use of the term "physician" simply because that comes from the world where I live and work and it sounds natural to me.

In a similar manner, I use the word "patient" to describe the person who is ill, rather than the term "client," which is a term preferred by some clinicians. "Patient" seems to better fit the original purpose of the text.

## Why Use the Three Function Approach?

Many other very good textbooks on medical interviewing are currently available.

Why choose this one?

The third edition of *The Medical Interview: The Three-Function Approach* provides learners or practitioners with a cognitive framework that is simple, logically compelling, and relatively easy to assimilate and master; yet, also robust enough to help us teach and understand higher-order processes of expert communication.

First conceived by Julian Bird, and later developed by me and others, this model offers learners a straightforward approach to conceptualizing essential core components of communication that is rich enough to address subtleties and complexities of expert interviewing.

The three functions address three core objectives of the clinician-patient communication process: (1) build the relationship; (2) assess and understand the patient's problems; and (3) collaborate for management of these problems. The model promotes a clear distinction between 28 core skills that can be developed in a relatively limited period of time and advanced applications of these basic skills.

Advanced applications of the basic skills are described in the second half of the book with respect to many complexities of interviewing that practitioners commonly address. Two specific higher-order Motivational Interviewing skills are presented, with a detailed case example. Whether basic core competencies or advanced and higher order, the Three Function Model serves as a useful template for conceptualizing the full range of communication processes and skills.

Differentiating basic skills from higher-order skills and presenting operational definitions of the basic skills helps learners remain clear-headed about what skills can be realistically attained with limited time and resources. When learners appreciate that higher-order skills require considerably more effort to master, they can avoid the frustration of trying to model the behaviors of truly expert, seemingly "facile" interviewers. The skilled interviewer, in fact, has perfected a finely tuned craft much as a skilled surgeon has developed his or her operating room ability. Acknowledging that such refined skills represent higher-order accomplishments can help learners realize the necessity for dedicated efforts, and practice over time, to achieve such proficiency.

This new text on the medical interview therefore seems worthwhile because it simplifies the task of learning to communicate with patients. By simplifying the task, the text strives to make the process more interesting and more relevant. Furthermore, by providing equal emphasis on each of the three separate functions of the interview, the text underscores the point that the first and third functions (i.e., the relationship and collaborative management aspects of interviewing) represent dimensions of medical care of equal importance to the second and more traditionally emphasized function of the interview (i.e., to assess and understand the patient's problem).

If this book helps even a few clinicians learn better communication skills, the effort to create it will have been worthwhile. If even a few patients benefit, the justification for the book will be self-evident.

*Steven A. Cole*

## References

1. There is an earlier online publication on BAP, Reims K, Gutnick D, Davis C, Cole S: Brief Action Planning: A White Paper, downloadable at www.CentreCMI.ca, January 2013.
2. Ibid
3. Polanyi M: *Personal Knowledge: Towards a Post-Critical Philosophy*, Chicago, 1974, University of Chicago Press.

# ACKNOWLEDGMENTS

Many patients, colleagues, mentors, and trainees have made significant contributions to this book. It is a pleasure to acknowledge my indebtedness and gratitude to them.

Julian Bird developed the original concept of the three function model in London in the mid-1970s and I owe him a considerable intellectual debt. The medical landscape is more efficient and more humane because of his creativity. He contributed a continuous stream of ideas to the model, especially when we worked so closely together in Birmingham, Alabama and during his visits over the years. He provided editorial input and direct contributions to the last two chapters on higher-order skills. For all that, and more, his stamp on the book is organic and indelible.

Aaron Lazare, Mack Lipkin Jr., and Sam Putnam developed a robust elaboration of the original three function concept[1] and their ideas contributed to the model presented here. Ulrich Grueninger, Michael Goldstein, Penny Williamson, and Dan Duffy also developed ideas that contributed significantly.[2]

Mack Lipkin, Jr., introduced me to the generative concepts and methods of learner-centered learning and I am also very grateful to him for his thoughtful and meticulous page-by-page commentary on an early version of the manuscript. Ruth Hoppe and David Steel also read sections of an early manuscript and offered valuable suggestions.

I would like to acknowledge, with warmth, my colleagues from the American Academy on Communication in Healthcare, with whom I learned and grew in the 1980s and 1990s when so many of the original concepts and skills of the three function approach reached higher levels of definition and depth. So many participants in those generative Faculty Development courses I attended touched my life and influenced my thinking, including: William Branch, William Clark, Dennis Cope, Douglas Drossman, Mary Lynn Field, Richard Frankel, Geoff Gordon, Craig Kaplan, Wendy Levinson, Mack Lipkin Jr, Rosalind Mance, Dennis Novack, Tim Quill, John Stoekel, Tony Suchman, Penny Williamson, and Sarah Williams.

I am very grateful to my colleagues in the Centre for Comprehensive Motivational Interventions (CCMI)—Connie Davis, Damara Gutnick, and Kathy Reims—who, along with Mary Cole, were so instrumental in helping me develop Brief Action Planning (BAP) and who now make our ongoing collaborative BAP work so generative. Oliver Cornell deserves special mention for his craftsmanship as our webmaster in creating the online program for BAP; Mary, Damara, and Connie also provided invaluable assistance in developing the online program, and Mary lent her camera-ready expertise to direct and produce the superb videos.

Mary Cole helped develop (e)TACCT,[3] the other foundation for Function Three. She and I presented earlier versions of (e)TACCT to Health Disparities Collaboratives on diabetes and cardiovascular disease for Federally Qualified Health Centers in 2001-2002.

Damara Gutnick was instrumental in suggesting and integrating "change talk" concepts into the theoretical structure of SAAP, Stepped Care Advanced Skills for Action Planning (see Chapter 18). She also contributed all the useful descriptive graphics for that complex and important chapter.

I want to cite Joseph Weiner with special attention, because his intellectual contributions to this third edition permeate many chapters integral to the entire volume. He helped define the new model in its overall conceptualization, not just as a coauthor of Chapters 2, 3, and 18, and author of 27A, but as close friend and intellectual colleague throughout the 8 years of its development. As core faculty at Hofstra North Shore LIJ School of Medicine, he and his colleagues are implementing a 4-year medical school curriculum built around the three function approach, as he himself helped to define it for this text.

The following each contributed chapters to the third edition and have improved it immeasurably: Thomas Campbell, Cecile Carson, William Clark, Mary Cole, Kathy Cole-Kelly, Connie Davis, Roxanne Gardner, Geoff Gordon, Damara Gutnick, Khati Hendry, Susan Lane, Steven Locke, Catherine Nicastri, Dennis Novack, David Steele, Guy Undrill, and Toni Walzer.

Mary Cole, my wife, partner, friend, colleague, fellow clinician, and co-researcher, through many years together, deserves heartfelt appreciation because she lived and breathed the concepts and ideas of this book with me, day and night, when she and we could have, might have, perhaps should have, been doing, thinking, and enjoying other things. Mary deserves very special thanks for her help and support through the trials and efforts of this book; not only for putting up with them and me but also for her very real assistance and contributions towards helping them reach better ultimate outcomes.

I've tried honestly and respectfully to acknowledge Mary's intellectual contributions to the ideas in this book; she is co-author of Chapters 5 and 21, but it is possible or indeed likely that some of her ideas permeate other chapters in ways that I do not fully recall or acknowledge. For those ideas, I want to thank her and acknowledge her ongoing support and intellectual contributions throughout my career to my work in subtle ways that are sometimes hard to specify and recall.

I dedicated this book to my wife, children, grandchildren, and parents. Along with my sister Peggy and hers, they are my family. I appreciate them and thank them for who they are to me and for me.

I would like to thank my editor at Elsevier, James Merritt, especially, and his colleagues Saravanan Thavamani, and Jacob Harte for their help and support and patience through the long process of developing the third edition of the text.

And finally, I owe a special debt of gratitude, more than words can express, to my patients. I feel deeply, that I learned more from them than from anyone else. I would like to say directly to them:

*"If any of you see or read this text, please know that I am so grateful to you for letting me into your lives and offering me the chance to help you. When I have been able to help, I not only felt sincerely enriched myself, but I also learned from you...I learned what I needed to know and grow to write this book."*

Although all of the above individuals can rightly claim credit for strengths found in the text, I assume sole responsibility for its deficits.

*Steven A. Cole*

## References

1. Lazare A, Lipkin M Jr, Putnam SM: Three functions of the medical interview. In Lipkin M Jr, Putnam SM, Lazare A, editors: *The medical interview: clinical care, education and research*, New York, 1995, Springer-Verlag.
2. Grueninger V, Goldstein M, Duffy D: Patient education in the medical encounter: how to facilitate learning, behavior change, and coping. In Lipkin M Jr, Putnam S, Lazare A, editors: *The medical interview: clinical care, education and research*, New York, 1995, Springer-Verlag.
3. Adapted from Mariana Hewson, TACT ("Tailored Approach for Caring Transculturally"), personal communication.

# CONTENTS

# Three Functions of the Medical Interview

# Learning to Interview Using the Three Function Approach: Introduction and Overview

## OVERVIEW

Chapter 1 provides:
1. A brief description of the three function approach.
2. The rationale and need for a clear, pragmatic model to guide teaching and learning.
3. An overview of the different sections of the text.

This book helps students and practicing clinicians learn and, ultimately, master the three core functions of the medical interview. Before anything else, the effective practitioner must be a good communicator. By using the interview as a clinical tool, the skilled clinician strives to accomplish the three broad objectives defined by the model: (1) to build an effective relationship; (2) to assess and understand the patient's problems; and (3) to collaboratively manage those problems.

The medical interview represents the clinician's core tool for assessing and managing all medical problems. To become proficient in medical interviewing, trainees and practitioners must work hard to master basic and complex techniques and must practice these techniques with patients. Teachers of interviewing typically guide their trainees in this journey by observing interviews and providing constructive and detailed feedback with suggestions for improvement and practice. This book has been written to assist teachers, learners, and practicing clinicians in these efforts.

The book is organized around the three core functions of the medical interview, first described by Bird and Cohen-Cole,[1] later modified by Lazare and colleagues,[2] and now updated for this edition to incorporate new evidence and innovative new conceptual approaches. In the current version, the three core functions of the interview are best understood as communication to:
1. Build the relationship.
2. Assess and understand.
3. Collaborate for management.

For the purposes of efficient and effective teaching and learning, the authors articulate a set of 30 explicit and pragmatic operationally defined skills. (See Table of Skills, Appendix 1.) Each of these 30 skills is clearly defined, can be demonstrated through real or simulated patient encounters or videotaped vignettes, and is practiced by trainees with feedback (in simulations, role-play, or with live patients). In the complex reality of the clinical encounter, these core skills serve as the evidence-based foundation for virtually limitless verbal and nonverbal variations that expert clinicians develop to enhance their own personal communication styles.

This interplay encompasses both the science and the art of medical interviewing. The core skills serve as the scientific basis supporting the practitioner's interpretative interpersonal style.

3

*Function one* concerns the relationship and employs skills focused on the emotional domain of the interview, including engagement, rapport, mutual respect, trust, expression of empathy, and development of the affective connection for a working alliance. *Function two* uses inductive and deductive information-gathering techniques to diagnose, assess, and understand patient problems as well as the patient as a person who is experiencing those problems. *Function three* relies primarily on education, patient activation, shared decision making, self-management support, and motivational skills to facilitate collaboration for management of patient problems.

Interview training programs in medical schools have undergone significant evolution in recent years. Previously, many of these courses were focused on history taking as the principal goal of the communication process; that is, a limited conceptualization of only one core function of the interview. The other two functions—the emotional domain and the collaborative management aspect of the encounter—were routinely omitted. Furthermore, even within the realm of the data-gathering domain, courses in medical interviewing often centered on the particular information students needed to collect by the end of the interview, rather than the process of the interview, or the specific interpersonal skills needed to gather the information efficiently. Furthermore, the objective of information gathering was generally unidimensional, focused on making the biomedical diagnosis, rather than multidimensional and focused on understanding the patient's problems in the context of his or her biopsychosocial reality.[3,4]

Traditional interviewing programs operated under the assumption, usually implicit, that the interpersonal skills necessary for effective interviewing were either "naturally" part of the students' repertoire or would develop through the process of accumulated medical experience. It has become clear, however, that the communication skills of medical students do not improve through years of medical training. In fact, research findings and clinical experience confirm that unless students have the benefit of explicit communication skills training, their "natural" communication skills do not improve and often deteriorate throughout the years of medical school and residency.[5,6] More often than not, a hidden curriculum in the clinical socialization process leads to an implicit and sometimes explicit cynical devaluation of the emotional and psychosocial aspects of medical practice.[7] Pejorative labeling of difficult patients (e.g., "crock, troll, gomer") is one manifestation of this type of devaluation.[8] This hidden curriculum leads clinicians into a coarse biomedical position that often misses broad psychosocial dimensions of the patient's illness and thus fails to integrate psychosocial management principles into a care plan.

On the other hand, recent research findings, along with contemporary changes in the culture of medical education, have facilitated the emergence of medical interviewing courses that focus specifically on developing interpersonal skills needed for efficient and effective medical communication.[9,10] Most medical schools in the United States and internationally now provide broad communication skills training programs.[11,12] Licensing examinations for U.S. medical students now have a clinical skills (CS) component requiring demonstration of interpersonal competencies. Nursing practitioner training, physician assistants programs, and virtually all allied medical training programs (e.g., occupational therapy, physical therapy, speech therapy) also include communication preparation and practice standards that routinely require mastery of interpersonal competencies. The Accreditation Council on Graduate Medical Education (ACGME) has identified interpersonal skills as one of the six core competencies for all graduate medical trainees, regardless of specialty.[13] Consequently, all ACGME-approved graduate medical education programs are required to have interpersonal training programs for accreditation and are required to provide documentation of competency of all their trainees in these skills. Similar developments have occurred with respect to the Liaison Committee on Medical Education concerning standards for medical student training.

Despite this explosion of interest and demand for interpersonal skills education, however, it is the authors' impression that most current courses still lack a pragmatic, yet comprehensive conceptual framework that can help learners organize the complexities of medical communication. This text provides such a tool to help organize teaching and learning.

This model provides an explicit and pragmatic overview of the communication process that helps trainees understand the larger goals of interview training while developing concrete skills associated with each of only three core functions. By identifying these three core functions of the interview and describing 30 specific operationally defined skills that serve each core function, the model assists learners as well as practicing clinicians develop a conceptual framework to master the techniques of good interviewing that will help them throughout their medical careers.

The book is organized so that each of the three core functions of the interview can be taught and learned separately. This format is artificial to some extent because, in practice, relationship building and collaborative management issues overlap with the assessment process, and vice versa. However, for the purposes of educational clarity the three functions are addressed separately.

Some programs may choose to focus on only one or two of the three functions discussed in this text. This book can easily be adapted for these approaches as well. For example, some courses may not examine collaborative management in basic courses. In this case, the sections of the book dealing with the third function could be excluded. Conversely, some programs (perhaps for more advanced learners) may themselves focus primarily on collaborative management. The book has been written so that different sections may be used separately, depending on the needs of the educational program for which it is assigned.

In Part I, Three Functions of the Medical Interview, the text begins with an elaboration of each of the three functions of the interview and a description of the specific skills (including basic nonverbal skills) useful for achieving each of the functional goals. This foundation is essential for all learners; that is, medical students, nurse practitioners and physician assistants, graduate physicians in training, as well as practicing clinicians.

Parts II, III, and IV are focused on the needs of students learning to interview patients for the first time. Chapter 6 asks and answers "Ten Common Concerns" for medical and other beginning students as they take their initial steps into the clinical venue. Chapters 7 to 14 present the common structural view of the interview. As described by Lipkin and associates,[14] the structural view of the interview identifies the concrete, sequential stages in which expert clinicians usually conduct an interview. This text builds upon previous descriptions of interview structure and presents an integrated view of the three functions of the interview (as described in this text) within the classic contextual structure of the medical interview. This section includes the Opening, Chief Complaint (and problem survey, patient perspective, and agenda setting), History of Present Illness, Past Medical History, Family History, Patient Profile and Social History, Review of Systems, and Mental Status. Part IV contains a new chapter for this edition describing the basic elements for the write-up (documentation) and the verbal presentation.

Chapters 16 and 17 in Part V focus on understanding patients' emotional responses to chronic illness. These two chapters review both normal and maladaptive patient reactions and present clinician communication strategies for both.

Part VI, Advanced Applications, more specifically addresses the needs of advanced trainees (e.g., residents) and practicing clinicians (e.g., physicians, nurse practitioners, physician assistants). Thirteen chapters cover wide-ranging evidence-based topics including (among others) stepped-care advanced skills for action planning, medical errors and apology, health literacy, chronic illness, risky drinking, interviewing the elderly, personality problems, and family interviewing. Four chapters in Part VII address other higher-order communication competencies, including nonverbal skills, use of the self in medical care, and using psychological principles in the interview. The final chapter in this section, on Integrating Structure and Function, has been revised substantially for this third edition and includes a discussion of higher-order communication processes and skills such as clinical inference and cognitive/communication flexibility and introduces six new principles ("rules") to guide highly skilled levels of communication.

In conclusion, the model has also found applications outside medicine, in the business community for programs on negotiation, and in journalism and correctional (police) work for programs on interviewing. This book can be adapted for use in these settings, as well as any other context requiring excellence in interpersonal communication.

## Summary

Chapter 1:
1. Provides a brief overview of the three-function approach.
2. Discusses the rationale and need for a pragmatic, clear conceptual model to organize teaching and learning.
3. Reviews the content of the different sections of the book.

### References

1. Bird J, Cohen-Cole SA: The three function model of the medical interview. An educational device. *Adv Psychosom Med* 20:65–88, 1990.
2. Lazare A, et al: Three functions of the medical interview. In Lipkin M, Jr, et al, editors: *The medical interview: clinical care, education, and research*, 3–19, New York, 1995, Springer.
3. Novack DH, et al: Medical interviewing and interpersonal skills teaching in US medical schools. Progress, problems, and promise. *JAMA* 269(16):2101–2105, 1993.
4. Stoeckle JD, Billings JA: A history of history-taking: the medical interview. *J Gen Intern Med* 2(2):119–127, 1987.
5. Poole AD, Sanson-Fisher RW: Understanding the patient: a neglected aspect of medical education. *Soc Sci Med Med Psychol Med Sociol* 13A(1):37–43, 1979.
6. Bellini LM, Shea JA: Mood change and empathy decline persist during three years of internal medicine training. *Acad Med* 80(2):164–167, 2005.
7. Lempp H, Seale C: The hidden curriculum in undergraduate medical education: qualitative study of medical students' perceptions of teaching. *BMJ* 329(7469):770–773, 2004.
8. Cohen-Cole SA, Friedman CP: The language problem: integration of psychosocial variables into medical care. *Psychosomatics* 24(1):52–55, 59–60, 1983.
9. Yedidia MJ, et al: Effect of communications training on medical student performance. *JAMA* 290(9):1157–1165, 2003.
10. Kalet A, et al: Teaching communication in clinical clerkships: models from the Macy initiative in health communications. *Acad Med* 79(6):511–520, 2004.
11. Washer P: *Clinical communication skills*, New York, Oxford Core Texts Series, 2009, Oxford University Press.
12. Makoul G, Schofield T: Communication teaching and assessment in medical education: an international consensus statement. Netherlands Institute of Primary Health Care. *Patient Educ Couns* 37(2):191–195, 1999.
13. Delzell JE, Jr, Ringdahl EN, Kruse RL: The ACGME core competencies: a national survey of family medicine program directors. *Fam Med* 37(8):576–580, 2005.
14. Lipkin M, Putnam SM, Lazare A: *The medical interview: clinical care, education, and research*, New York, Frontiers of Primary Care, 1995, Springer-Verlag.

# Three Functions: The Basic Model

Steven Cole ■ Julian Bird ■ Joseph S. Weiner

## OVERVIEW

Chapter 2 provides:
1. A description of the basic model.
2. A detailed discussion and justification (with evidence) for the importance of each of the three core functions.

The three function model of the medical interview was created to help students and practicing clinicians master a core set of basic and advanced skills to facilitate empathic, efficient, and effective communication with their patients. The set of 30 discrete competencies described in this text provide an evidence-based foundation from which trainees and clinicians in practice can develop further higher-order skills as well as their own personal communication styles.

The text describes three functions that address all the core tasks of the medical encounter: (1) build the relationship; (2) assess and understand patient problems; and (3) collaborate for management. Each function is associated with a specific set of operationally defined communication behaviors that can help the clinician achieve objectives related to each specific function. The book describes each interviewing behavior in detail and demonstrates how these skills can be used in the communication process. This chapter describes the core concepts in more detail and discusses the logic and the evidence supporting their importance for efficient, effective medical practice.

## Function One: Build the Relationship

The first function of the interview addresses the physician's primary task: to build and maintain an effective clinician-patient relationship.[1,2] An effective partnership serves as the foundation for every medical encounter, regardless of whether the encounter concerns acute emergency care or an episode within a long-term relationship over time. Conversely, a troubled clinician-patient relationship leads to inefficient assessment and problematic management.[3] The experienced medical practitioner uses relationship-building skills from the first moment of the interview throughout the assessment and management process to engender trust and forge a working alliance.

In general, clinicians build rapport and trust by communicating a sense of personal caring. The most efficient and profound pathway to rapport comes via attention to the *emotional* domain of patients' problems. The illness experience, for example, pain, discomfort, disability, and the threat of death, invariably provokes numerous and sometimes complex emotional reactions for patients and their families. Illness usually leads to feelings of anxiety about the unknown, sadness or depression about losses or potential losses, and anger about the impact of illness on quality of life.

No one escapes these emotional issues, neither providers nor patients. All patients must deal with the emotional domain of illness. The child with juvenile-onset diabetes must cope with the lifelong burden of chronic illness and the impact on peer relationships, school adjustment, and family life. The young mother with multiple sclerosis faces a future of uncertain disability with frightening implications for her ability to care for her children in the way she would like. The middle-aged executive with coronary artery disease has to deal with a life-threatening illness that may affect income, career opportunities, and family life. Furthermore, coping with illnesses such as coronary artery disease usually entails the additional challenge of attempting to accomplish major lifestyle changes (e.g., stopping smoking, adjusting to healthier diets, starting to exercise). The terminal cancer patient and family must find ways to deal with the inevitability of death with its associated emotional turmoil.

Each emotionally charged illness leads to unique reactions in different individuals. The manner in which clinicians respond to patients' emotions will influence the quality of rapport and affect patient satisfaction and self-management, adherence, adaptation, as well as the physiologic course and outcome of the illness itself. The evidence supporting these assertions is strong.[3-8] Mumford and associates, for example, reviewed 34 controlled studies of emotionally supportive or educational interventions after surgery or myocardial infarctions. Patients in the experimental groups suffered fewer physical and emotional complications of illness and they were discharged from hospitals an average of 2 days earlier than were patients in the control groups.[9] Other studies indicate that patients who are more satisfied with their physicians are more likely to adhere to treatment recommendations and that physicians who are more skilled in the emotional domain of patient interaction are likely to have more satisfied patients.[10,11] Health care providers who have been trained in interviewing skills have been shown to be better able to detect and manage emotional distress in their patients who in turn report better emotional outcomes.[12] Similarly, patient centeredness on the part of the physician, partnership, and participatory decision making between the physician and the patient have been shown to lead to improved physical outcome in hypertension, diabetes, and arthritis.[8]

In general, research documenting the relevance of physician-patient relationships to the outcome of illness emanates from a theoretical perspective called the biopsychosocial model of illness.[13] This view of illness asserts that psychological and social variables play a key role in the development, course, and outcome of all illnesses. Persuasive scientific evidence supports this model: meta-analysis of 27 prospective studies demonstrates that psychosocial stress predicts the subsequent onset of upper respiratory infections;[14] meta-analysis of more than 300 studies indicates that acute and chronic stress is associated with significant impairments of multiple measures of immune functioning;[15] depression or depressive symptoms are associated with a two- to fivefold increase in post-MI and post-CABG complications or death;[16,17] depression predicts subsequent development of coronary artery disease, cerebrovascular disease, and diabetes;[16] low social support has been associated in prospective studies with subsequent death, even after controlling for other health-related variables such as previous health status, smoking, visits to the doctor, and social class; meta-analysis of 18 prospective studies shows that stress is associated with onset and course of inflammatory bowel disease.[18] Numerous other studies and reviews of similar data are available.[7,18-23]

A basic tenet of the biopsychosocial model of illness is that physicians who are both aware of the psychosocial dimensions of illness and skilled in the assessment and management of these variables will deliver optimal patient care.

**The three function model of the medical interview has been carefully designed to serve as the vehicle for applying the biopsychosocial model in actual clinical practice.**

Elaboration of the first function explicitly addresses the need for clinicians to attend to the psychological, emotional, and relational aspects of their communication with patients. Because the emotional domain of medical practice plays such a key role in patient outcome, students and practicing clinicians will inevitably improve the care they provide by learning the explicit communication skills that improve competencies related to this function.

To be sure, most students and medical practitioners already possess intuitive abilities to respond to patients' emotions. In many situations, helping a patient who is anxious or sad may simply require the use of "natural" empathic skills. As Peabody pointed out in a classic article, originally published in JAMA in 1927:

> One of the essential qualities of the physician is interest in humanity, for the secret of the care of the patient is caring for the patient.[24]

On the other hand, numerous studies, clinical observations, and physicians' responses to surveys indicate that this intuitive ability may not be sufficient. The intensity of busy practices and the wide variety of patients' emotional responses understandably demand more knowledge and skill in the emotional domain of clinician-patient relationship building than many practitioners naturally possess without additional training. For example, although approximately 20% of medical patients suffer from significant psychiatric disorders (primarily anxiety, depression, and substance abuse), studies indicate that, in general, their primary care physicians do not recognize half of these disorders.[25] Undergraduate or graduate medical training that does not explicitly address the recognition and management of the emotional aspects of general medical illness may, therefore, not prepare trainees adequately for their future practice of medicine. Training in communication skills has been shown to be effective in improving detection and management of psychiatric illness in primary care as well as overall clinician-patient rapport.[12,26]

The first function of the three function model of the medical interview focuses on the emotional domain of clinical practice. Five skills can be demonstrated and practiced to help learners master basic approaches to this core and sometimes-difficult aspect of interviewing. Although there are certainly many ways to build trust and a working alliance, students who learn to respond to patients' emotions using the five basic interventions described in this book will be better able to rely on their own intuitive inclinations and abilities as they become more expert clinicians. Furthermore, research indicates that physicians who are better able to respond to patients' emotional distress report higher satisfaction of their own.[10]

Students and practitioners interested in learning more sophisticated strategies for helping patients cope with emotions (including supportive, insight-oriented, cognitive, or behavioral strategies) can appropriately build these higher-order skills upon the foundation of the basic skills described in this text.[27]

## Function Two: Assess and Understand the Patient's Problems

The second function of the interview concerns the need to obtain information to assess and understand the patient's problems. Experts rate the interview as more important than either the physical examination or laboratory investigations to make accurate diagnoses. Perhaps three fourths of all diagnoses can still be made based on the history alone, despite the technologic innovations of modern medicine.[28] The skillful clinician uses data-gathering skills to assess and understand the patient's problems, arrive at diagnostic formulations, and develop collaborative management strategies.

Collecting accurate information in a time-efficient manner is recognized as a universal goal for medical practice. Occasionally, these two goals (accuracy and brevity) may be in opposition. For example, in an effort to be efficient, physicians may rush their patients and miss important information. When Beckman and Frankel recorded interviews between primary care physicians and their patients, they found that in 69% of interviews, physicians interrupted their patients within the first 18 seconds of the encounter. Of even greater concern, these interruptions led to decreased accuracy of the physicians' understanding of the patients' problems and to incomplete collection of data. In 77% of the interviews the patients' reasons for coming to the physicians were not fully elicited.[29]

This seminal and widely cited study was published in 1984. Since that time, many medical schools developed communication skills training programs to address these obstacles, and the medical literature continued to encourage practicing physicians to address these issues in their own practices. To establish the extent to which this new emphasis on medical interviewing may have altered common (negative) habits of interrupting patients, the Beckman-Frankel study was repeated fifteen years later in another city, with a much larger number of patients and physicians and a more systematic methodology. Unfortunately, the results were virtually identical, indicating the continued existence of these tendencies and the continuing need for basic communication skills instruction at all levels of training and practice.[30]

The goal of the second function of the interview is collection of accurate, sufficient, and relevant data, as efficiently as possible. Understanding the patient's "explanatory model" of his or her symptoms, realizing the impact of illness on the patient's quality of life, and appreciating the patient's expectations and preferences for the encounter all contribute to achieving optimal outcomes through the collaborative management process (Function Three).[2,31-33] Reliance on a small set of evidence-based skills contributes to the clinician's goal to assess and understand. Eight core skills of Function Two are described in detail in Chapter 4.

## Function Three: Collaborate for Management

Clinicians rely on the third function of the interview to collaborate for management: to educate patients for shared decision making, to support patient self-management, and to motivate patients for adaptive health behaviors. Because the third function addresses all of these separate but related objectives, it is clearly the most complex of the three functions of the interview, served by 14 basic skills and two advanced skills.

Patients often do not understand their clinicians. For example, patients who were asked to discuss their illness and its treatment (even immediately after leaving their physicians' offices) could correctly identify only about 50% of critical information.[34] Additional research demonstrates that about 50% of patients do not know the medications they are supposed to take. This lack of fundamental information may be attributable in part to inadequate patient education by physicians and the health care team.[35] It seems reasonable that clinicians who learn to communicate better will have patients who understand more about their illness, who know the treatment recommendations better, and who will be more likely to adhere to treatment recommendations. A recent meta-analysis of 167 studies indicated that patients of physicians with better communication skills had, on average, 20% higher rates of adherence. Patients of physicians who had been exposed to communication training had 1.62 higher likelihood of improved adherence.[11,36]

Patient nonadherence is another major problem in current medical practice. Hundreds of studies indicate that between 22% and 72% of patients do not follow their doctors' recommendations. The percentage of nonadherent patients varies according to illness category (e.g., 23% nonadherence in medications for acute illness vs. 45% for illness prevention) and outcome measured (e.g., 54% nonadherence to appointments for prevention and 72% nonadherence to diets). It is worth noting, however, that these numbers, in general, do not vary according to the educational level or socioeconomic status of the patient.

Many physicians spend a great deal of time trying to educate or motivate patients, but few practitioners have received any training in strategies to do this efficiently or effectively. There is good evidence that such training can improve physician skill, patient knowledge, patient satisfaction, and, ultimately, patient adherence and, most importantly, physical outcome.[11]

Recent evidence has underscored the relationship between certain lifestyle behaviors (e.g., overeating, alcohol consumption, tobacco use, lack of exercise) and negative health consequences. Physicians are becoming increasingly involved with attempts to influence patients' high-risk health behaviors. To achieve effectiveness in such areas, physicians can benefit from training in the empirically validated strategies that help patients change these behaviors.[37]

This text raises communication strategies regarding education, patient self-management support, and motivation to a level of importance equal to that of relationship building and assessment. To be sure, the ultimate impact of a clinician's rapport-building or assessment skills on patient care may be entirely undermined by his or her inability to achieve patient adherence to treatment recommendations. Therefore, a concrete and pragmatic set of educational, self-management support and motivational strategies is recommended, in this text, for all medical, nurse practitioner, and physician-assistant education. Learners interested in developing higher-order skills in this area will be directed to other sources for future learning (www.ComprehensiveMI.com; www.CentreCMI.ca).

## Summary

Chapter 2:
1. Provides a description of the basic model.
2. Provides a detailed discussion and justification (with evidence) for the importance of each of the three core functions.

## References

1. Tresolini C: *The Pew-Fetzer Task Force: health professions education and relationship centered care*, San Francisco, 1994, Pew Healthy Professions Commission.
2. Suchman AL, Hinton-Walker P, Botelho RJ, editors: *Partnerships in healthcare: transforming relational process*, Rochester, 1998, University of Rochester Press.
3. Mauksch LB, et al: Relationship, communication, and efficiency in the medical encounter: creating a clinical model from a literature review. *Arch Intern Med* 168(13):1387–1395, 2008.
4. Roter D, Hall JA: *Doctors talking with patients/patients talking with doctors: improving communication in medical visits*, ed 2, Westport, Conn., 2006, Praeger, pp xvi, 238.
5. Pedersen R: Empirical research on empathy in medicine-A critical review. *Patient Educ Couns* 76(3):307–322, 2009.
6. Switankowsky I: Empathy as a foundation for the biopsychosocial model of medicine. *Hum Healthy Care* 4(2):E5, 2004.
7. Zanbelt LC, et al: Medical Specialists' patient-centered communication and patient-reported outcomes. *Med Care* 44(4):330–339, 2007.
8. Stewart MA: Effective physician-patient communication and health outcomes: a review. *CMAJ* 152(9):1423–1433, 1995.
9. Mumford E, Schlesinger HJ, Glass GV: The effect of psychological intervention on recover from surgery and heart attacks: an analysis of the literature. *Am J Public Health* 72(2):141–151, 1982.
10. Suchman AL, et al: Physician satisfaction with primary care office visits. Collaborative Study Group of the American Academy on Physician and Patient. *Med Care* 31(12):1083–1092, 1993.
11. Roter DL, Hall JA: Communication and adherence: moving from prediction to understanding. *Med Care* 47(8):823–825, 2009.
12. Roter DL, et al: Improving physicians' interviewing skills and reducing patients' emotional distress. A randomized clinical trial. *Arch Intern Med* 155(17):1877–1884, 1995.
13. Engel GL: The need for a new medical model: a challenge for biomedicine. *Science* 196(4286):129–136, 1977.

14. Pedersen A, Zachariae R, Bovbjerg D: Influence of psychological stress on upper respiratory infection—A meta-analysis of prospective studies. *Psychosom Med* 72:823–832, 2010.
15. Segerstrom SC, Miller GE: Psychological stress and the human immune system: a meta-analytic study of 30 years of inquiry. *Psychol Bull* 130(4):601–630, 2004.
16. Rozanski A, et al: The epidemiology, pathophysiology, and management of psychosocial risk factors in cardiac practice: the emerging field of behavioral cardiology. *J Am Coll Cardiol* 45(5):637–651, 2005.
17. Blumenthal JA, Lett HS: Depression and cardiac risk. *J Cardiopulm Rehabil* 25(2):78–79, 2005.
18. Camara RJ, et al: The role of psychological stress in inflammatory bowel disease: quality assessment of methods of 18 prospective studies and suggestions for future research. *Digestion* 80(2):129–139, 2009.
19. Grippo AJ, Johnson AK: Stress, depression and cardiovascular dysregulation: a review of neurobiological mechanisms and the integration of research from preclinical disease models. *Stress* 12(1):1–21, 2009.
20. Zupancic ML: Acute psychological stress as a precipitant of acute coronary syndromes in patients with undiagnosed ischemic heart disease: a case report and literature review. *Prim Care Companion J Clin Psychiatry* 11(1):21–24, 2009.
21. Karasek R: The stress-disequilibrium theory: chronic disease development, low social control, and physiological de-regulation. *Med Lav* 97(2):258–271, 2006.
22. Takkouche B, Regueira C, Gestal-Otero JJ: A cohort study of stress and the common cold. *Epidemiology* 12(3):345–349, 2001.
23. Gwaltney JM, Jr, Hayden FG: Psychological stress and the common cold. *N Engl J Med* 326(9):644–645; author reply 645-646, 1992.
24. Peabody FW: Landmark article March 19, 1927: The care of the patient. By Francis W. Peabody. *JAMA* 252(6):813–818, 1984.
25. Mant A: Is it depression? Missed diagnosis: the most frequent issue. *Aust Fam Physician* 28(8):820, 1999.
26. Jenkins V, Fallowfield L: Can communication skills training alter physicians' beliefs and behavior in clinics? *J Clin Oncol* 20(3):765–769, 2002.
27. Novack DH: Therapeutic aspects of the clinical encounter. *J Gen intern Med* 2(5):346–355, 1987.
28. Peterson MC, et al: Contributions of the history, physical examination, and laboratory investigation in making medical diagnoses. *West J Med* 156(2):163–165, 1992.
29. Beckman HB, Frankel RM: The effect of physician behavior on the collection of data. *Ann Intern Med* 101(5):692–696, 1984.
30. Marvel MK, et al: Soliciting the patient's agenda: have we improved? *JAMA* 281(3):283–287, 1999.
31. Yedidia MJ, et al: Effect of communications training on medical student performance. *JAMA* 290(9):1157–1165, 2003.
32. Eisenthal S, et al: "Adherence" and the negotiated approach to patienthood. *Arch Gen Psychiatry* 36(4):393–398, 1979.
33. Kleinman A, Eisenberg L, Good B: Culture, illness, and care: clinical lessons from anthropologic and cross-cultural research. *Ann Intern Med* 88(2):251–258, 1978.
34. Stewart M: Patient recall and comprehension after the medical visit. In Lipkin M, Jr, editor: *The medical interview: clinical care, education, and research*, NY. P, 1995, Springer, pp 525–529.
35. Kravitz RL, et al: Recall of recommendations and adherence to advice among patients with chronic medical conditions. *Arch Intern Med* 153(16):1869–1878, 1993.
36. Zolnierek KB, Dimatteo MR: Physician communication and patient adherence to treatment: a meta-analysis. *Med Care* 47(8):826–834, 2009.
37. Whitlock EP, et al: Evaluating primary care behavioral counseling interventions: an evidence-based approach. *Am J Prev Med* 22(4):267–284, 2002.

# Function One: Build the Relationship

Steven Cole ▪ Julian Bird ▪ Joseph S. Weiner

## OVERVIEW

Chapter 3 reviews:
1. The importance of the relationship for optimal care
2. Nonverbal communication skills
3. Empathic communication
4. Reflection
5. Legitimation
6. Empathic Communication to Deepen Understanding (ECDU) (ECDU = Reflection + Legitimation + Exploration)
7. Support
8. Partnership
9. Respect
10. The acronym P(E)ARLS can be used to aid learners to remember five skills to build the relationship.
11. Rule #1: Respond to Patient's Feelings as Soon as They Appear

The clinician-patient relationship stands as the cornerstone of all medical care. The first function of the interview, Build the Relationship, relies upon a set of emotional response skills and stands as uniquely important among all the communication skills practitioners can develop.

Patients expect their doctors and caregiving clinicians to be knowledgeable and technically competent. But they also want and need their doctors to be good listeners, supportive, and emotionally available. Clinicians with good relationship skills will have patients who are more satisfied and who will be more likely to adhere to treatment recommendations.[1] Furthermore, the practitioner with good relationship skills will cope with emotionally troubling situations more easily and will, in general, find the clinical practice of medicine more enjoyable. Such a physician will be able to give more to patients emotionally and will, in turn, get more satisfying responses from them.[2,3] Clinicians with good relationship skills will have patients who are much less likely to sue them when unexpected bad outcomes occur or even when mistakes are made.[4-6]

This chapter describes a group of basic skills that help build the clinician-patient relationship: (1) nonverbal skills; (2) reflection; (3) legitimation; (4) support; (5) partnership; and (6) respect. These skills build rapport through engendering patient trust, facilitating the physician-patient working alliance, and communication of empathic caring. Once learned, these skills can be integrated into the student's or practitioner's natural response set. This can then provide the foundation for interested learners to master higher-order skills for continued (and more challenging) relationship building or for helping patients cope better with emotional distress.[7-11]

## Nonverbal Skills

The nonverbal behavior of the physician contributes significantly to the overall quality of the doctor-patient relationship.[12] Appropriate body posture (forward lean), body movements, facial expression, tone and rate of speech, touch, and the space between doctor and patient can convey an attitude of concern and warmth far beyond the impact of any specific words that may be uttered. Quiet, attentive listening conveys interest and builds rapport more powerfully than virtually any other action or utterance the physician can make.[12,13]

Physicians should, therefore, strive for consistency between their verbal and nonverbal behavior. For example, if there is a disjunction between the doctor's verbal statements of concern and his or her nonverbal behavior (which may, for example, indicate boredom or contempt), the nonverbal message will usually prevail in the patient's mind.[14]

An emerging body of research supports the importance of doctors' nonverbal behavior. Doctors who establish appropriate eye contact are more likely to detect emotional distress in their patients.[15] Doctors who perform better on tests of nonverbal sensitivity have patients who are more satisfied.[1] Doctors who lean forward and have an open body posture also have more satisfied patients.[12,13,16]

In addition, the nonverbal behavior of the patient is a key or window into his or her emotional life. Patients express their emotional states through facial expressions, body posture, movement, tone and inflection of voice, and physical manifestations of autonomic nervous system reactivity (e.g., sweaty palms or a flushed face). Skilled physicians who are interested in their patients' emotional states will look for these signs and consider their importance at every stage of the communication process.

In general, clinicians should establish and keep comfortable eye contact with patients throughout the interview. This is essential to facilitate active and effective listening as well as to observe new emotional cues. As with all rules, there are exceptions; angry, suspicious, or paranoid patients may perceive steady eye contact as provocative.

Thoughtful attention to the use of space also facilitates rapport. Vertical space between the doctor and patient (e.g., not standing while the patient sits) should be minimized and horizontal space (e.g., not too close or too far) should be carefully planned. Chapter 25 on nonverbal communication discusses all of these issues in more depth.

## Empathy

Empathy starts with an individual's appreciation, understanding, and acceptance of someone else's life situation. The communication of this understanding and acceptance completes the empathic process and becomes, in virtually every situation, the most helpful, meaningful, and comforting intervention one person can have with another. A parent soothes an upset child by letting the child know that the distress is understood, appreciated, and accepted. Friends and lovers do the same. Similarly, a physician can best build rapport and respond to patients' emotions and thoughts by communicating empathy.[16-23]

Communicating an empathic understanding of a patient's predicament is clearly the most important relationship-building skill the clinician can possess. There are many ways to communicate empathy effectively. The challenge of learning empathic skills lies in the ability to both master basic interventions and integrate these into a natural interpersonal style that feels genuine to the clinician and patient.

In addition, nonverbal behaviors can sometimes communicate empathy more effectively than concrete statements. A sympathetic look, attentive silence, or simple touch (e.g., a hand on the arm or shoulder) can all effectively tell a patient that the clinician hears his or her distress and is in tune with it.

Unfortunately, many medical students and, indeed, practicing physicians believe that empathic understanding and the ability to communicate empathically are "basic" (i.e., "inborn") human traits that cannot be taught. However, research indicates the contrary. Without specific training in empathic communication, medical students and medical residents commonly demonstrate little growth in their empathic abilities (over the course of training) and occasionally even decreased levels of empathy in their relationships with patients over time. Although many studies have suggested a rather sharp decrease in empathic communication over the course of medical training,[24] other research indicates more complex results,[25] and a recent meta-analysis indicated very modest changes, at best, in either direction.[26]

On the other hand, targeted training efforts have been shown to improve empathic skills. Randomized, controlled trials indicate that students and practicing physicians who have participated in training programs or communication workshops have improved empathy skills, including consequent improvement in patient outcome when measured.[8,27-30]

Most physicians already possess considerable and intuitive empathic abilities, but the challenges of medical practice require the development of additional skills, such as expressing empathy under time pressures, often with patients they have never before met.

This chapter describes two operational components of empathic communication, *reflection* and *legitimation,* which can be used to facilitate and focus the physician's response to patients' emotional distress. "Reflection" refers to the physician recognizing and naming the emotional or cognitive response of the patient, and "legitimation" refers to the physician's confirming that the response is understandable and acceptable.

## REFLECTION

Reflection is a straightforward concept drawn from Rogerian psychology.[31] It refers to a physician's statement of an observed feeling or thought of the patient. For example, when the clinician notices that a patient begins to look sad when discussing the illness of a parent, the clinician can "reflect" this feeling by saying something like the following:

> **PHYSICIAN:** *You look sad right now.*
>
> or
>
> **PHYSICIAN:** *I can see this is upsetting to you.*
>
> or
>
> **PHYSICIAN:** *This is hard to talk about.*

This type of reflective comment usually helps the provider communicate empathic concern for the patient's emotional situation. In actual practice, such comments function as facilitators and usually give patients "permission" to talk more about the feelings or thoughts they experience. Physicians can then listen attentively as patients go on to explain and clarify more about what they are experiencing.

The specific words are much less important than the fact that the clinician has interrupted the factual exchange of information to notice and respond to the patient's emotional state. This is a critically important event in the building of a relationship and demonstrates to the patient that the doctor is concerned about the patient as a person.

An example of a reflective comment might occur just after a clinician notices that a patient looks sad or teary eyed and might say the following in a supportive tone of voice:

> **PHYSICIAN:** *I can see that you seem a bit upset right now.*

Sometimes clinicians are reluctant to use reflective comments to encourage the patient to express feelings more deeply. They may feel that this will open a "Pandora's box" of emotions, or that empathic comments will push patients to express feelings that they might otherwise wish to keep private. To the contrary, it is generally helpful and supportive to allow patients the opportunity to express verbally the feelings that are near the surface of awareness. Such interventions help develop rapport and actually contribute to the overall efficiency of the interview. Furthermore, despite the belief that such attention to the emotional domain of patient care increases interview time, research indicates the contrary: after training, empathic communication by primary care physicians improved numerous outcomes of importance (e.g., recognition of emotional disorders, patient satisfaction, disclosure of information, and decreased emotional distress) *without increasing overall interview time.*[27-29]

In general, initial reflective comments should be presented in a manner that is the least threatening to a patient and in terms he or she is likely to accept. Lazare[14] has correctly pointed out that the premature use of terminology indicating levels of emotion deeper than the patient is ready to acknowledge may interfere with rapport or, even worse, lead to the patient experiencing guilt or shame. For example, it is usually better to tell the angry patient something like, "You seem a bit frustrated," rather than, "You seem very angry." Similarly, a depressed patient should be told initially, "I can tell you're down," rather than, "You seem to be in despair." Or when a patient who disputes a clear diagnostic result, like a biopsy that shows lung cancer, the physician may say, "This is hard to believe," rather than, "You're in denial."

If patients at this point indicate that they do not wish to discuss their emotional or cognitive reactions, physicians should, of course, respect these desires. However, it is important that the physician not confuse his or her own desire to avoid emotional issues with the inference that it is the patient who wishes to avoid these topics. If the physician does not acknowledge the patient's thoughts or feelings, the patient will feel unconfirmed and less understood. Such feelings undermine doctor-patient rapport and also interfere with subsequent attempts to collect data, understand the patient, and collaboratively manage problems. In addition to the pragmatic usefulness of reflection for the task of data collection, patients who feel understood by their physicians are generally more satisfied and feel better.[15] This leads to better doctor-patient rapport, a more satisfying relationship for physicians, better detection of psychiatric illness,[13] better physical outcome,[16] and fewer lawsuits.[17,18]

The following suggestion stands as one of the cardinal "rules" of good interviewing proposed in this text:

**Rule #1: Respond to patient's feelings as soon as they appear.**

Recognizing a feeling as soon as it appears facilitates the interview process. The patient feels that the clinician understands his or her emotional condition and this recognition builds trust. If the clinician ignores the patient's emotional state, the patient's feelings will not go away. The feelings will linger and may interfere later with efficient progression of the encounter. The patient may feel that the clinician doesn't want to hear about feelings, that feelings may not "be appropriate" for medical interviews or, even worse, that the clinician simply doesn't care. Recognition of a patient's feelings represents an empathic opportunity to deepen the relationship as well as to elicit important information that might not otherwise be obtainable.[20,32]

It is useful for physicians to understand that one reflective comment is often insufficient to acknowledge emotions adequately. Reflective comments can be used several times as a patient discusses and experiences feelings that may change slightly in focus, form, or intensity as they are expressed. In fact, as a patient ventilates emotional reactions, the specific feeling expressed may change in quality and degree. For example, a patient who seems irritated at first may later express disappointment, or vice versa. If the physician listens carefully, the initial feeling can be acknowledged and subsequent ones reflected as they emerge.

As discussed, the clinician is best advised to start emotional reflections titrated to surface, less intense levels (simple reflection) and move to deeper emotional levels using more complex reflections as rapport deepens and the patient seems ready. Consider this dialogue:

PHYSICIAN: *You look upset today. (simple reflection)*

PATIENT: *I am. I've been waiting an hour for you and I'm late for work now.*

PHYSICIAN: *Okay. I understand; you're angry (complex reflection). I apologize. This should not happen and I will make every effort to make sure it doesn't happen again.*

As pointed out, attention to patients' feelings usually does not require significant time that interferes with efficient care. However, occasionally emotional issues do become too complex to address in the time available. The physician should then acknowledge the significance of the feelings and make arrangements to deal with the emotional issues at a later, but mutually acceptable, date. Alternatively, a suitable alternate approach (e.g., a psychiatric, psychologist, or social work referral) could be arranged.

## LEGITIMATION

Legitimation, or validation, is closely related to reflection but indicates an intervention that specifically communicates acceptance of and respect for the patient's emotional experience. After a physician has carefully listened to the patient's discussion of an emotional reaction, the physician should let the patient know that the feelings are understandable and make sense to the physician. The following are examples of validating comments:

PHYSICIAN: *I can certainly understand why you'd be upset under the circumstances.*

or

PHYSICIAN: *Anyone would find this very difficult.*

or

PHYSICIAN: *Your reactions are perfectly normal.*

or

PHYSICIAN: *This would be anxiety provoking for anyone.*

or

PHYSICIAN: *Of course you're angry. Anyone would be.*

With respect to validating the feelings of someone who is angry, it is important to realize that the physician does not have to agree with the reasons for the anger. It is important to first try to understand this anger from the patient's point of view and then communicate this realization to him or her. This can be difficult to do if the physician disagrees with or feels threatened by an angry patient. Nevertheless, reflective and validating comments can play the same helpful role with angry patients as they do with sad or anxious patients. For example, if the patient is annoyed because he or she has been waiting too long (an occurrence that happens all too frequently), the physician may appropriately apologize and does not necessarily have to provide an "excuse."

PHYSICIAN: *I can see that you are frustrated because you've been waiting so long. I understand why you are angry. I am truly sorry.*

In a more threatening situation, when the physician feels accused of making a mistake but does not think a mistake has been made, the following type of comment can be helpful:

PHYSICIAN: *I understand that you feel a mistake has been made. I know this has made you very angry. I need to let you know that I do not agree with you about a mistake, but I can understand why you feel so angry. Can I ask you why you think a mistake was made?*

In this type of situation, it would be important for the physician to go on to make an effort to assess and understand why the patient had the impression a mistake had been made (using Function Two skills as described in Chapter 4).

Unfortunately, there are times when physicians, of course, do make mistakes. Maintaining rapport in these situations is complex and is discussed in detail in Chapter 28. Chapters 17 and 25 also discuss strategies for communicating with patients with troubling emotions or behaviors.

## Empathic Communication to Deepen Understanding (ECDU)

Effective empathic communication develops trust and builds the relationship. On the other hand, empathic communication can also be used as a powerful bridge to Function Two (assess and understand the patient). Consider the example below of a patient who may be hearing bad news of breast cancer for the first time (see also Chapters 27 and 27A on Bad News). Not only must the physician skillfully present the information in a way to help the patient manage his or her emotions at the moment, but the physician should also use empathic skills to assess and understand the meaning of the illness to the patient:

PATIENT: *Oh my, that's terrible. [she cries]*

PHYSICIAN: *[after a moment of allowing the patient to cry] I see how upset you are.* (**reflection**)

PATIENT: *I feel like a baby, crying. I'm sorry.*

PHYSICIAN: *There's no need to apologize. Patients often cry when they hear this diagnosis.* (**legitimation**)

PATIENT: *They do?*

PHYSICIAN: *Yes. However, people cry for different reasons. What upsets you most about hearing this news?* (**exploration**)

PATIENT: *This is one more thing on my plate. Who will take care of my kids when I go for treatment?*

　　or

PATIENT: *Will I die?*

　　or

PATIENT: *I'm concerned about how my husband will react to this. He's ill himself.*

PHYSICIAN: *Let's talk about your concerns, as well as how we will treat the cancer. Is that okay?*

Thus, empathy (reflection and legitimation) followed by exploration becomes a dynamic, shared experience between the patient and physician. Empathic communication elicits the specific concerns of the patient, allowing the physician to not only become even more empathic (i.e., understanding, accepting) of the patient's suffering, but it also enables the physician to deliver more targeted, focused care directed to the explicit, expressed concerns of the patient.

This general model for empathic communication to deepen understanding (ECDU):

$$ECDU = Reflection + Legitimation + Exploration$$

is a reasonable approach for more complex or chronic emotional issues that do not lend themselves to static, cross-sectional, one- or two-sentence interventions.

Consider one more example of a patient who is upset about being laid off from work:

PHYSICIAN: *I know you're pretty upset about being laid off.* (**reflection**)

PATIENT: *I sure am.*

PHYSICIAN: *Well, that's something that's terrible for anyone.* (**legitimation**)

PATIENT: *Yeah, I know.*

PHYSICIAN: *I wonder, what is the worst part of this for you?* (**exploration**)

The exploration part is critical because the patient could be depressed, angry, nonadherent to medical regimens, anxious about finances, drinking too much, irritable with spouse or children, or anything else. Without focused inquiry the physician really has no idea about the impact on the patient's life and medical care.

## Personal Support

Statements of personal support enhance rapport. The physician should make explicit efforts to reassure the patient that he or she is there and wants to help. Of course, this must be an honest statement, or it will not be effective. As genuine caring develops in the physician for the patient, limited self-disclosure is also appropriate. Statements like the following indicate personal support:

PHYSICIAN: *I want to help in any way I can.*

or

PHYSICIAN: *Please let me know what I can do to help.*

or

PHYSICIAN: *I care about you and helping you feel better.*

These statements of direct personal support encourage patients to feel that the physician wants to help and cares, leading to improved rapport and solidification of the doctor-patient relationship.

## Partnership

Patients are more satisfied with physicians and are more likely to adhere to treatment recommendations when they feel a sense of partnership with their physicians.[33] Increasing the participation of a patient in his or her treatment improves coping skills and increases the likelihood of a good outcome.[1] When physicians decide to promote this type of partnership, they can make such statements as these:

PHYSICIAN: *Once I have reviewed our options, I'd like us to work together to develop a treatment plan that works for you.*

or

PHYSICIAN: *After we've talked more about your problems, I'm confident we can work together to find some solutions.*

## Respect (Affirmation)

The physician's respect for patients and their problems is implied by attentive listening, specific nonverbal signals, eye contact, and genuine concern. However explicit, respectful comments also help build rapport, improve relationships, and help patients cope with complex situations.

For the purposes of this text, an intervention communicating respect refers to an appreciative statement about a specific patient behavior. Such statements of respect will, in general, reinforce the behavior and make it more likely to happen again. Well-timed, repeated demonstrations of authentic respect will foster a positive relationship and promote the patients' capacity for coping. In addition, such statements generally make patients feel better about themselves.

Physicians can usually find something to affirm in all their patients. Almost everyone does something well. This holds true even for patients with troubling or difficult behaviors (see Chapter 25). Doctors can help their patients by focusing on one or more of their patients' successful coping skills. This can also improve patient satisfaction and adherence. The following are examples of respectful statements:

**PHYSICIAN:** *I'm impressed by how well you're coping.*

or

**PHYSICIAN:** *You're doing a good job handling the uncertainty.*

or

**PHYSICIAN:** *Despite your feeling so bad, you're still able to carry on at home and at work. That is quite an accomplishment.*

Like all discussed interventions, statements of affirmation must be honest or they will be more destructive than helpful. When these sentiments reflect true feelings of the physician, they are powerful facilitators of communication and rapport between doctors and patients.

## P(E)ARLS

The acronym P(E)ARLS can be used to aid learners to remember five skills to build the relationship.

Partnership

(Empathy), expressed through reflection and legitimation

Affirmation (respect)

Reflection

Legitimation

Support

## Summary

Chapter 3 discusses:

1. Importance of the relationship in medical care
2. Nonverbal communication
3. Communication of empathy
4. Reflection
5. Legitimation
6. Empathic Communication to Deepen Understanding (ECDU)
   (ECDU = Reflection + Legitimation + Exploration)
7. Support
8. Partnership
9. Respect
10. The acronym P(E)ARLS can be used to aid learners to remember five skills to build the relationship.
11. Rule #1: Respond to Patient's Feelings as Soon as They Appear

### References

1. Roter DL, Hall JA: Communication and adherence: moving from prediction to understanding. *Med Care* 47(8):823–825, 2009.

2. Suchman AL, et al: Physician satisfaction with primary care office visits. Collaborative Study Group of the American Academy on Physician and Patient. *Med Care* 31(12):1083–1092, 1993.
3. Suchman AL, Hinton-Walker P, Botelho RJ, editors: *Partnerships in healthcare: transforming relational process*, Rochester, 1998, University of Rochester Press.
4. Cole S: Reducing malpractice risk through more effective communication. *Am J Manag Care* 485–489, 1997.
5. Frank GW: Malpractice claims and physicians' communication patterns. *JAMA* 277(21):1682, 1997.
6. Beckman H: Communication and malpractice: why patients sue their physicians. *Cleve Clin J Med* 62(2):84–85, 1995.
7. Hojat M, et al: Empathy in medical education and patient care. *Acad Med* 76(7):669, 2001.
8. Fernndez-Olano C, Montoya-Fernndez J, Salinas-Sánchez AS: Impact of clinical interview training on the empathy level of medical students and medical residents. *Med Teach* 30(3):322–324, 2008.
9. Stepien KA, Baernstein A: Educating for empathy. A review. *J Gen Intern Med* 21(5):524–530, 2006.
10. Griffin JW: Teaching and learning empathy. *Nat Clin Pract Neurol* 2(10):517, 2006.
11. Switankowsky I: Empathy as a foundation for the biopsychosocial model of medicine. *Hum Health Care* 4(2):E5, 2004.
12. Roter DL, et al: The expression of emotion through nonverbal behavior in medical visits. Mechanisms and outcomes. *J Gen intern Med* 21(Suppl 1):S28–S34, 2006.
13. Hall JA, et al: Nonverbal sensitivity in medical students: implications for clinical interactions. *J Gen Intern Med* 24(11):1217–1222, 2009.
14. Mast MS, et al: Physician gender affects how physician nonverbal behavior is related to patient satisfaction. *Med Care* 46(12):1212–1218, 2008.
15. Goldberg DP, et al: Training family doctors to recognize psychiatric illness with increased accuracy. *Lancet* 2(8193):521–523, 1980.
16. Halpern J: What is clinical empathy? *J Gen Intern Med* 18(8):670–674, 2003.
17. Mercer SW, Reynolds WJ: Empathy and quality of care. *Br J Gen Pract* 52(Suppl):S9–12, 2002.
18. Coulehan JL, et al: "Let me see if I have this right ...": words that help build empathy. *Ann Intern Med* 135(3):221–227, 2001.
19. Branch WT, Jr, et al: The patient-physician relationship. Teaching the human dimensions of care in clinical settings. *JAMA* 286(9):1067–1074, 2001.
20. Suchman AL, et al: A model of empathic communication in the medical interview. *JAMA* 277(8):678–682, 1997.
21. Spiro H: What is empathy and can it be taught? *Ann Intern Med* 116(10):843–846, 1992.
22. Salzman GA: Empathy: can it be taught? *Ann Intern Med* 117(8):700–701, 1992; author reply 701.
23. Platt FW: Empathy: can it be taught? *Ann Intern Med* 117(8):700, 1992; author reply 701.
24. Hojat M, et al: The devil is in the third year: a longitudinal study of erosion of empathy in medical school. *Acad Med* 84(9):1182–1191, 2009.
25. Pedersen R: Empirical research on empathy in medicine-A critical review. *Patient Educ Couns* 76(3):307–322, 2009.
26. Colliver JA, et al: Reports of the decline of empathy during medical education are greatly exaggerated: a reexamination of the research. *Acad Med* 85(4):588–593, 2010.
27. Roter D, Hall JA: *Doctors talking with patients/patients talking with doctors: improving communication in medical visits*, ed 2, Westport, Conn., 2006, Praeger, Xvi, 238 p.
28. Gerrity MS, et al: Improving the recognition and management of depression: is there a role for physician education? *J Fam Pract* 48(12):949–957, 1999.
29. Roter DL, et al: Improving physicians' interviewing skills and reducing patients' emotional distress. A randomized clinical trial. *Arch Intern Med* 155(17):1877–1884, 1995.
30. Kalet A, et al: Teaching communication in clinical clerkships: models from the macy initiative in healthy communications. *Acad Med* 79(6):511–520, 2004.
31. Carkhuff RR: *Helping and human relations; a primer for lay and professional helpers*, New York, 1969, Holt, v.
32. Branch WT, Malik TK: Using 'windows of opportunities' in brief interviews to understand patients' concerns. *JAMA* 269(13):1667–1668, 1993.
33. Dye NE, DiMateo MR: Enhancing cooperation with the medical regime. In Lipkin M, Jr, editor: *The medical interview: clinical care, education, and research*, NY. P, 1995, Springer, pp 134–136.

# Function Two: Assess and Understand

## OVERVIEW

Chapter 4 discusses skills and rules to assess and understand:
1. Nonverbal listening behavior
2. Questioning style: open-ended questions and the open-to-closed cone
3. Rule #2: Let the patient complete the opening statement.
4. Facilitation
5. Clarification and direction
6. Checking/summarizing
7. Rule #3: When in doubt, check.
8. Survey problems: What else?
9. Avoid leading questions.
10. Elicit the patient's perspective: Ideas, Concerns, and Expectations ("ICE").
11. Explore the impact of the illness on the patient's quality of life.

*Listen to the patient, he is telling you the diagnosis.*

SIR WILLIAM OSLER

The second function of the interview addresses the need to assess and understand the patient's problems. "Assess and understand" refers not only to the process of identifying biomedical diagnoses, but also to a method for appreciating the psychosocial aspects of a patient's illness. This approach becomes especially important for the management of chronic illnesses. Understanding the more complete biopsychosocial aspects of a chronic illness helps guide management decisions in the short run, and ultimately, improves outcomes over time. Gaining this appreciation requires the ability to elicit information from the patient and listen carefully to the answers. The importance of skillful data collection is underscored by the widely accepted understanding that the medical history contributes 60% to 80% of the information needed for accurate diagnoses as well as for the psychosocial background needed for effective management planning.

This chapter describes a range of skills that has been shown to enhance the ability of clinicians to collect information from patients accurately and efficiently. In the actual practice of medicine, experienced practitioners guide data collection through an iterative process of diagnostic reasoning. Awareness of illness profiles and pattern recognition guides interviewing strategies of clinicians in practice.[1] Nevertheless, even without this knowledge base and clinical experience, students can develop good interviewing habits to enhance data-gathering accuracy and efficiency by focusing on the basic skills described in this chapter.[2,3]

## Nonverbal Listening Behavior

The clinician's nonverbal behavior has a powerful effect on the flow of information. Appropriate nonverbal signals are essential. Patients will usually continue speaking when they feel their physician is listening. Physicians who look at their patients and maintain an attentive and interested body posture will be more likely to instill confidence and trust than doctors who retreat behind a desk, slouch in a chair, drink coffee while talking, or try to read or write in the chart while also trying to listen.[4-7]

Appropriate eye contact is an essential first ingredient for collecting information from patients. In general, to listen well to a patient and to watch for emotional cues, the clinician must look directly at the patient. In addition, an attentive body posture is crucial; for example, an open body position, a forward lean of the head, and a forward lean of the body all indicate receptivity to the patient and a willingness to listen. Although these recommendations may seem straightforward and obvious, they are commonly neglected in actual practice, and the student who begins a career with attention to such nonverbal cues will learn good habits for a lifetime of practice.[8,9]

## Questioning Style: Open-Ended Questions and the Open-to-Closed Cone

Open-ended questions are particularly crucial in the opening of the interview and for opening up new topics as they arise. Open-ended questions are defined as questions that cannot be answered in one word. A considerable body of literature supports the use of open-ended questioning as the most efficient and effective vehicle to gain an accurate and complete understanding of patients' problems.[7,10-13]

An open-ended question invites the patient to use his or her own judgment in deciding what topics and problems to emphasize. Open-ended questions require patients to generate responses other than a simple "yes" or "no," or any other one word response. The following are examples of open-ended questions:

> PHYSICIAN: *What symptoms brought you to the hospital?*
>
> or
>
> PHYSICIAN: *How can I be of help to you today?*

In contrast, closed questions can be answered with one word. The following are examples of closed questions:

> PHYSICIAN: *Does your head hurt?*
>
> or
>
> PHYSICIAN: *Are you short of breath?*
>
> or
>
> PHYSICIAN: *Does the pain go down your leg?*

Open-ended questions invite patients to describe their problems by using their own vocabulary and their personal experience of the symptoms. Such questioning is much more likely to lead to the clinician gaining an accurate understanding of patients' subjective experience of illness. In contrast, premature reliance on closed questioning usually leads to inaccurate or incomplete understanding.

Open-ended questioning is particularly useful because it allows a patient to inform the clinician about the problem as the patient sees it. Such questioning indicates willingness to listen to the patient's story. By using open-ended questioning in the beginning of the interview, the practitioner can learn more about the patient's perception of the problem, the major concerns about the problem, the context of the problem, and perhaps the deeper meaning of the problem to the patient. Such information will be invaluable in developing diagnostic hypotheses and management strategies.

After an initial nondirective phase, during which the clinician has allowed the patient to speak freely about the problems as the patient sees them, the clinician must ask progressively more focused questions to explore specific diagnostic hypotheses. This subsequent graduated narrowing of focus (after initial open-ended inquiries) can be considered an "open-to-closed cone."[7,13,14]

Consider the example of a young man with headaches. After the patient indicates that headaches are his major problem, the physician may choose one of two very different approaches: the physician may explore the problem of the headaches in an open-ended manner or, alternatively, rely on closed-ended inquiries to learn more about specific physical symptoms. The closed-ended approach might include many detailed questions about the location of the pain, intensity, timing, quality, and so on. These are important questions and need to be asked but should be reserved until after the initial, more open-ended exploration has been completed.

The following dialogue demonstrates an open question, followed by a series of premature closed questions for clarification.

> PHYSICIAN: *What can I do for you today?*
>
> PATIENT: *I've been having terrible headaches.*
>
> PHYSICIAN: *I'm sorry. Where is the pain?*
>
> PATIENT: *The pain is all over.*
>
> PHYSICIAN: *Is the pain sharp or dull?*
>
> PATIENT: *Dull.*
>
> PHYSICIAN: *Does the pain come and go, or is it there all the time?*
>
> PATIENT: *It comes and goes. But when the headache comes, it may be there for several days.*

In this sequence of closed-ended questioning, the clinician has not learned as much as might be gained from more open-ended inquiries at the early stage of the assessment process. A more open-ended inquiry is usually more efficient in leading to accurate diagnostic hypotheses. Consider the following, alternative strategy to the same opening problem.

> PHYSICIAN: *What can I do for you today?*
>
> PATIENT: *I've been having terrible headaches.*
>
> PHYSICIAN: *Can you tell me some more about these headaches?*
>
> PATIENT: *Well, they come on slowly and get worse and worse over several days. They seem to come only in the hay fever season when my allergies get worse.*

Experienced physicians develop diagnostic hypotheses from the first moments of meeting a patient.[3] These hypotheses are formulated by fitting patterns of the patient's complaints and physical signs into entities of known illness categories. By allowing the patient the opportunity to describe his or her own complaints in a nondirected way, the skilled physician can more efficiently develop diagnostic hypotheses and recognize patterns that are relevant for the particular patient's problems.[1]

In the preceding open-ended example, the patient's description of the symptoms allows the clinician to narrow the set of diagnostic possibilities considerably, even within the first few moments of the interview. The open-ended inquiry has suggested an allergic etiology for the headaches rather than numerous others. In contrast, the closed-ended inquiry was significantly less efficient. Although beginning medical students will not be able to recognize the hundreds of patterns that will soon become second nature for them, it will be particularly useful for students to learn good habits of open-ended questioning early in their careers.

In addition, open-ended questioning usually provides the clinician the opportunity to learn also about the important environmental precipitants or stress factors that may influence the development of symptoms. For example, this same complaint of headaches might lead to the following:

PHYSICIAN: *Can you tell me some more about your headaches?*

PATIENT: *Well, they only started about 3 weeks ago and seem to come on when I'm in the library late at night studying for exams.*

This information can help the clinician understand the environmental context of the symptoms, which will help in the formulation of diagnostic hypotheses and treatment strategies. The context of late-night headaches may suggest problems with fatigue or excessive caffeine intake. In addition, the mentioning of exams suggests the possibility of stressful life situations that may be related to the headaches. This leads to Rule #2 of interviewing:

# RULE #2: LET THE PATIENT COMPLETE THE OPENING STATEMENT

Beckman and Frankel's classic report in 1984,[15] replicated in 1999,[16] documents the importance of allowing the patient to complete his or her opening statement. Although most medical interviews do begin with open-ended questioning, in at least 75% of interviews, physicians typically interrupt their patients before they get the chance to complete the initial opening statement, generally within the first 18 seconds of the interview! Most patients have at least three different problems that they would like to discuss with their physicians. Once interrupted, however, patients do not get the chance to present all these problems to the clinician. Clinicians, on the other hand, who do let their patients complete their opening statements, have access to a more complete and accurate list of their patients' problems and experience a significant reduction in the frequency of late-arising problems. Of note, most patients who were allowed to complete their opening statements did so in less than 90 seconds.[16]

## Facilitation

Any comment or behavior on the interviewer's part that encourages the patient to keep talking in an open-ended manner can be considered facilitative. The preceding example, "Tell me more about your headaches," is one very effective type of facilitative comment. Another would be a head nod to indicate attention. A comment like "uh-huh" or "go on" accomplishes similar ends. Attentive silence can also be facilitative in that the clinician's quiet attention usually encourages the patient to keep talking. Finally, repeating the last few words that the patient has said often invites him or her to keep talking.

Most interviewers do not use facilitation enough. This is a skill that needs to be intentionally practiced many times for the interviewer to learn to appreciate its striking efficiency and effectiveness. In general, whenever a patient brings up a new problem, the interviewer should use nondirective facilitative interventions (several times) to allow the patient to tell the story in his or her own words so as to provide the most useful and accurate information.

For the purposes of illustration, the same young man with headaches can be considered. The clinician can use several facilitating comments, including nonverbal responses (such as attentive silence) to encourage the nondirective flow of information.

PHYSICIAN: *Can you tell me some more about the headaches?*

PATIENT: *Well, they come on slowly over a period of days and seem to come on only in the hay fever season when my allergies get worse.*

PHYSICIAN: *You say they only come in hay fever season?*

PATIENT: *Well, I guess I might get a headache in the winter or summer, but this is quite rare. Spring and fall tend to be the time the allergies and the headaches come.*

PHYSICIAN: *Okay … (pause and attentive silence)*

PATIENT: *This headache now has gone on for 5 days and I'm having trouble at work. I don't sleep so well either. These allergies are just getting out of hand.*

In this example, the clinician used two facilitating interventions (repetition of the patient's last words, and "Okay") to encourage the patient to provide useful information for assessment and management, before moving forward with more directive questioning in the open-to-closed-cone.

## Clarification and Direction

To understand clearly what patients mean to convey and to piece together a coherent narrative of a patient's problem, the clinician must make use of clarifying and directive questions. Even during the nondirective phase of the interview, the clinician may find the need to interrupt the patient's flow of information to clarify jargon or ambiguities or direct the process. For example:

PHYSICIAN: *You say the allergies have gotten out of hand. Can you help me understand what you mean when you talk about your allergies?*

PATIENT: *Well, every spring and fall I sneeze a lot, and my eyes run and itch. My head feels congested and sometimes hurts.*

Clinicians may also need to interrupt patients to gain an appreciation for the chronology of the problem. For example:

PHYSICIAN: *Can you tell me when these allergies started?*

PATIENT: *I've been having them all my life to some degree, but they seem much worse in the last 2 or 3 years.*

After such a clarification, the clinician should return to open-ended facilitation, which, as before, will encourage the patient to elaborate on the problem(s) in his or her own words, choosing to highlight issues and concerns of importance to him or her.

PHYSICIAN: *So they've been getting worse in the last 2 or 3 years? (pause)*

PATIENT: *Yes. I got married 3 years ago, changed jobs, and had a baby. My life is different now. I can't seem to get enough rest. That probably has something to do with the headaches.*

The patient has introduced several new subjects at this point and has come to a natural pause. The patient seems to be waiting for the clinician to make a decision about where to direct the interview. The clinician can choose to let the patient discuss the changes in his life or direct the interview back toward the headaches or allergies. At the beginning of an interview, when significant psychosocial factors are raised, it is usually preferable to attend to them, at least briefly. After an initial acknowledgment, if the clinician decides to return to the physical symptoms, this can be done with directing comments.

PHYSICIAN: *It sounds like you've been under a great deal of stress lately.*

PATIENT: *You can say that again. I just never seem to get time for myself.*

PHYSICIAN: *This sounds like it could be a problem in itself. Why don't we talk about the headaches for a few more minutes and then come back to the stress situation.*

# Checking/Summarizing

Checking or summarizing the story by periodically restating what it seems the patient has said is probably the most important information-gathering skill, and it is the least used.[9] Language is replete with complex meanings that can be easily misinterpreted. Furthermore, clinicians often have incorrect information about their patients. A clinician's memory may not be accurate, or attention may wander when the patient says something important. Even experienced physicians can collect inaccurate information from patients. It is therefore essential for the clinician to check the accuracy of information that is received. This is generally very brief, but it is a powerful and important intervention. Continuing with the example discussed above, the clinician can say something like this:

> **PHYSICIAN:** *Let me check to see if I understand what you have told me so far. You've been having spring and fall allergies all your life, but these have gotten much worse in the last 2 or 3 years since you've been under a lot more stress. You sometimes get headaches with these allergies. The headaches tend to come on slowly and develop over several days. You're having one of these headaches now, and it's getting so bad that you are having trouble at work and sleeping at night.*

This type of checking (or summarizing) by restatement accomplishes multiple important functions. It gives the clinician a few moments of time to review what has been heard and what needs to be explored next. It allows the clinician the opportunity to check the accuracy of what he or she thinks the patient actually said. Checking feels reassuring to the patient because he or she realizes the doctor is interested in gaining an accurate understanding of the problem, and this promotes trust as well as the patient's experience of the physician as caring. It also allows the patient the opportunity to correct any misinformation that is presented. Patients' understanding and recollection of symptoms often develops in an articulate form only during the process of being interviewed. Thus, checking can play a generative role by inviting further clarification and elaboration of the problem by the patient.

Finally, checking helps the student learner avoid the humiliation of presenting misinformation to a supervisor and having it later "corrected" by the patient in front of the student (and others) when the supervisor checks it out with the patient directly. (Unfortunately, this is an all too common experience!)

For all these reasons, checking is probably the most important data-gathering skill available to the physician and should be used frequently in the course of routine interviewing.

Beginning interviewers, in particular, find checking useful to help manage their own anxiety while trying to conduct an efficient interview. There are so many different questions that medical students need to learn that they commonly "freeze" and find it hard to know in which direction they should go. They find it hard to remember what they have just heard as they think about what they must ask next. This common problem for learners has led to the development of the third "rule" for any and all interviewers who feel lost or simply uncertain about where or how to proceed next.

# RULE #3: WHEN IN DOUBT, CHECK

Checking offers a safe, effective, efficient, and generative way to get out of trouble. If an interviewer becomes confused, lost, or uncertain of how to proceed, he or she can always say something like:

> **PHYSICIAN:** *I'd like to take a few moments now to make sure that I have understood you correctly. You told me that...*

This checking comment invites the patient into a partnership to reconsider the information that has been received. Thus, checking by restatement is an essential skill for experienced interviewers as well as for beginning students. In this text, we use the term "checking" and "summarizing" interchangeably. Summarizing, however, usually refers to relatively longer forms of checking nearer the end of an interview.

## Survey Problems: "What Else?"

Many interviewing texts do not emphasize the importance of surveying problems. George Engel, an internist, psychoanalyst, and one of the pioneers in the development of medical interviewing, has particularly emphasized this skill.[17] He has stated that he believes the question, "What else is bothering you?" to be the most important question he asks his patients.[A]

Patients often are anxious or embarrassed about discussing their most serious worries (e.g., "Do I have AIDS?" or "Why am I impotent?") and may leave their chief concern until the end of an interview, when the physician is ready to terminate the session. Sometimes, if the physician directs the interview too strongly, patients may be too anxious to remember to discuss all their concerns, or there are simply too many to get to.

The physician should survey problems in the early stages of every interview. It is useful and efficient in the long run for the physician to hear the complete list of the patient's problems before going into a detailed exploration of any of them. This may help prevent a situation, for example, in which a patient's presenting complaint is a headache, but the patient does not mention symptoms of angina-like chest pain until the end of the interview. This type of late-arising or "end-of-the-interview" problem can develop because of patient anxiety about bringing up important symptoms earlier or simply because of patient unawareness of the critical importance of some symptoms. At the end of the interview, for example, the patient may say something like, "Oh, by the way, doctor … is this chest pain important?"

Late questions create difficulties for physicians because they are unpredictable, add anxiety, and require time and attention that may not already have been allocated for this patient. Such situations are common. Studies indicate they occur in up to 20% to 35% of interviews.[18] Use of surveying techniques can decrease these problems significantly.

Surveying problems allows the patient and the physician to get an understanding of the medical landscape and then decide which territory to explore first. This increases the efficiency of the interview and allows the patient and physician together to make informed decisions about how to spend the available time.

In practice, it is recommended that the physician begin surveying problems shortly after eliciting and briefly exploring the patient's chief complaint. (The chief complaint is defined as the patient's response to the clinician's first open-ended question: "What problem brought you here today?") The chief complaint is reviewed in detail in Chapter 8. For example:

> PHYSICIAN: *Now that I've heard a little about your headache, your allergies, and some of your recent stresses, I'd like to make sure I know something about all your other problems before we get back to them one at a time. What else is bothering you?*

"What else is bothering you?" is a more effective question than, "Is there anything else bothering you?" The former, open-ended question invites the patient to come up with other problems and suggests that the clinician is expecting more information from the patient. The latter form is a closed-ended question and, depending on tone and inflection, can actually be used to cut off discussion. An example of a question that may "seem" to survey problems and ask about other symptoms, but actually closes off discussion, might be something like:

> PHYSICIAN: *You don't have any other problems, do you?*

Surveying problems should proceed until the patient indicates that there are no other problems. The clinician should continue asking, "What else is bothering you?" until the patient indicates that all the problems have been mentioned.

## Avoid Leading (Biased) Questions

Because of the social power differential in a medical interview, patients tend to be strongly influenced by the wording of a clinician's question, especially if the wording implies that a certain kind of answer is expected. Such a question is called a "leading question." Leading questions can result in significant and sometimes dangerous misinformation, such as in the following example:

PHYSICIAN: *The pain doesn't go down your arm, does it?*

PATIENT: *No, not really.*

Because the patient usually wants to please the clinician, a leading question will usually elicit the answer the clinician expects. In the preceding example, a patient may, in fact, overtly confirm the clinician's expectation that the pain does not go down the arm. This information might not be entirely true, however, as implied by the patient's ambiguous response, "not really."

Sometimes the bias may be less obvious and yet just as powerful. For example, "How helpful was the medication I gave you?" may be a problematic question if the patient thinks the clinician is hoping for a positive response. By adding the phrase, "that I gave you," the clinician may link the medication to the person of the clinician in a way that the patient may have difficulty separating. The patient may overemphasize the positive if he or she thinks that is what the clinician wants to hear. Even if the medication had a mixed benefit, if the patient thinks the clinician wants to hear a positive response, the patient may say something like, "It was pretty helpful."

To try and minimize bias, this last question might be rephrased in the following manner:

PHYSICIAN: *What effects, good and bad, did the medication have?*

Phrasing the question in this way, the clinician can eliminate the bias that might lead the patient to incomplete or inaccurate statements in the attempt to give the clinician what the patient thinks is expected.

## Elicit the Patient's Perspective: Ideas, Concerns, and Expectations ("ICE")

### Explore the Patient's Ideas about the Meaning of the Illness

At times the patient's ideas about the meaning of the illness are quite clear. A patient with headaches in the allergy season may think his headaches are directly related to pollen. However, patient ideas about the meaning of illness may not be clear. For example, the patient with some rather obscure abdominal pain might be concerned that cancer could be causing the pain. Alternatively, the concern might be social embarrassment from the passing of flatus. Unless the clinician knows the patient's ideas about the meaning of the symptom (i.e., the patient's "explanatory model"), the clinician will be inefficient in his or her care and may not be able to meet the patient's needs.[22]

The clinician should directly ask the patient what he or she thinks could be causing the symptom. For example:

PHYSICIAN: *Could you tell me what you think might be causing this stomach pain?*

PATIENT: *I don't know. You're the doctor. That's why I came to you.*

PHYSICIAN: *Of course I am the doctor, and I will do what I can to help. But it will help me if you could tell me what thoughts have crossed your mind about what could be causing these problems.*

Some patients may be unwilling to discuss their own ideas about the meaning of the illness, even with encouragement. However, when given an opportunity, many patients will be able to discuss their fears and ideas directly with the clinician. This discussion can contribute to the efficiency of the clinician-patient interaction, as well as to the ability of the clinician to reassure the patient. It can also enhance patient satisfaction. For example:

PATIENT: *Well, I know it's probably nothing. But my father died of colon cancer, and I'm kind of worried that I might have the same problem.*

PHYSICIAN: *I'm glad you could tell me that. It will help me understand your problem. After we talk about your pain and perhaps do some tests, I will do what I can to reassure you about your concern about cancer.*

### Elicit the Patient's <u>Concerns</u> about the Problems

It is important for the clinician to elicit the patient's concerns about his or her problems. Without understanding the patient's particular concerns, the clinician may not be able to efficiently provide the care that is most needed.

PHYSICIAN: *Mr. Burke, I would like to know what concerns you most about the pain in your stomach?*

PATIENT: *It just hurts so much.*

PHYSICIAN: *Okay, I will look into that and work on the pain. Is there anything else?*

PATIENT: *Well, yes … my father had a pain in his stomach for a long time … and then it turned out to be cancer of the pancreas.*

## ELICIT THE PATIENT'S <u>EXPECTATIONS</u>

<u>Sometimes the patient's expectations of the clinician are</u> quite clear. Clinicians who elicit patient expectations early in the interview achieve higher levels of patient satisfaction and increased efficiency and effectiveness. Asking directly about the patient's expectations generally increases rapport in the relationship, improves efficiency in the interview, and achieves a more satisfied and more adherent patient in the long run.[19-21] If the clinician knows what the patient wants, the clinician will have an easier time satisfying the patient. Patient expectations can be elicited directly:

PHYSICIAN: *In what ways do you think I can be of most help to you?*

or

*What were you hoping I could do to help you?*

## Explore the Impact of the Illness on the Patient's Quality of Life

To understand a patient's illness and facilitate coping, the clinician must evaluate the impact of the illness on the patient's quality of life. This is especially true for chronic illness. This information forms part of the history of the present illness. The clinician should explore the impact of the illness on the patient's general functioning. This includes the impact on (1) interpersonal relationships (especially spouse, significant other, and family), (2) work, (3) sexual relationships, and (4) emotional stability.

After the clinician has developed the narrative thread, he or she will already have obtained a great deal of information about the impact of the illness on the patient's quality of life. This is especially true if the clinician has responded to the emotions the patient has manifested. The clinician should then complete the quality-of-life evaluation:

PHYSICIAN: *I'm interested in hearing more about how this problem has affected your life in general.*

PATIENT: *What do you mean?*

PHYSICIAN: *Let me explain. I'd like to hear about the impact this problem has had on your overall life, your home situation, your work, and things like that.*

PATIENT: *Okay. It's been hard. My work has fallen down because I've had to be out so much. I've been very tense, and I think I'm starting to take things out on my family.*

PHYSICIAN: *It sounds difficult.*

PATIENT: *Yes, it has been. I'm a data analyst for a large computer company. I have a lot of responsibility and a lot of deadlines to meet. I've been falling behind.*

PHYSICIAN: *You also said you've been tense and taking it out on your family. Can you say some more about that?*

PATIENT: *I'm worried and tense all the time. I yell at the kids a lot, and I can't really talk to my wife.*

PHYSICIAN: *How has this affected your sex life?*

PATIENT: *Well, I've been out of sorts lately, and sex has been one of the first things to go.*

Throughout the evaluation of the quality of life, the form of the questions can make a great difference in the patient's willingness to talk openly about psychosocial problems. This is especially true for topics like sexual adjustment, about which patients may be embarrassed or sensitive. For example, it is usually much more productive for the clinician to ask *how* a symptom has affected someone's life (open-ended question) rather than whether a symptom *has* had an effect (closed question). For example, the following closed question may not be the most effective way to explore the issue of impact of illness on sexual functioning:

PHYSICIAN: *Has this pain changed your sex life? (closed question)*

PATIENT: *Not really.*

In general, the following open-ended form of this question is usually considerably more generative and productive:

PHYSICIAN: *How has this pain affected your sex life? (open-ended question)*

PATIENT: *Well, things have kind of slowed down a little.*

Although this distinction may seem subtle, this style difference makes a significant difference in the way a patient responds to the clinician's inquiries. When asked the open-ended question, *how* has a symptom affected his or her life, a patient usually feels encouraged to talk more freely because the clinician clearly expects a positive response and, in that sense, has given "permission" to the patient to discuss a problem(s) that he/she might otherwise be reluctant to reveal. In contrast, when a clinician asks a closed question, simply whether or not a symptom *has* changed a patient's sexual life, the patient may feel defensive and embarrassed to admit a problem. As students gain experience in eliciting this quality-of-life information, it becomes clear that different patients respond in different ways, even when suffering from similar illnesses. For example, some patients are most distressed by the loss of sleep, others by pain, and others by a change in sexual function. Family responses to illness are also quite different. When facing similar illness situations, one family might become more closely bonded and another might threaten to disintegrate.

Thus, by talking with patients about how a set of symptoms affects their quality of life, the clinician attempts to develop a picture of the overall impact of the illness on general functioning and adaptation. This inquiry enables the clinician to learn of the most distressing aspects of an illness for one specific patient and his or her family. Research indicates that clinicians who inquire about the impact of symptoms are more likely to recognize emotional distress in their patients.[7,23]

Treatment planning that takes quality-of-life issues into consideration is much more likely to be realistically accepted and followed by patients. For example, targeted interventions can be designed specifically to assist patient adaptation in the particular areas most problematic to the patient. This understanding is essential for optimal collaborative management.

## Conclusion

Gathering accurate data is the central task of patient assessment. Numerous problems exist in the current communication patterns of many clinicians. Inefficient and ineffective interviewing can lead to misinformation, incomplete information, and frustrating or lengthy visits. Skillful use of basic data-gathering skills such as open-ended questioning and the open-to-closed cone, facilitation, and checking can lead to increased efficiency, with improved patient and clinician satisfaction and clinical outcome. Use of these data-gathering skills for exploration of patient's expectations, patient's ideas about the meaning of illness, and general quality-of-life issues are all also essential to understand patients and their illnesses, in the service of effective treatment planning and improved outcomes.

## Summary

Chapter 4 discusses skills and rules to assess and understand:
1. Nonverbal listening behavior
2. Questioning style: open-ended questions and the open-to-closed cone
3. Rule #2: Let the patient complete the opening statement.
4. Facilitation
5. Clarification and direction
6. Checking
7. Rule #3: When in doubt, check.
8. Survey problems: What else?
9. Avoid leading questions.
10. Elicit the patient's perspective; Ideas, Concerns, and Expectations ("ICE")
11. Explore the impact of the illness on the patient's quality of life.

### References

1. Elstein AS, Shulman LS, Sprafka SA: *Medical problem solving: an analysis of clinical reasoning*, Cambridge, Mass., 1978, Harvard University Press. Xvi, p 330.
2. Mandin H, et al: Helping students learn to think like experts when solving clinical problems. *Acad Med* 72(3):173–179, 1997.
3. Kassirer JP: Teaching clinical medicine by iterative hypothesis testing. Let's preach what we practice. *N Engl J Med* 309(15):921–923, 1983.
4. Mast MS: On the importance of nonverbal communication in the physician-patient interaction. *Patient Educ Couns* 67(3):315–318, 2007.
5. Laemmel K: [Nonverbal aspects of the physician-patient relationship]. *Praxis (Bern 1994)* 87(27-28):915–917, 1998.
6. DiMatteo MR, Hays RD, Prince LM: Relationship of physicians' nonverbal communication skill to patient satisfaction, appointment noncompliance, and physician workload. *Health Psychol* 5(6):581–594, 1986.
7. Goldberg DP, et al: Training family doctors to recognize psychiatric illness with increased accuracy. *Lancet* 2(8193):521–523, 1980.
8. Hall JA, et al: Nonverbal sensitivity in medical students: implications for clinical interactions. *J Gen intern Med* 24(11):1217–1222, 2009.

9. Roter D, Hall JA: *Doctors talking with patients/patients talking with doctors: improving communication in medical visits*, ed 2, Westport, Conn., 2006, Praeger. Xvi, p 238.
10. Roter DL, Hall JA: Physician's interviewing styles and medical information obtained from patients. *J Gen Intern Med* 2(5):325–329, 1987.
11. Maguire P, et al: Helping cancer patients disclose their concerns. *Eur J Cancer* 32A(1):78–81, 1996.
12. Hopkinson K, Cox A, Rutter M: Psychiatric interviewing techniques. III. Naturalistic study: eliciting feelings. *Br J Psychiatry* 138:406–415, 1981.
13. Cox A, Hopkinson K, Rutter M: Psychiatric interviewing techniques II. Naturalistic study: eliciting factual information. *Br J Psychiatry* 138:283–291, 1981.
14. Gask L, et al: Improving the psychiatric skills of the general practice trainee: an evaluation of a group training course. *Med Educa* 22(2):132–138, 1988.
15. Beckman HB, Frankel RM: The effect of physician behavior on the collection of data. *Ann Intern Med* 101(5):692–696, 1984.
16. Marvel MK, et al: Soliciting the patient's agenda: have we improved? *JAMA* 281(3):283–287, 1999.
17. Engel GL, Morgan WL: *Interviewing the patient*, London, Philadelphia, 1973, W. B. Saunders. Xv, p 129.
18. White J, Levinson W, Roter D: "*Oh, by the way...*": *the closing moments of the medical visit. J Gen Intern Med* 9(1):24–28, 1994.
19. Eisenthal S, Lazare A: Evaluation of the initial interview in a walk-in clinic. The clinician's perspective on a "negotiated approach." *J Nerv Ment Dis* 164(1).30–35, 1977.
20. Eisenthal S, Koopman C, Lazare A: Process analysis of two dimensions of the negotiated approach in relation to satisfaction in the initial interview. *J Nerv Ment Dis* 171(1):49–54, 1983.
21. Eisenthal S, et al: "Adherence" and the negotiated approach to patienthood. *Arch Gen Psychiatry* 36(4):393–398, 1979.
22. Kleinman A, Eisenberg L, Good B: Culture, illness, and care: clinical lessons from anthropologic and cross-cultural research. *Ann intern Med* 88(2):251–258, 1978.
23. Roter DL, et al: Improving physicians' interviewing skills and reducing patients' emotional distress. A randomized clinical trial. *Arch Intern Med* 155(17):1877–1884, 1995.

### Endnotes

A. Grand Rounds presentation, Chapel Hill, 1976, University of North Carolina.

# CHAPTER 5

# Function Three: Collaborate for Management

Steven Cole ■ Mary DeGenaro Cole ■ Damara Gutnick
■ Connie Davis

## OVERVIEW

This chapter presents Function Three, Collaborate for Management, and the two structured tools which support it: (e)TACCT, an educational device, and Brief Action Planning (BAP), a self-management support tool based on the principles and practice of Motivational Interviewing (MI).

The third function of the interview concerns collaborative management. Regardless of whether the focus of medical concern is acute, chronic care, or prevention, a collaborative management style facilitates optimal outcomes. Building on both a trusting relationship (Function One) and understanding (Function Two), collaborative management (Function Three) focuses on the skills of education, self-management support (SMS), and motivational interviewing (MI). Readers will note that four different terms or grammatical structures are used to describe Function Three throughout this text: "collaborate for management," "collaborative management," "manage collaboratively," and "collaboratively manage." While there may be subtle differences among the four terms, we consider all four so similar that they are used interchangeably.

The evidence indicates that neither education nor SMS skills come naturally or easily. Numerous studies demonstrate that physicians, in general, are not very effective in educating their patients or motivating them to adopt healthy behaviors. The majority of patients with chronic illness fail to recall important elements of their treatment recommendations and, in general, patients understand only about 50% of the information presented to them.[1,2] High levels of patient nonadherence to essential medication or lifestyle modification is worrisome: 22% to 74% of patients are nonadherent, rates seeming to vary depending on the severity and chronicity of the medical problem(s) and types of treatment recommendations.[3-5]

This chapter presents two pragmatic tools, eTACCT (Tailored Approach for Caring and Counseling Transculturally) and Brief Action Planning (BAP), to help clinicians become more efficient and more effective in educating patients and to use basic SMS and MI skills to encourage adaptive health behaviors.

Fourteen basic Function Three skills are addressed in this chapter. Two advanced MI skills (elicit and resolve ambivalence, and develop the discrepancy) are presented in Chapter 18. Motivational interviewing is a highly specialized, refined, and complex type of self-management support that has been shown to be particularly effective for patients with persistent unhealthy behaviors.[6,7]

This chapter also discusses the importance of the spirit of MI,[8] which refers to four underlying clinician attitudes demonstrated to help motivate patients to change. The four attitudes of the spirit of MI include compassion, acceptance, partnership, and evocation (CAPE). These attitudes are discussed in some detail in this chapter because of their general utility: understanding and applying them across all patient encounters deepens engagement and rapport while increasing commitment to change and improving outcomes.

*An interactive, automated e-learning platform on the website www.ComprehensiveMI.com supports mastery of the eight core competencies of Brief Action Planning (BAP), as well as the Spirit of Motivational Interviewing. Purchasers of this text receive access to Part One of this training at no cost via www.studentconsult.com. Part One of the web program covers the first five core competencies, one of three high-definition video demonstrations, one of three two-part "real-play" field exercises, and one of three automated computer-scored quizzes to assess mastery. Information about further access to the complete BAP web training program, other supporting materials for BAP, and more advanced training for comprehensive motivational interventions is available at www.ComprehensiveMI.com and a companion website, www.CentreCMI.ca.*

## Education About Illness: Use (e)TACCT

Patient education is not as simple as it may at first appear. Many factors interfere with the successful transfer of information from clinician to patient, such as patient anxiety, use of overly technical language, low health literacy, and simple misunderstandings. Consequently, many patients are not well informed about their illnesses and recommended treatments. Even after clinicians believe that they have educated their patients, most patients have retained only about 50% of the relevant information.[2]

This chapter presents a new tool, (e)TACCT, which can enhance the clinician's effectiveness as an educator.

---

**BOX 5.1 ■ (e)TACCT**

(e)TACCT
____ (e) elicit patient's baseline understanding of the problem.
____ (T) Tell the patient the core message.
    (A) Ask the patient for his or her understanding of the condition and his or her reaction.
____ (C) Care by responding to the emotional impact (using Function One skills).
____ (C) Counsel the patient about the details of the educational message.
____ (T) Tell-back: Ask the patient to "Tell-back" the core details of the message.

---

### USING (E)TACCT: ELICIT BASELINE UNDERSTANDING

Before providing any educational message, clinicians should elicit a patient's ideas about the problem and baseline understanding of any area of concern. For example:

PHYSICIAN: *What is it that most concerns you about your symptoms?*

PATIENT: *Well, I've been weak and dizzy and urinating a lot. That's what happened when my mother first got sugar diabetes. I'm worried that's what I may have now.*

PHYSICIAN: *Okay. That's helpful to know. I'd also like to know what else you know about diabetes....*

### USING (E)TACCT: TELL THE CORE MESSAGE

After eliciting the patient's expectations and explanatory model(s), and while paying attention to communicating in plain language, the practitioner should provide the core message briefly and succinctly. The patient will be very anxious while listening to diagnostic information, and will only remember information that is delivered in short, discrete bundles. One or two sentences should be all that is said in providing the initial information. For example:

> PHYSICIAN: *Mr. Brown, the tests confirm that you have diabetes.*

> or

> PHYSICIAN: *Mrs. Jones, your blood pressure is high.*

These short sentences are sufficient for the first piece of information. Patients will usually then have more specific questions or will demonstrate an emotional response.

Giving life-threatening bad news is far more delicate and complicated, but it should also be short and succinct. The specific challenge of giving or "sharing" bad news is discussed in more detail in Chapters 27 and 27A. It is usually best to include some hopeful statement along with the bad news. Because of the gravity of the situation, comments indicating continued attention and support and realistic hope are especially important. For example:

> PHYSICIAN: *Mr. Wright, I'm sorry to have to tell you that I have some bad news for you today … but I want you to know there is a lot we can do for you. Unfortunately, your biopsy confirmed that there is a cancer in your colon.*

## USING (E)TA**CC**T: <u>ASK</u> ABOUT THE PATIENT'S KNOWLEDGE OF THE ILLNESS

Many patients already know a great deal about their illness. Unless the clinician actually inquires about this knowledge, however, telling the patient something he or she already knows may waste time. Patients may also have a great deal of misinformation. This should be elicited early in the interview (if it has not already been elicited), so it can be corrected before it has a deleterious effect. The clinician can say something like:

> PHYSICIAN: *Before I go into more detail about high blood pressure, its causes, and what can happen if we don't control it, perhaps you can tell me what you already know about high blood pressure and its treatment.*

## USING (E)TA<u>CC</u>T: <u>CARE</u> ABOUT PATIENTS' EMOTIONAL RESPONSES AND CONCERNS

Patients often respond emotionally to new diagnostic information. This is particularly true if they are receiving bad news. At times, this response may be only nonverbal. They may become especially silent and look sad, fearful, or anxious. They may weep or ask a lot of questions.

The clinician should make it clear to the patient that the expression of feelings is acceptable and understandable. Clinician statements of reflection and legitimation are usually appropriate here, as is nonverbal support, such as attentive silence, holding the patient's hand, or passing a box of tissues. If the patient has just heard bad news, the physician should provide realistic hope along with emotional support. For the patient who is visibly shaken, the physician can say something like:

> PHYSICIAN: *I see how upsetting this news is for you. I'm going to do everything I can to help you through this and I'm going to be here for you. I want you to remember that there's a lot we can do to fight this thing together.*

Even when a diagnosis is not immediately life threatening, the patient often has an emotional reaction that should be acknowledged. By acknowledging this emotion, the practitioner allows the patient to verbalize fears about the illness. This will ultimately increase efficiency in the interview and enable the clinician to better support the patient. All the skills of Function One (communicating empathy through reflection, legitimation, support, partnership, and respect) may be useful during this educational process.

## USING (E)TACCT: <u>COUNSEL</u> ABOUT THE DETAILS

Only after the clinician has provided the basic message, established the patient's baseline knowledge, and responded to the patient's emotions can the clinician effectively elaborate on the details of the core message, whether about diagnosis, acute management, chronic care, and so on. If the practitioner attempts to deliver important educational messages before these other important steps have occurred, the patient will generally not be able to "hear" what the doctor says. The practitioner should take pains to use language consistent with the patient's health literacy, making sure to use terms that the patient will understand and short sentences that clarify each point. The physician should stop frequently to check the patient's understanding (tell-back) and ask for questions, as described in the next section.

Clinicians should also use visual aids, such as charts, graphics, or drawings, to communicate complex treatment options (see Chapter 20).

## USING (E)TACCT: <u>TELL-BACK</u> TO CHECK THAT THE PATIENT UNDERSTANDS

Checking a patient's understanding is the clinician's most important educational skill. A clinician cannot be sure that a patient understands what he or she has been told unless the clinician actually closes the loops and explicitly checks for comprehension. For example, the clinician can say:

> PHYSICIAN: *I would like to make sure that I have been able to make this information clear. Would you mind telling me back what we just discussed about your condition?*

> or

> PHYSICIAN: *I would like to make sure that I have explained the treatment possibilities to you clearly. Would you mind reviewing your understanding of these options?*

Similarly, after the patient has demonstrated appropriate understanding, the clinician should check what questions the patient may have about the information provided:

> PHYSICIAN: *What questions do you have about what we discussed?*

This question is most useful if it is presented in this positive manner, assuming that the patient does have questions. If the clinician asks, "Do you have any questions?" the patient may respond, "No," simply out of social embarrassment. The physician should anticipate that the patient or family will have further questions that will arise after the initial news has been delivered and should make plans for early follow-up to answer these additional questions.

# Brief Action Planning

Clinicians can work collaboratively with their patients to comanage illnesses by using Brief Action Planning (BAP), a highly structured, evidence-informed self-management support tool based on the principles and practice of Motivational Interviewing (MI).[7,9-11,A] Brief Action Planning has been published by the American Medical Association and the Commonwealth Fund (in its Tool-Kit for the Medical Home) and can be found in the 11th edition of *Bates' Guide to the Physical Exam and History Taking*.[2] It has been used in programs of the Centers for Disease Control, the Robert Wood Johnson Foundation, Health Resources Services Administration, Indian Health Service, the Institute for Healthcare Improvement, and many others. Brief Action Planning can also be considered an application of MI.[3]

The evidence is clear that patients who actively self-manage their own illnesses experience better health outcomes.[12] In supporting patient self-management, the practitioner gives up the traditional medical role of telling the patient what he or she *should* do, but rather shares information with the patient and then asks the patient what he or she *wants* or *is willing* to do. This approach is generally much more effective for motivating positive health behavior change and adherence than the more traditional "education and exhortation" approach. Confrontational, highly directive, and authoritarian approaches to behavior change tend to build resistance and are often counterproductive, especially in patients with persistent unhealthy behaviors.[13] Allowing patients the freedom to work on whatever is important to them builds patient self-efficacy, which in the long run is the most important factor in adopting healthy lifestyles and behaviors consistent with optimal self-care.[14]

The core competencies of BAP are structured around three foundation questions and five related skills. The BAP Flow Chart (Figure 5.1) and BAP Guide (Appendix 2) illustrate all eight BAP competencies, which are described in detail in the following.

## 1. QUESTION ONE: ELICIT IDEAS FOR CHANGE.*

Brief Action Planning begins with Question One:

> **PHYSICIAN:** *Is there anything you would like to do for your health in the next week or two?*

In actual clinical practice, Question One can be asked at different points throughout the encounter, sometimes early in a meeting, sometimes midway through, and sometimes toward the end. Regardless of timing, however, we believe that Question One or a functional equivalent should be part of most routine medical visits. In some acute or urgent care situations, however, there may not be sufficient time to use Brief Action Planning effectively.

From a purely grammatical point of view, Question One is closed. It can be answered either "yes" or "no." Despite this formal grammatical classification, however, in actual practice, Question One functions as a remarkably generative open question. In contrast to the typical closed question, which constricts a discussion, closing off conversation, Question One typically opens things up, generating and facilitating new productive talk about change. Even when a patient answers with a one word "yes" or "no" or something in-between such as, "I'm not sure," the clinician can, almost always, smoothly and seamlessly introduce or transition to a continuing dialogue about change.

In practice, Question One is highly motivating. Our collective experience to date suggests that, depending somewhat on clinical context, about 50% of patients who are asked Question One go on to develop an action plan for health with relatively little need for more advanced motivational interventions; and about two thirds of these patients complete their action plan for health at least some of the time or more.[B]

Although Question One can be answered "yes" or "no," there are typically three kinds of responses from patients to Question One (see the BAP Flow Chart).

### "Yes" Response

Patients answer Question One with a straightforward "yes" response and go on to generate an idea and specific action plan for health in relatively brief periods of time (3 to 5 minutes).

### "Not Sure" Response

Patients ask for more information or suggestions before developing an action plan. Clinicians can use a behavioral menu (discussed below) to help educate and motivate patients who are not

---

*A YouTube video, "Brief Action Planning" (available at the following url http://www.youtube.com/watch?v=w0n-f6qyG54), demonstrates Question One and the first two skills of BAP.

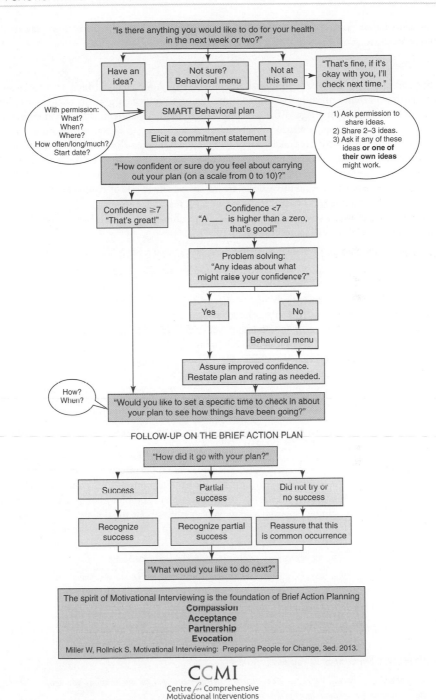

**Figure 5.1** Brief Action Planning Flow Chart. *(Developed by Steven Cole, Damara Gutnick, Connie Davis, Kathy Reims)*

sure to select a domain of their own choosing and go on to develop a specific action plan related to that domain.

## "Not Now" Response

Patients are complex, resistant, emotional, or ambivalent about change. Such patients usually present with persistent unhealthy behavior. Clinicians often find such patients challenging, frustrating, and difficult to manage. Effective motivation of these patients typically requires the strategic use of more complex relationship-building skills, skills for assessment and understanding, and/or higher-order motivational interviewing skills (Chapter 18). Mastery of higher-order motivational interviewing skills requires specific and focused intensive training.[C] Without this training, clinicians must rely on their own personal intuitive skills of persuasion. With ambivalent patients, unfortunately, these intuitive skills are rarely effective, and if confrontational in tone, can be counterproductive and create even more intense resistance to change.[13]

When a patient answers yes to Question One, the clinician can help him or her develop a specific action plan by asking something like:

> PHYSICIAN: *Can you say some more about what you would like to start doing?*

Then the clinician can move forward with the next structured step of BAP (SMART planning, see the following).

Alternatively, in lieu of an entirely non-focused Question One, the clinician may choose to probe the patient's readiness to start working on an issue of particular focus or concern. For example, if a patient has been discussing his or her problems with smoking, the clinician might use a functional derivative of Question One related to the behavior of concern, for example:

> PHYSICIAN: *Now that we have talked about your smoking for a while, is there anything you would like to do about your smoking in the next week or two?*

In practice, Question One usually generates a thoughtful process of self-reflection, and most patients begin talking about something meaningful they would like to do for their health.

## 2. SMART BEHAVIORAL PLANNING

Once a general behavioral domain has been specified, the clinician can ask the patient if he or she would like to make the plan more specific by asking questions such as what, where, when, where, how long, and how often? The more specific the plan, the more likely it will be carried out.[15,16] One process of helping patients become very specific about the details of a plan is called SMART behavioral planning. Plans should be specific, measurable, achievable, relevant, and time specific.

The following dialogue represents an example of SMART planning.

> PHYSICIAN: *Is there anything you'd like to do for your health in the next week or two?*

> PATIENT: *Well, you know, I think it's about time that I started to get some exercise. This might even help me lose weight.*

> PHYSICIAN: *That sounds like a good idea. Is that something you would like to make a plan to do?*

> PATIENT: *Sure. What do you mean, "plan?"*

> PHYSICIAN: *Okay. Making a plan means getting very specific about what you would like to do ... like when, where, how often, how long ... things like that?*

> PATIENT: *Sure. I think I can start exercising this weekend. I used to walk three times a week, and I think I can start that again on Saturday.*

> PHYSICIAN: *Do you know which three days you'll exercise?*

PATIENT: *Well … if I walk on Saturday and Sunday, I can usually find at least one other day of the week to walk.*

PHYSICIAN: *Great. Do you know* where *you're going to walk and for* how long?

PATIENT: *Yes. I'll walk about one mile around my neighborhood, on Saturday and Sunday morning, and then on one other day in the week.*

This process of specification, for most patients, can usually be completed in 3 to 5 minutes. Although clinicians always struggle with intense time pressures, the time to develop a specific action plan is usually a good investment because the more specific the plan, the more likely it will be carried out. The process of working through and describing the SMART details of the plan allows the individual to mentally work through potential barriers and increases the chances of success. It is more effective for behavior change than repeated exhortations and directives, which often occupy a considerable portion of a contemporary clinical visit, yet generally speaking, have been shown to be relatively ineffective and, with refractory unhealthy behaviors, can increase resistance and become counterproductive.[13]

## 3. ELICIT THE COMMITMENT STATEMENT

When SMART planning is complete, the clinician should elicit a commitment statement. Eliciting a commitment statement refers to a request from the clinician that the patient restate the action plan in his or her own words. Patient commitment statements are the best predictors of subsequent behavior change.[17,18] Some clinicians may feel awkward asking patients to repeat what they seemingly just went over. However, "closing the loop" solidifies the plan by encouraging patients to use their own words. The subsequent feeling of commitment using one's own words is much greater than if the clinician told the patient what he or she should do. Asking the patient to put the plan into writing may be even more effective.[19] For example:

PHYSICIAN: *Okay. Now that you have a plan you would like to carry out, please go over the details one last time to make sure we both understand what you are planning to do.*

PATIENT: *Okay. I am going to walk two times a week, on Saturday and Sunday morning, hopefully with my husband, for a mile around my neighborhood.*

## 4. QUESTION TWO: SCALE FOR CONFIDENCE

Once the patient has completed the commitment statement, the clinician can move on to Question Two of BAP. Question Two, Scale for Confidence, asks the patient to consider the degree of likelihood that he or she will be able to actually carry out the plan.

PHYSICIAN: *Okay. That sounds like a great plan. What is your level of confidence you can carry out the plan, on a 0-to-10 scale, in which 10 means you are very confident you can carry out the plan, and 0 means you are sure you will not be able to carry out the plan?*

Patients who report a confidence level of 7 or greater have a high likelihood of carrying out the plan.[14] On the other hand, patients whose confidence level is less than 7 may have a harder time sticking to the plan. If the patient reports a confidence level less than 7, the clinician can engage the patient in collaborative problem solving, described below.

## 5. QUESTION THREE: ARRANGE ACCOUNTABILITY

If the confidence level is 7 or greater, the clinician can then move on to Question Three. Question Three focuses on arranging accountability. Patients who feel accountable in some way to another person or tracking system will have a greater likelihood of actually carrying out the plan.[20]

It is worth noting that as patients elaborate specifics of a plan, confidence levels, and account-ability, they may volunteer positive adjustments to their plan along the way. Each time the patient has the opportunity to repeat the plan, he or she may shape it in ways that are more realistic and more powerful for that particular patient.

With respect to accountability, different approaches may be necessary or helpful. For patients with chronic illnesses followed by one clinician or team, the action plan can be entered into the paper chart or electronic medical record and follow-up visits become the most logical form of accountability. Some patients, however, may be seen only one time by a specialist or may be seen in an emergency room without personal follow-up. It is still possible to use Brief Action Planning effectively. In such cases, patients may arrange accountability by reporting to friends or family, or develop a form of self-accountability by keeping a calendar. For more typical follow-ups within a team structure, Question Three would be delivered like this:

> **PHYSICIAN:** *Would you like to set up a time to come back to review how your plan has been going?*

# Behavioral Menus and Problem Solving

In addition to the five discussed BAP competencies, behavioral menus and problem-solving skills are also useful for many clinical encounters.

## 6. THE BEHAVIORAL MENU

Sometimes patients who express an interest in doing something to improve their health often also ask for or benefit from education or suggestions from the clinician. As clinicians offer a behavioral menu of relevant choices, clinicians should also encourage patients to introduce ideas of their own at any time, which would be perfectly acceptable to the clinician.

In actual practice, if the patient seems to be a "not sure" individual needing more informa-tion or ideas, the clinician can ask if he or she would like this input and, if so, offer ideas tailored to the patient's particular condition, such as diabetes, obesity, depression, arthritis, and so on.

There are three elements involved in presenting behavioral menus to patients who need or request more information along these lines:

1. Ask the patient if he or she is interested in hearing ideas (ask permission).
2. Present a range of potential action ideas.
3. Suggest that hearing other ideas may in fact trigger new ideas from the patient.

The dialogue could go something like this:

> **PHYSICIAN:** *It sounds like you would like to start doing something, but you are not really sure what to do. Would it be helpful if I offered some suggestions?*
>
> **PATIENT:** *Sure, why not?*
>
> **PHYSICIAN:** *Well, some people in your situation try to get a little more exercise, or work on eating better or focus on taking their medications regularly as prescribed. Perhaps one of these ideas makes sense for you, or maybe you can think of something else that you would prefer to work on?*

Many preprinted behavioral menus are available (Figure 5.2) or clinicians can create their own. Use of a printed behavioral menu is recommended when possible because the intervention gains strength through the use of visual as well as verbal channels of communication.

It is important to give patients the opportunity to suggest ideas of their own. Clinicians are often surprised at the views and proposals patients develop for themselves. One patient may want

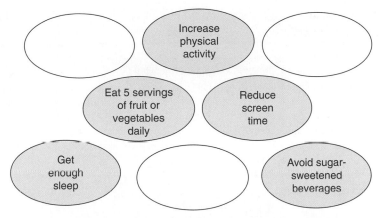

Adapted from Stott et al, Family Practice 1995; Rollnick et al, 1999, 2010

CCMI
Centre For Comprehensive
Motivational Interventions

**Figure 5.2** Visual Behavioral Menu Example.

to clean his car, whereas another might want to go fishing with his father, and someone else believes a short vacation would contribute to his/her health. If a patient comes up with an idea himself or herself, the clinician should work with the patient to develop a concrete realistic action plan for that idea, even if the patient's idea may seem entirely unrelated to the specific illness at hand. This may require something of a paradigm shift for both the clinician and the patient. But accomplishing any action plan builds self-efficacy, which can then lead to more active action planning for health in general.[21]

## 7. PROBLEM SOLVING

Some patients develop a plan that appears reasonable and achievable, yet when asked to declare a confidence level, they report a number less than 7. In these cases, clinicians should work with patients to problem solve ways to overcome barriers to implementing the plan or to revise the plan in such a way that a confidence level of 7 or higher can be attained. Sometimes this is the point in the conversation at which it becomes clear that the initial plan was created to please the physician or is something the patient feels like he or she *should* do but is not actually *interested* in doing; therefore, creating a completely different plan may be the next best step.

As stated, action plans associated with confidence levels of 7 or greater have a greater likelihood of success.[22-24] Therefore when a patient declares a confidence level below 7, the clinician should attempt to work with him or her to find a way to bring a plan up to 7 or higher. The conversation should emphasize the strengths suggested by any number (strength-based counseling), however low, rather than the deficits of a low number that could be higher. The dialogue might go something like this:

> **PHYSICIAN:** *A confidence level of 5 is terrific. It's much higher than 0 or 1. So you do have a lot of confidence that you might actually be able to do something. But I should also tell you that plans with confidence levels of 7 or greater have a higher chance of being carried out. I wonder if there is anything you might be able to change to get your confidence level up to 7 or more; perhaps making your plan a little less ambitious, or perhaps finding someone to help you keep to your plan might help....*

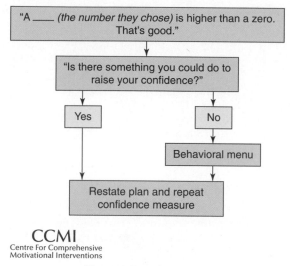

**Figure 5.3** Problem-Solving.

**PATIENT:** *Okay. I understand. Let me change the exercise plan to two times a week and I will ask my husband to help me remember. In fact, I'm going to ask him to walk with me! That will be good for him too, and give us the chance to spend some time together.*

**PHYSICIAN:** *Does that change your confidence level?*

**PATIENT:** *Yes. I would give this plan an 8 now.*

The discussion around confidence levels usually leads to collaborative problem solving, resulting in realistic action planning with higher likelihoods of success. Figure 5.3 illustrates the dialogue around problem solving.

## 8. FOLLOW-UP

Follow-up is an essential aspect of Brief Action Planning and may be especially powerful if it occurs with the clinician who participated in developing the plan itself.

The follow-up involves three core elements.

1. Nonjudgmental inquiry
2. Reassurance if the plan was not completed successfully
3. Checking into the patient's ideas and desires about most appropriate next steps

An inquiry about the previous plan should be made relatively early in the visit, especially if the patient does not volunteer this information himself or herself. This inquiry should be nonjudgmental, without inducing guilt or shame, accepting the possibility that the patient may not have carried out the plan as intended. For example:

**PHYSICIAN:** *I wonder how things went with your action plan?*

**PATIENT:** *I didn't do any of the plan at all. I don't know what happened. I just didn't do it. I'm kind of embarrassed.*

**PHYSICIAN:** *This happens with lots of people. You don't need to feel embarrassed. What's important is what you'd like to do next. Would you like to talk about what you learned the last few weeks about the action plan you set for yourself and had trouble completing? Or would you* *like to talk about something entirely different? Or perhaps you'd like to set up an entirely new action plan?*

If the patient actually did accomplish part or all of the plan we suggest a very patient-friendly and generous three-tiered measurement plan for assessment at follow-up. The plan was accomplished:

1. Little or none of the time
2. Some of the time
3. 50% of the time or more

This three-tiered metric facilitates and encourages the following type of positive, "reframing" dialogue on follow-up:

PHYSICIAN: *So, I wonder how things went with your exercise plan?*

PATIENT: *Well, not so well, if I have to tell you the truth.*

PHYSICIAN: *That's Okay. Lots of people have some trouble with their action plans. What happened?*

PATIENT: *I tried to do my walking three times a week like I said I would, but I just couldn't make it that third time. But I did do it two times a week.*

PHYSICIAN: *You know, that actually puts you in our highest category for follow-up. You did your action plan 50% of the time or more. So I think you should feel good about what you accomplished.*

PATIENT: *Okay. That does make me feel much better!*

PHYSICIAN: *So, now, I wonder if you would like to set some new goals for yourself for the next few weeks?*

In general, attention to follow-up creates opportunities for ongoing behavior change. If omitted, it can be interpreted by the patient as lack of interest or lack of caring on the part of the clinician.

It is also important to consider how other health care team members can be included in follow-up. Medical office assistants are often in an ideal situation to take on parts or all of the steps of BAP.

Figure 5.4 demonstrates the three response patterns of follow-up.

## The Eight Core Skills of Brief Action Planning

To review what has just been covered, the eight foundation motivational competencies of Brief Action Planning are:

1. Question One: Elicit patient ideas for change
2. Offer a behavioral menu when needed or helpful
3. SMART behavioral planning
4. Elicit the commitment statement
5. Question Two: Scale for confidence
6. Problem solving to increase confidence level when necessary
7. Arrange accountability
8. Follow-up

## Four Essential Attributes of a Brief Action Plan

A brief action plan has four essential elements.

1. The plan is patient centered. The plan is what the patient wants to do, not what the clinician tells the patient to do or wants the patient to do.

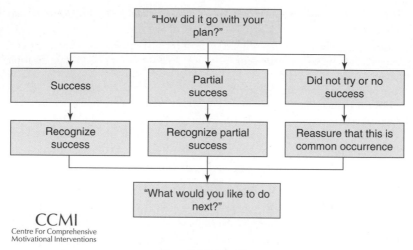

**Figure 5.4** Follow-Up.

2. The plan is very concrete, clear, specific, and measurable. (It is not general or vague, like "Lose weight" or "Get some exercise.")
3. The patient's confidence in the plan is 7 or greater on a 0-to-10 scale.
4. The plan is associated with specific follow-up.

## Spirit of Motivational Interviewing

There are four attitudes underlying the spirit of MI that clinicians should incorporate into their general approach to patient care and that have been shown to maximize the potential for change. The four components are compassion, acceptance, partnership, and evocation.[8]

*Evocation* refers to the concept that ideas for behavior change must emanate from the patient and cannot be demanded by the clinician. The practitioner can facilitate behavior change through empathy, strategic questioning, and suggestions through a behavioral menu, as well as providing the supportive environment to help the patient who is striving to improve health behaviors. The chance of success is greatest, however, when the specific ideas for change actually come from the patient himself or herself.

*Partnership* (or collaboration)[6] stands as the cornerstone of Function Three and is also one of the three core attitudes of the spirit of MI. Partnership suggests that the clinician and the patient are equals in the change process. Again, the clinician cannot tell the patient what he or she "should" do. The clinician should share ideas for change as an equal with the patient.

*Acceptance*[7] may be the most complex element of the spirit of MI. The four components of acceptance include accurate empathy, absolute worth, affirmation, and autonomy support. Respect for autonomy suggests that the clinician should respect the patient's decision whether or not to change. As long as the medical team provides necessary information in an understandable and usable manner for the patient and the team provides an empathic environment, the practitioner should make it clear that the patient is the "expert" on his or her own health and has the right to make his or her own decision whether or not to change. Whichever way the patient decides to go, the medical team should respect this decision without communicating disappointment or disapproval and avoid inducing feelings of embarrassment or guilt.[25,26]

*Compassion* refers to one of the four central components of the underlying *spirit* of MI by which the interviewer acts benevolently to promote the client's welfare, giving priority to the client's needs.

Three (evocation, partnership, autonomy support) of the four attitudes related to the spirit of MI can be assessed reliably when listening to or observing actual clinician-patient encounters. Clinicians scoring high on "spirit" measures have been shown to be more effective in motivating positive behavior change in their patients than clinicians demonstrating lower scores on "spirit" measures.[13]

## WHAT ABOUT THE PATIENT WITH PERSISTENT UNHEALTHY BEHAVIOR WHO SAYS "NO" TO QUESTION ONE?

Advanced skills useful for motivating patients with persistent unhealthy behavior are discussed in detail in Chapter 18. For the purposes of this chapter on basic skills, however, clinicians should indicate to these patients their interest and willingness to discuss behavior change whenever the patient feels ready to do so.

## Conclusion

This chapter reviews the educational and self-management support (or motivational) strategies of Function Three, Collaborate for Management. These six skills of (e)TACCT and eight competencies of BAP provide learners with the foundation they need to build satisfying and successful physician-patient partnerships to comanage the complex and challenging illnesses that they will face throughout long careers of practice.

## Summary

This chapter presents Function Three, Collaborate for Management, and the two structured tools which support it: (e)TACCT, an educational device, and Brief Action Planning (BAP), a self-management support tool.

### References

1. Kravitz RL, et al: Recall of recommendations and adherence to advice among patients with chronic medical conditions. *Arch Intern Med* 153(16):1869–1878, 1993.
2. Stewart M: Patient recall and comprehension after the medical visit. In Lipkin M, editor: *The medical interview: clinical care, education, and research, e.a,* New York, 1995, Springer.
3. DiMatteo MR: Variations in patients' adherence to medical recommendations: a quantitative review of 50 years of research. *Med Care* 42(3):200–209, 2004.
4. DiMatteo MR, et al: Patient adherence and medical treatment outcomes: a meta-analysis. *Med Care* 40(9):794–811, 2002.
5. DiMatteo MR: Enhancing patient adherence to medical recommendations. *JAMA* 271(1):79, 83, 1994.
6. Hettema J, Steele J, Miller WR: Motivational interviewing. *Annu Rev Clin Psychol* 1:91–111, 2005.
7. Cole S DC, Cole M, Gutnick D: Motivational interviewing and the patient-centered medical home: a strategic approach to self-management support in primary care. In Steidl J, editor: *Transforming patient engagement: health information technology and the medical home,* Washington, D.C, 2010, Patient Centered Primary Care Collaborative.
8. Miller WR, Rollnick S: *Motivational interviewing: preparing people for change,* ed 2, New York, 2002, Guilford Press, Xx, p 428.
9. American Medical Association: *Physician resource guide to patient self-management support,* Chicago, 2008, American Medical Association.

10. Cole S DC, Cole M, Gutnick D: Motivational interviewing and the patient centered medical home: a strategic approach to self-management support in primary care. In Steidl J, editor: *Transforming patient engagement: health it in the patient centered medical home*, Washington, D.C., 2010, Patient Centered Primary Care Collaborative, pp. 20–25.
11. Cole SBJ: *UB-PAP (ultra-brief personal action planning): an innovative tool to support patient self-management, motivate healthy behavior change and improve adherence*, New York City, 2009, Institute of Psychiatric Services.
12. Bodenheimer T, et al: Patient self-management of chronic disease in primary care. *JAMA* 288(19):2469–2475, 2002.
13. Miller WR, Rose GS: Toward a theory of motivational interviewing. *Am Psychol* 64(6):527–537, 2009.
14. Lorig KR, Holman H: Self-management education: history, definition, outcomes, and mechanisms. *Ann Behav Med* 26(1):1–7, 2003.
15. Bodenheimer T, Handley MA: Goal-setting for behavior change in primary care: an exploration and status report. *Patient Educ Couns* 76(2):174–180, 2009.
16. Strecher VJ, et al: Goal setting as a strategy for health behavior change. *Health Educ Q* 22(2):190–200, 1995.
17. Amrhein PC, et al: Client commitment language during motivational interviewing predicts drug use outcomes. *J Consult ClinPsychol* 71(5):862–878, 2003.
18. Aharonovich E, et al: Cognition, commitment language, and behavioral change among cocaine-dependent patients. *Psychol Addict Behav* 22(4):557–562, 2008.
19. Cialdini RB: *Influence: science and practice*, ed 5, Boston, 2009, Pearson Education, Xii, p 259.
20. Glasgow RE, Emont S, Miller DC: Assessing delivery of the five "As" for patient-centered counseling. *Healthy Promot Int* 21(3):245–255, 2006.
21. Bandura A: Self-efficacy: toward a unifying theory of behavioral change. *Psychol Rev* 84(2):191–215, 1977.
22. Lorig K: *Living a healthy life with chronic conditions: for ongoing physical and mental health conditions. Canadian ed*, Boulder, Colo., 2007, Bull Pub. Company, Vii, p 398.
23. Lorig K, Fries JF, Gecht-Silver MR: *The arthritis helpbook: a tested self-management program for coping with arthritis and fibromyalgia*, ed 6, Cambridge, Mass., 2006, Da Capo Lifelong, Xiii, p 386.
24. Lorig K: *Patient education: a practical approach*, ed 3, Thousand Oaks, Calif., 2001, Sage Publications, Xvi, p 246.
25. Lazare A: The suffering of shame and humiliation in illness. *NLN Publ* (15-2461):227–244, 1992.
26. Lazare A: Shame and humiliation in the medical encounter. *Arch Intern Med* 147(9):1653–1658, 1987.

## Endnotes

A. www.ComprehensiveMI.com
B. Clinical experience from more than 500 patients from physician internal medicine, nurse practitioner rheumatology, nurse practitioner geriatrics, psychiatry, psychology, and telephonic social workers in Employee Assistance Programs or chronic disease management. Cole S, et al: *UB-PAP (Ultra-Brief Personal Action Planning): An Innovative Tool to Support Patient Self-Management, Motivate Healthy Behavior Change and Improve Adherence*, in *Institute of Psychiatric Services*. 2009: New York City.
C. www.ComprehensiveMI.com; www.motivationalinterview.org

# Meeting the Patient

# CHAPTER 6

# Ten Common Concerns

## OVERVIEW

This chapter answers ten common questions of early medical trainees and presents six general principles to help guide professional behavior. These six principles are listed below.

1. If you feel uncomfortable touching a patient, do not touch the patient (other than what is absolutely necessary for the physical examination).
2. Any sexual relationship between a medical practitioner and a patient is always an abuse of power and should never occur.
3. Do not answer medical questions if you are not part of the medical team. Refer questions politely back to the primary medical team.
4. Respond to an emotion as soon as it appears. (Rule #1 of Interviewing; see Chapter 3). When in doubt about how to respond to an emotion, use reflection and legitimation (see Chapter 3, Function One).
5. Never promise a patient absolute confidentiality.
6. Communicate all clinically relevant information a patient may have told you back to the treatment team. Do it yourself.

Most medical trainees eagerly anticipate their first contacts with patients. Despite recent trends to introduce patient contact early in the curricula, most medical students still spend at least 1 year, and sometimes more than that, in classroom settings before they get a chance to talk with patients as clinician caregivers. Therefore courses on clinical methods, physical diagnosis, or the doctor-patient relationship usually come as a great relief to students because they will finally be getting a taste of what "real" medicine will be like for them.

Most physicians remember their first interviews with patients in considerable detail because these early encounters mark the beginnings of their professional lives in a very real, as well as symbolic, way. These first contacts with patients often remain some of the most poignant and memorable ones of their careers.

Anticipation of these encounters brings reasonable and expected excitement as well as anxiety. Students are almost always anxious before they meet their first patients. Although somewhat variable from trainee to trainee, sources of this anxiety are numerous, understandable, and predictable.

Students feel worried about how their patients will react. Will patients feel like "guinea pigs?" Students often feel uncomfortable because they feel that their interviews will invade patients' privacy and dignity. Virtually overnight, students have been given the right, and indeed the expectation, to ask intimate questions of others (including patients of the opposite sex who are their parents or grandparents age) that they would never dream of otherwise asking ... about sexuality, about bowel and bladder habits, about life and death issues, etc. And, as if that weren't enough, when students are learning the basic elements of the physical examination, they must further impose upon patients to ask them to expose themselves and to undergo sometimes uncomfortable and occasionally even painful examination. Students feel awkward or even guilty asking anyone to go through this experience for them, viewing it as an indignity or humiliation and typically ask themselves, "Why would a patient want to go through this, just for my education?" These concerns become even more troubling if the patient is seriously ill, in pain, or suffering from a terminal illness.

Students who feel anxious about these practice interviews, however, should rest assured that they are in good company and for good reasons. Developing proficiency in medical interviewing involves far more than simply mastering a new set of difficult and complex skills. It demands the assumption of a new and dramatically different social role and identity. In putting on the white coat for the first time, or simply entering into the social status of physician or clinician (for those who do not "wear" the white coat itself), the trainee steps into an entirely new relational world that forever changes the way he or she interacts with people who now become "patients" or "significant other/families." This seemingly simple, symbolic change marks a momentous interpersonal change. Suddenly, students take powerful charge of dyadic interactions, requesting others to undress and follow their leadership, and those others, virtually without objection, accommodate to this control quite often with both respect and gratitude.

Learning to function in this new and powerful social role understandably makes most medical trainees both uncomfortable and anxious. There are many questions learners ask themselves and their instructors as they begin this part of their training. This chapter discusses ten common concerns.

The Ten Concerns

1. Why should the patient want to talk to or be examined by a student?
2. Is a student interview or examination a humiliation or indignity for the patient?
3. How should I dress? Should I wear a white coat?
4. Should I introduce myself as "doctor"? If I do that, am I not deceiving the patient?
5. If the patient is in pain or emotional distress, should I continue with the interview?
6. Should I shake the patient's hand? Under what circumstances is it acceptable to touch a patient?
7. If the patient asks me questions, should I answer the questions if I know the answers? What should I do if I do not know the answers?
8. What do I do if the patient starts crying or if the patient gets angry with me?
9. What should I do if the patient promises to tell me some important secrets if I agree to maintain his or her confidence?
10. What should I do if the patient tells me something his or her doctor does not know? For example, what if the patient tells me that he or she is depressed or suicidal?

## 1. WHY SHOULD THE PATIENT WANT TO TALK TO OR BE EXAMINED BY A STUDENT?

Students usually find it difficult to understand the reasons that a patient agrees or even may want to be interviewed or to be examined by a student. Students may wonder what the patient could possibly gain from this encounter.

As a matter of fact, most patients are quite willing to be interviewed and examined by respectful students. Patients, as a general rule, understand that students need to learn about illness through practicing on real patients, and patients often derive altruistic satisfaction from allowing themselves to be such subjects. Patients who agree to practice interviews and exams do not feel like guinea pigs. More commonly, patients interviewed or examined by students feel that they are making a genuine and active contribution by assisting in the training of physicians or other medical practitioners. In fact, participating in such educational activities can play a profound role in the psychologic adaptation of the severely ill or incapacitated. The feelings of uselessness that are associated with illness can be meaningfully counteracted for some patients by their sense of genuine contribution to the education of future medical practitioners. Thus, even if students do nothing other than practice and learn, patients actually do benefit from this exercise by being allowed to "give" something of real value to these practitioners in training. In addition, some patients also feel they can make additional contributions by offering clinical advice to trainees or recounting personal experiences that they feel will help students become better or more caring clinicians. Trainees, for their part, almost always find this additional information interesting, useful, and sometimes profoundly moving. The following case illustrates a typical example of a mutually beneficial patient-trainee interaction.

> Mr. Braverman, a 68-year-old Vietnam War veteran, was hospitalized for severe chronic obstructive pulmonary disease (COPD) and heart failure, and gave permission for Robert Henry to practice a medical interview. The interview turned out to be a moving and important learning experience for Robert because he learned about Mr. Braverman's posttraumatic stress disorder (PTSD) from his Vietnam war exposures and how the PTSD and COPD both get worse during national disasters like 9-11 and school shootings. Mr. Braverman in turn benefitted from Robert's empathic and genuine concern. However, of even more direct clinical importance, when Robert asked about quality of life and impact of illness, Mr. Braverman reported there was virtually no sexual intimacy in the last 10 years with his wife because he had erectile difficulties and both he and his wife thought sex would be dangerous for his heart. No doctor had actually asked him about sexual adjustment over the last 10 years, so he assumed that it probably was better to leave well enough alone. Robert brought these findings back to his preceptor and the medical team. Also of importance, Mr. Braverman told Robert and the preceptor that he was very glad that the student (compared with all previous physicians) had finally brought up this issue because it had been deeply troubling for him and his wife for a very long time.

Thus there are many ways that students can and do, in fact, give patients something quite important, just by learning. The simple fact that the trainee learns from what the patient gives is sufficient, in and of itself, but there is more. The concern, interest, and attention provided by the student offers significant emotional comfort to the patient as well. Although it is intangible and not measurable, this emotional dimension to the student-patient interaction is important and can be dramatic. Furthermore, the practice physical examination can also feel like an emotional gift. Thus students would do well to recognize that most patients are quite willing and even eager to be interviewed and examined, even if it is just for practice.

To be sure, it is also true that some patients will not want to be interviewed or examined. Therefore, before beginning any practice interview, students should ask their assigned patients if they are willing to be interviewed. If the patients indicate that they do not want to be interviewed, these wishes should be respected. In such situations the students should politely thank the patients and leave. The students should check with their supervisors for guidance in how to proceed further.

## 2. IS A STUDENT INTERVIEW OR EXAMINATION A HUMILIATION OR INDIGNITY FOR THE PATIENT?

Some students feel awkward because they think patients will feel humiliated when subjecting themselves to an interview by a student. Students have this fear partly because of the implied power of the role of the physician or medical practitioner. Students may feel uncomfortable assuming this power, thinking they do not deserve it because they are not able to offer "true" medical assistance, because they are only practicing skills and not functioning as a member of the patient's care team. As pointed out previously, however, few patients experience this practice encounter as an embarrassment or humiliation. Most experience it as the opportunity for them to make a contribution, for which they are often actually grateful.

## 3. HOW SHOULD I DRESS? SHOULD I WEAR A WHITE COAT EVEN THOUGH I AM NOT A DOCTOR? DOESN'T THIS INTRODUCE AN ARTIFICIAL SEPARATION AND INEQUALITY INTO THE RELATIONSHIP? IF I WEAR A WHITE COAT, ISN'T THAT DECEIVING THE PATIENT?

In general, students should dress in the same attire as the other physicians or medical practitioners in their institution. If most of the other providers wear whites, students should wear whites. Dressing in the same manner as their colleagues indicates respect for the patient and, symbolically, the role soon to be assumed.

To be sure, dressing as a physician distinguishes students from patients and introduces an inequality into the student-patient relationship. However, this distinction and inequality are both appropriate. Students will be interviewing patients and asking them to divulge some of the most intimate details of their lives. Patients will be asked to undress and to allow themselves to be physically examined. These requests and inequalities are accepted and expected parts of the doctor-patient relationship, and the white coat, when used conventionally, helps respectfully demarcate the boundaries of these different roles.

As discussed below, students should clearly introduce themselves as student doctors, or a nurse practitioner student or a physician's assistant student. This helps ensure that patients will not be deceived.

## 4. SHOULD I INTRODUCE MYSELF AS "DOCTOR"? IF I DO, AM I NOT DECEIVING THE PATIENT?

Most beginning students are uncomfortable with introducing themselves as "doctor." This discomfort is understandable because many patients do not understand the differences among students, interns, residents, and attending physicians. As a general rule, students should always make their status and level of training clear. The following examples illustrate ways this can be achieved:

> STUDENT: *Hello. My name is John Smith. I am a medical student taking a course on how to interview patients. I was given your name as someone who might be willing to talk with me about your illness. Would that be all right with you?*

Another alternative, for students in a clerkship situation, could be to say something like the following:

> STUDENT: *Hello. My name is Bill Stevens, and I am a student doctor working with Dr. Jones. Do you mind if I ask you a few questions about your problems before you see Dr. Jones?*

In practice, this type of introduction works easily and well for most students and their patients. Patients, on the other hand, often wonder how they should address medical students. Is it appropriate for patients to call the student "doctor," or should patients use a student's first name? There is no clearly appropriate label that conveys the character of the student physician-patient relationship. Most such relationships closely resemble true doctor-patient relationships. They resemble such relationships much more closely than they resemble anything else. Thus it is no surprise that many patients prefer to address their student doctors as "doctor." This is perfectly appropriate, especially if the patient understands that the student is not a licensed physician. Sometimes patients ask students what they want to be called. It is common for students to want to be called by their first names and it is acceptable in these cases for patients to do so. Similarly, some students prefer to leave this choice to the patients. However, if students would like to be called "doctor," patients can be told something such as the following:

> **STUDENT:** *I am a student doctor now and would prefer for you to call me "Doctor Jones." I will be finished with my training in another year. I hope this is acceptable to you.*

Nurse practitioner students and PA students can comfortably have patients call them Mr. or Mrs. or by their first names, whichever they prefer.

## 5. IF THE PATIENT IS IN PAIN OR EMOTIONAL DISTRESS, SHOULD I CONTINUE WITH THE INTERVIEW?

If the patient is in pain or emotional distress, the wishes of the patient must be respected. First, the student must acknowledge the pain or distress. The student may say something like the following:

> **STUDENT:** *You seem to be in distress.*

> or

> **STUDENT:** *You seem to be in a lot of pain right now.*

These comments are appropriate and will let the patient know that his or her suffering has been noticed. Students can and should directly ask whether anything can be done to help. Often patients appreciate a glass of water, a change of the position of the bed, or some other small intervention.

After discomfort has been acknowledged and offers of assistance have been made, the student should ask the patient whether the interview can be conducted or should be postponed. If the patient wants the student to go away, this desire should be respected. Most often and to the surprise of most students, the patient wants to continue the interview or examination. Once pain or distress has been acknowledged, the patient will usually feel comforted by the concern and attention of the student and will prefer to continue.

## 6. SHOULD I SHAKE THE PATIENT'S HAND? UNDER WHAT CIRCUMSTANCES IS IT ACCEPTABLE TO TOUCH THE PATIENT?

Most physicians and medical practitioners in the United States offer a hand to their patients in greeting when they introduce themselves. This practice generally works well for beginning students. However, some male students from other cultures have expressed discomfort with this practice because they have been taught that it is rude to offer a hand to a woman, even for a social or professional greeting. These students have been taught that respectful behavior requires a gentleman to wait for a woman to offer him her hand before he attempts to shake hands. Students who are uncomfortable with shaking hands in greeting will do better to wait for patients to offer a hand to them. Students who are uncomfortable about touching a patient in any way are better advised to avoid the touch than to force themselves into physical contact out of a belief that it may be good for the patient.

Touch is a powerful and supportive technique in medicine. In situations of great distress, physicians and other medical practitioners commonly and appropriately touch a patient's forearm or put an arm around a patient's shoulders. Experienced clinicians routinely use limited physical contact to reassure their patients and enhance rapport. Most patients feel comforted by sensitive and appropriate physician physical touch. However, some patients do not want to be touched at all, and some practitioners find that any type of touch (other than the physical examination) provokes anxiety. In general, students (and all practitioners) should adhere to the following rule:

**Principle One: If you feel uncomfortable about touching a patient, do not touch the patient.**

Discomfort with touching communicates itself to patients through nonverbal channels, and such a touch becomes an anxiety-producing intervention for the patient rather than a support.

Some students and clinicians may be overly familiar with their patients and touch them too much. Observing the patient is critical. A patient who is uncomfortable with being touched will give some signal, usually nonverbal, that the touch is not appreciated. For example, he or she will back away, stiffen up, or become quiet. The clinician must be vigilant to watch for these signs and respond to them appropriately, generally by backing away respectfully.

Touch can also be emotionally or sexually seductive. Physicians and other medical providers should be aware of the tremendous power they wield over their patients. Illness causes patients to regress psychologically and physically and thus elevates the role and importance of the clinician (especially physicians) in patients' minds. The resulting emotional dependency can be overwhelming. Often, patients are not able to use their most rational thought processes; patients in this situation may relate to their physicians as children relate to their parents. Inappropriate touch can be part of an emotionally seductive clinician-patient relationship that can harm patients by fostering dependency rather than adaptive coping.

Sexual seductiveness can be communicated by touching patients. Tragically, this can lead to sexual relationships between clinicians and patients. Because of the inherently unequal power in the provider-patient relationship and the psychological dependency fostered by the context of illness, patients may not be able to make mature decisions about sexuality with their physicians or other practitioners. Students and providers must remember the following ethical principle:

**Principle Two: Any sexual relationship between a medical practitioner and a patient is always an abuse of power and should never occur. This is exploitative and unethical behavior as well as grounds for claims of clinician misconduct.**

## 7. IF THE PATIENT ASKS ME QUESTIONS, SHOULD I ANSWER THEM IF I KNOW THE ANSWERS? WHAT SHOULD I DO IF I DO NOT KNOW THE ANSWERS?

In general, students practicing an interview or physical examination with someone else's patients should avoid answering any questions about a patient's individual condition. In the heady moments of finally being regarded as an expert, students might be tempted to answer some medical question that they think they understand well. It is important to resist this temptation. Students may have an incomplete understanding of the medical issue and generally will not understand the personal meaning of the question to the patients they are interviewing or examining. Because the students will breeze into and out of the patients' lives in a few hours, the students will not be able to observe the impact of whatever information they give the patients. Some seemingly innocuous question and answer might have great import and impact for any unique patient. The following statement is important for students practicing an interview:

**Principle Three: Do not answer medical questions if you are not part of the medical team. Refer questions politely back to the primary medical team.**

This rule does not necessarily hold for patients of students who are serving clinical clerkships. Such students sometimes become patients' primary source of information. When students assume the role of educators, however, they should be confident of the information they give to their patients and sensitive to the emotional impact of the information they transmit. Any uncertainty should be reviewed carefully with supervisors.

## 8. WHAT DO I DO IF THE PATIENT STARTS CRYING OR IF THE PATIENT GETS ANGRY WITH ME?

Nothing makes some trainees (and even some more experienced clinicians) more uncomfortable than the expression of emotion by patients. What should students do when patients start crying? This will be a common occurrence, and trainees need to start learning how to respond in a way that is helpful and supportive to patients.

An attitude of interest and respect will almost always be comforting to patients, regardless of what the students do or say. Students can best start supportive communication of respect and caring nonverbally through attentive silence, without any conscious effort spent (at first) on thinking about what to say. Just listen.

Some students are so uncomfortable with sadness that they communicate this anxiety to patients. Students (or physicians) display this anxiety about patients' emotions in several ways: by changing the subject quickly to something without emotional content or by premature reassurance. This discomfort is usually interpreted by patients as meaning that the practitioners do not want the patients to show any more emotion. Patients usually honor this perception and cooperate by suppressing the expression of further emotion.

When students have some verbal strategy in mind to deal with situations in which patients are anxious, the students' own anxiety will be less and the students will be able to help patients more. The following general rule has proved useful:

Principle Four: Respond to an emotion as soon as it appears. (Rule #1 of Interviewing; see Chapter 3). When in doubt about how to respond to an emotion, use reflection and legitimation (see Chapter 3, Function One).

Comments like the following are appropriate:

STUDENT: *I can see that you are very upset by this situation.*

or

STUDENT: *I understand this is very troubling.*

In general, such reflective comments encourage patients to discuss some details of the troubling situation. This information can usually be followed by legitimating comments such as the following:

STUDENT: *I can certainly understand why this has taken such a toll on you.*

or

STUDENT: *Anyone would have trouble dealing with this.*

What about when patients get angry? This is even more difficult to manage. The natural responses to anger are to withdraw or attack. Neither response is particularly helpful in developing rapport with angry patients. Of more help is reflection, even of an angry emotion. For example, students can say something such as the following:

STUDENT: *This conversation seems to irritate you.*

Again, this type of reflective comment will usually lead patients to discuss more of the particular details of their situations. Subsequent to this discussion a legitimating comment may be appropriate:

STUDENT: *I can certainly understand why this situation has made you so frustrated.*

This difficult topic will be discussed further in Chapter 17 (Understanding Chronic Illness: Maladaptive Reactions)

## 9. WHAT SHOULD I DO IF THE PATIENT PROMISES TO TELL ME SOME IMPORTANT SECRETS IF I AGREE TO MAINTAIN HIS OR HER CONFIDENCE?

Because most students demonstrate a high degree of emotional interest in their patients, it is not unusual for patients to discuss personal information that they may not want to be shared with the rest of the medical team. However, this request cannot be accepted.

**Principle Five: Never promise a patient absolute confidentiality.**

If a patient asks for confidentiality, the student should indicate that his or her status as a trainee makes it impossible to give a promise of complete confidentiality. The student may have to share this sensitive information with a supervisor or the patient's treatment team if it is clinically relevant.

In general requests for complete confidentiality represent opportunities for students to enhance the care a patient receives, as long as the patient is told the limits of the confidentiality and the information is handled sensitively and appropriately after it has been received by the trainee.

## 10. WHAT SHOULD I DO IF THE PATIENT TELLS ME SOMETHING HIS OR HER DOCTOR DOES NOT KNOW? FOR EXAMPLE, WHAT IF THE PATIENT TELLS ME THAT HE OR SHE IS DEPRESSED OR SUICIDAL?

For the same reason that patients sometimes ask for confidentiality from trainees who interview them, they also sometimes reveal clinically relevant and urgent or emergent information. Despite any request for confidentiality, students/trainees are obligated ethically and legally to communicate clinically relevant information to the treatment team.

**Principle Six: Communicate all clinically relevant information back to the treatment team. Do it yourself.**

Students can advise patients to tell this new information directly to the treatment team themselves, but this is not sufficient. If the patients have not already told these problems to their team, they cannot be relied on to do it now. The only way to ensure that the team will become aware of the problem is for the students to tell the team themselves.

## Summary

This chapter answers ten common questions of early medical trainees and presents six general principles to help guide professional behavior. These six principles are listed below.

1. If you feel uncomfortable about touching a patient, do not touch the patient.
2. Any sexual relationship between a medical practitioner and a patient is always an abuse of power and should never occur.
3. Do not answer medical questions if you are not part of the medical team. Refer questions politely back to the patient's primary medical team.
4. Respond to an emotion as soon as it appears. (Rule #1 of Interviewing; see Chapter 3). When in doubt about how to respond to an emotion, use reflection and legitimation (see Chapter 3, Function One).
5. Never promise a patient absolute confidentiality.
6. Communicate all clinically relevant information a patient may have told you back to the treatment team. Do it yourself.

# Structure of the Interview

# CHAPTER 7

# Opening the Interview

## OVERVIEW

This chapter discusses a five-step approach to opening the interview:
1. Introduction
2. Establish goals
3. Obtain patient consent
4. Establish initial rapport
5. Establish patient comfort

The next eight chapters review traditional structural elements of the medical interview. Despite this emphasis on structural elements, the student should remember that each of the three functions of the interview may be used appropriately during any particular phase or structure of the interview, depending on the condition of the patient and the topics being discussed. For example, when reviewing information about the patient's family medical history (function two), if a patient breaks down in tears when discussing his or her parent's death, the interviewer should take time to respond appropriately to the emotions revealed at that moment (function one). Similarly, during the physical examination, a patient may ask a question about moles on the skin, and the clinician may find it appropriate to provide education at that point (function three).

To deal systematically with the wealth of information to collect and to both give and build emotional rapport, the skilled clinician needs to maintain a rough organizational plan for the interview, which will cover all the relevant structural and functional elements. As described by Lipkin and others,[1-4] the specific dynamic interaction of each patient and physician with the particularities of the medical condition requires the interviewer to weave a complicated mosaic of both structural elements and functional interventions to achieve all the goals of the interview (see Chapter 33 on integrating structure and function). This chapter discusses the beginning structure of the encounter between the patient and the clinician.

The opening of the interview can be broken into five components. There are of course many different ways a skilled clinician can open an interview with a patient. The following format represents just one approach that is usually effective in laying the groundwork for a therapeutic clinician-patient encounter.

The nonverbal greeting occurs before the actual verbal introduction. The physician or student should establish good eye contact and (most commonly) extend a friendly hand in greeting. The verbal message follows. For example:

**STUDENT:** *Good morning, Mr. Cummings. My name is Bill Sams. I am a student doctor.*

## Establishing Goals of the Interview

In general, effective interviews begin with an explicit statement or acknowledgment of goals. Sometimes these may need to be negotiated between the doctor and the patient if their objectives differ. For the purposes of the student in a clinical methods class, there needs to be a brief statement about the purposes and the expectations for the interview. This can be done in many ways. For example:

> **STUDENT:** *Good morning, Mr. Cummings. My name is Bill Sams, and I am a student doctor learning how to interview patients. Your doctor gave me your name.*

## Obtaining Patient Consent to Your Interview Plan

For most interviews in actual practice, patient consent is implied by the patient's presence in the physician's office or hospital. However, in some situations explicit patient consent should be obtained. Similarly, the student in a clinical methods class should obtain the patient's consent to proceed with the interview. For example:

> **STUDENT:** *Good morning, Mr. Cummings. My name is Bill Sams, and I am a student doctor learning how to interview patients. Your doctor gave me your name. Would you be willing to talk with me for a few minutes?*

The interview can proceed as planned after the patient gives verbal permission. In the unlikely event that the patient does not want to be interviewed, the student should politely thank the patient and leave the room. Even when patients have previously given their permission for a student interview, some change their minds. Students should respect these wishes and not pressure such patients into agreeing to the interview.

## Establishing Initial Rapport

Establishing rapport may be the most important part of the interview. The doctor-patient relationship begins at the moment the physician and the patient see each other, even before any words are uttered. The patient and the physician will each make many judgments about the other before they establish verbal contact. Body posture, eye contact, interest level, and numerous other nonverbal cues will communicate important information to both the patient and the doctor. In general, the key to rapport is to demonstrate interest in the patient as a person. This can be demonstrated by showing concern and attention. Appearing hurried, bored, exhausted, or distracted can seriously undermine the relationship with the patient.

In addition to demonstrating interest, learners should recall Rule #1 from Chapter Three: which helps establish and maintain rapport:

**Respond to patients' emotional reactions whenever they occur.**

For example, if the patient shows some emotional reaction even as the physician first meets him or her, this can be acknowledged in the very beginning of the interview. If the patient is writhing in pain, the physician can acknowledge this before beginning an explanation about the purposes of the intended interview. Sometimes this acknowledgment can occur as part of the introduction itself. In a student interview, the student could say something like the following:

> **STUDENT:** *Hello. I am John Downing, a student doctor. You seem to be in pain. Is there anything I can do for you?*

Of course, there are numerous ways for physicians to respond appropriately to patients' emotions. Some of these modes have already been discussed in Chapter 3. Reflection is one of the most effective interventions. The student can comment on observed patient feelings, including pain, frustration, and sadness. These comments let patients know that their feelings have been noticed and that the feelings count for something. Such reflective comments usually help patients discuss their feelings and build doctor-patient rapport. The following are all examples of reflective comments that might be made in the very beginning of interviews:

> STUDENT: *I see that you seem quite uncomfortable.*

> or

> STUDENT: *You appear to be in great pain.*

> or

> STUDENT: *I can tell that you seem a bit down.*

When students or physicians make initial reflective comments about patients' emotions, especially early in the interview, some care must be taken to name feeling states that are relatively nonjudgmental and near the surface. No in-depth interpretations should be made. Physicians should not begin interviews with heavily interpretive statements such as "You seem quite enraged" or "You are obviously despondent." Patients may experience such statements as intrusive, derogatory, or humiliating.

In practice, patients are forgiving of physicians who are genuinely trying to empathize with their distress, even if the physicians are slightly "off base" in their initial understanding. In such instances patients are quite willing to correct initial misunderstandings. For example, if the physician makes an incorrect statement about patient distress, the patient usually makes a simple clarification of the situation:

> STUDENT: *You seem to be in pain right now.*

> PATIENT: *Actually, I'm mostly upset because I can't get my doctors to tell me what's the matter with me.*

> STUDENT: *I can understand why that might be disturbing. Would you be willing to tell me some more about that?*

If the patient demonstrates an emotion and the student quite properly acknowledges the feeling, the student can continue reflecting and legitimating feelings, as described in Chapter 3, until the patient is ready to proceed with the rest of the interview.

Occasionally, a patient assigned to a student for a practice interview might complain directly about "being a guinea pig." Although this is unusual, students should be aware that this affective complaint does occur and should be responded to like any other demonstration of emotion. Because the student is the target of the emotion, the patient's affect may generate sufficient anxiety in the student that it may be difficult to respond. Reflection and legitimation can also be useful in this instance:

> STUDENT: *Do you mind if I ask you a few questions?*

> PATIENT: *Another student? I've had so many people asking me questions, I don't know whether I'm coming or going.*

> STUDENT: *It sounds like you feel that you've been put through the mill. You may just not want to talk to another student.*

> PATIENT: *That's right. I haven't had a chance to rest since I was admitted, with all the doctors and nurses coming in all the time.*

> STUDENT: *I can certainly understand how you might not want to talk to another student. If you'd rather I leave, that's perfectly all right.*

> PATIENT: *No. That's all right. You can ask me some questions. What do you want to know?*

Many such initially resistant patients will be quite interested and willing to proceed with the interview if their initial feelings are simply recognized and accepted. Those patients who continue to be reluctant to be interviewed must have their wishes respected.

# Establishing Patient Comfort

After the introduction, statement of purpose, acquisition of patient consent for the interview, and establishment of initial rapport, the student should establish patient comfort before beginning the rest of the interview. This intervention indicates the student's concern for the patient's comfort and indicates the student's willingness to help if possible. Establishing comfort is accomplished by a simple question such as the following:

> STUDENT: *Before I ask you about your illness itself, I want to check—how are you feeling right now?*

This gives the patient the opportunity to tell the student how he or she is feeling at the moment. The response might be a physical or emotional answer, but the student has been given an important piece of information about the patient. If the patient is hot or cold, in pain, or thirsty, the student should ask whether he or she can do anything to help. If the patient responds with an emotional response such as "I am scared that I have cancer," the student can proceed with relationship skills to help the patient express and cope with these feelings (see Chapter 3).

In summary, the opening of the medical interview has five important components. There are many ways to open medical interviews, but the structure reviewed in this chapter represents one effective approach. The separate steps are summarized below.

## STEPS FOR AN EFFECTIVE OPENING

> INTRODUCTION: *Hello, I am John Smith, a student doctor. Dr. Jones gave me your name.*
>
> ESTABLISH GOALS: *Dr. Jones suggested that I talk with you about your illness to help me learn how to interview patients.*
>
> OBTAIN PATIENT CONSENT: *Is that okay with you?*
>
> ESTABLISH INITIAL RAPPORT: *You seem to be in pain.*
>
> ESTABLISH PATIENT COMFORT: *How are you feeling right now?*

# Summary

This chapter discusses a five-step approach to opening the interview:

1. Introduction
2. Establish goals
3. Obtain patient consent
4. Establish initial rapport
5. Establish patient comfort

## References

1. Lipkin M: The interview. In Feldman M, Christensen J: editors: *Behavioral Medicine in primary care,* ed 3, Stamford, CT, 2007, Appleton-Lange, pp 1–10.
2. Lipkin M, Jr: The medical interview as core clinical skill: the problem and the opportunity. *J Gen Intern Med* 2(5):363–365, 1987.
3. Williamson PR, et al: The medical interview and psychosocial aspects of medicine: block curricula for residents. *J Gen Intern Med* 7(2):235–242, 1992.
4. Lipkin M, et al: Performing the interview. In Lipkin M Jr, Putnam S, Lazare A, editors: *The medical interview: clinical care, education, and research,* New York, 1995, Springer.

# CHAPTER 8

# Chief Complaint, Problem Survey, Patient's Perspective, and Agenda Setting

## OVERVIEW

This chapter describes elicitation of:
1. The chief complaint
2. The problem survey and
3. The patient's perspective (ICE = ideas, concerns, and expectations).
4. Agenda setting is then discussed.

After the introduction, the opening of the interview, and the development of initial rapport, the clinician usually proceeds directly to the chief complaint, the problem survey, and elicitation of the patient's perspective (ideas about the illness, concerns about the illness, and expectations about the visit). The physician then engages the patient in a process of collaborative agenda setting.

## 1. Eliciting the Chief Complaint

The chief complaint is the primary reason for the patient's seeking medical attention. By convention, this is stated in the patient's own words and usually recorded in the medical record in quotation marks. Most commonly, the clinician asks a question like the following:

**CLINCIAN:** *What brought you here today?*

or

**CLINCIAN:** *How can I help you?*

or

**CLINCIAN:** *What is bothering you now?*

Student clinicians in an interviewing course will not be able to diagnose or treat a patient's problem, so a more appropriate question eliciting the chief complaint would be something like:

**STUDENT:** *What problem brought you to the hospital (or clinic)?*

The patient's answer will be recorded verbatim in the medical record as the patient's chief complaint. For example:

**PATIENT:** *I couldn't catch my breath.*

Occasionally patients will answer this question with a medical diagnosis rather than a description of symptoms. For example, a patient might respond in the following manner:

**PATIENT:** *It was my emphysema.*

or

**PATIENT:** *They told me it was an embolus.*

If patients provide a diagnosis rather than a symptom, they can be asked to describe exactly what they experienced themselves that made them seek medical attention. For example:

> STUDENT: *I understand that you were told that you had an embolus, but I would like to know exactly what you experienced that led you to come to the doctor.*

In response to this type of direct question, patients will usually be able to provide a statement concerning the symptoms that they experienced. For example:

> PATIENT: *Oh, I got really short of breath.*

## RESPONDING TO EMOTIONS

Occasionally patients will provide information in a chief complaint that is highly charged with emotion. When this occurs, it is usually best to respond to this emotion when it first becomes apparent. (Rule #1, see Chapter Three). For example, a patient might say something such as the following:

> PATIENT: *I was so short of breath I thought I was dying.*

When this degree of emotional intensity accompanies a report of symptoms, the student can respond effectively by using any one of many different interventions. However, brief reflective comments can be appropriate and supportive. For example:

> PATIENT: *I am sure that must have been very frightening.*

This type of comment usually invites the patient to discuss his or her feelings in more detail. For example:

> PATIENT: *I've never been so scared. I just couldn't get my breath. It was terrible.*

After a patient acknowledges and discusses some significant feelings, the student can indicate his or her acceptance of these feelings in many ways. One effective technique is the use of direct, validating (or legitimating) comments. For example:

> STUDENT: *I can certainly understand your fear. I'm sure I would have felt the same way myself.*

## INITIAL FACILITATION

The use of facilitating comments is an open-ended method of encouraging a patient to keep talking without interfering or influencing the direction of the patient's comments. Facilitation can be verbal or nonverbal. Examples of minimal and nonintrusive facilitation include head nodding or saying "uh-huh" or "yes" in response to a patient's comments. Such interventions, although minimal, let the patient know that the interviewer is listening and encourage the patient to keep talking. (See Chapter Four).

Use more specific facilitations to directly ask the patient to continue:

> PHYSICIAN: *Please tell me more.*

or

> PHYSICIAN: *Please go on.*

When a patient rambles or discusses many different themes together in a disjointed manner, the clinician can help guide the interview in a more efficient way by using facilitation to direct the patient:

> PHYSICIAN: *Before you tell me about the headache, can we first concentrate on the chest pain? Please tell me a bit more about the chest pains you've been having.*

The patient will usually respond to such focusing, (but open-ended) facilitation by discussing the points that are most important to him or her as a patient. This provides the clinician with crucial information that could not be obtained as easily by more closed-ended questions that focus on the clinician's concerns. The patient will generally respond in his or her own words about the symptoms of the chest pain that were most troubling. The psychosocial context might also emerge. For example, the patient might say something like the following:

> **PATIENT:** *Well, last Sunday I was almost finished mowing the lawn when I suddenly got short of breath and I noticed a heavy, tight feeling in my chest.*

Continued facilitation is still appropriate if the patient is talking about relevant symptoms. Thoughtful and attentive silence can also serve as a potent facilitator. If this is uncomfortable or feels socially inappropriate, the interviewer can provide a more direct facilitative comment:

> **PHYSICIAN:** *Could you tell me some more about the heavy, tight feeling?*

This type of facilitation will usually encourage the patient to talk more about the symptoms of interest.

> **PATIENT:** *Well, I've never really had anything like it before. It hurt, but it was more like an ache than a sharp pain. I thought it might be gas, but I couldn't get it to go away. And then I noticed that the tight feeling spread to my back and down my left arm.*

## CHECKING

> **Checking is a key and underused assessment skill.**
> **Remember Rule #3: When in doubt, check.**

Checking is the clinician's attempt to summarize the information that he or she has just received from the patient. (See Chapter Four) This single intervention is one of the most important data gathering skills for several reasons. It is the only way for the clinician to check the accuracy of what he or she thinks the patient has just said. Interviewers may at times misunderstand the meaning of what the patient has said or even specific data that patients have given them. Checking allows the clinician a chance to correct any misunderstandings. Checking also communicates a sense to the patient that the clinician is listening and trying to understand. Such efforts usually contribute to overall rapport.

In addition to other uses, checking provides a therapeutic "breathing space." When a lull occurs in the interview or the clinician needs to make a decision about which direction to proceed, checking can be used to review what has already been covered. The clinician can use these pauses to gracefully consider alternative strategies for the rest of the interview. The nature of the patient's response to the checking may itself help the clinician decide on the course of the rest of the interview. The clinician may use checking in the following manner:

> **PHYSICIAN:** *Let me take a moment to make sure that I've understood you correctly. You said that you were just finishing mowing the lawn last Sunday when you noticed the sudden onset of a sharp pain in your chest and had trouble breathing.*

## 2. The Problem Survey

The survey of problems is an extremely important part of the interview and, like checking, is often overlooked. (See Chapter Four). A skillful survey of problems can dramatically increase the efficiency of the interviewing process. In the survey of problems the clinician attempts to briefly scan the full range of a patient's problems. To begin the survey, the clinician asks the following key question:

> **PHYSICIAN:** *What else is bothering you?*

> or simply

> **PHYSICIAN:** *What else?*

Completing the survey of problems in the early stages of the interview is important because otherwise clinicians sometimes lose valuable time by focusing on problems that are not the most clinically significant or the most distressing to patients. The survey usually does not take long, and it allows the clinician to determine the full range of the patient's problems. After the clinician (1) elicits the chief complaint, (2) responds to the initial emotions, (3) facilitates the open-ended expression of more details about the chief complaint, and (4) checks what he or she has heard, the clinician should proceed with the survey of problems.

> **PHYSICIAN:** *Now that you have told me what problem brought you to the hospital initially, I want to ask you about your other problems. I will come back to the chest pain in a few moments. What other problems do you have?*
>
> **PATIENT:** *Well, I have had some prostate trouble.*

As with the original chief complaint, the clinician should follow this new complaint with open-ended facilitative interventions to collect more details about the problem, respond to emotions that are connected with this problem, and check the information obtained after several comments have been made by the patient.

> **PHYSICIAN:** *Can you tell me some more about the prostate problem?*
>
> **PATIENT:** *Well, I dribble, and it takes a long time to finish. I'm afraid I might need an operation.*
>
> **PHYSICIAN:** *So, in addition to this chest pain you have a problem with urinating. You take a long time to pass your water, and there is some dribbling. You're also concerned that you might need an operation. What other problems do you have?*
>
> **PATIENT:** *I also have trouble with migraine headaches.*
>
> **PHYSICIAN:** *Can you say more about the headaches?*
>
> **PATIENT:** *I have had them all my life. Sometimes they are so bad I can't stand it and I have to miss work and go to the emergency room for a shot. I haven't had one in 3 months now.*
>
> **PHYSICIAN:** *So, you have this chest pain, prostate trouble, and migraine headaches. I want to hear more about each of these problems. But now I still would like you to tell me what other problems you may have.*

Many patients are reluctant to tell clinicians about some problems that are particularly sensitive. Sometimes patients are so anxious about these problems that they postpone discussing them to the end of the interview, when the clinician may not be willing or able to spend more time. The source of the patient's anxiety may be an overwhelming health concern such as the fear of cancer. For example, the patient in the preceding dialogue might be afraid that the stomach pain he has been experiencing is cancer. If the fear of cancer is strong, he might avoid bringing the pain up at all because of anxiety. At the end of the interview the anxiety of not discussing the abdominal pain might be stronger than the anxiety of discussing it. This can lead to an unpleasant tension when the clinician is about to leave the room, as the patient awkwardly says something like the following:

> **PATIENT:** *Doctor, could I ask you something else? I've been having some terrible stomach pains.*

This type of interaction can be troubling for both patients and clinicians. It can lead to tension in the relationship. More important, the clinician may simply not have the time at the end of the interview to deal with this new problem adequately. The new problem may be quite important; sometimes it is the patient's hidden or unconscious chief complaint. In addition to the type of problem mentioned in the dialogue, patients often leave sexual, psychiatric, or interpersonal problems to the end of the interview, either because of the anxiety, embarrassment, or even humiliation they may arouse or because patients fear that the clinician may not consider these problems important or "medical." Studies indicate that these "doorknob," "end of the interview," or "Oh, by the way, doctor…" statements occur in up to 20% of interviews.[1-3] Permitting this covert complaint to remain uncovered until the end of the interview usually leads to inadequate care and certainly to inefficient care. A simple survey of problems usually eliminates this difficulty.

## PROBING TO COMPLETENESS

The survey of problems is not complete until the clinician has probed to completeness. The interviewer should continue asking, "What else?" until the patient convincingly indicates that all the problems have been mentioned. (See Chapter Four). It is important for the clinician to indicate that he or she is not rushed in this task and sincerely wants to hear at least briefly about all of the patient's problems. The clinician must give the patient full attention and watch closely for nonverbal messages from the patient about uncomfortable topics. If the patient demonstrates ambivalence about talking about some problems, the clinician should do what he or she can to encourage the patient to talk about these more anxiety-provoking problems. For example:

> PATIENT: *Well, now that you mention it, there is something else that has been on my mind …* *(pause)*
>
> PHYSICIAN: *Okay … go on … I would like to hear about it.*

The clinician should continue this type of interested inquiry until the patient clearly indicates that all problems have been mentioned.[4,5]

Some clinicians may wonder why it is so important to elicit all the patient's problems. Some clinicians may believe that sexual, psychiatric, and interpersonal problems may be beyond the scope of the medical practitioner to manage. Furthermore, the information necessary for the clinician to understand, let alone manage, these problems may take a great deal of time to elaborate. Although these are all understandable concerns, students must realize that a patient's sexual, psychiatric, and interpersonal problems do belong in the interview: they have a direct effect on the course and outcome of a patient's illness, on health care use, on the patient's coping with illness, on the quality of life, and on overall life adjustment.[2]

Clinicians do not need to be experts on all these sensitive issues to take some history about them. If there is not time in one interview to address all the concerns that arise out of a thorough survey of problems, some of the topics can be postponed to another interview. It is still important and efficient in the long run to take a complete survey of problems for every new patient seen and to survey the patient at least briefly during follow-up visits.

Some patients with significant psychiatric and psychosocial problems bring up problems such as impotence, family conflict, fears of dying, and work problems, in addition to problems such as chest pain, migraine headaches, and prostate trouble. The clinician, in collaboration with the patient, can decide which problems to investigate and in which order of priority they can reasonably be investigated. Some problems may need to wait until another visit to be investigated and some problems may need to be referred to outside experts or agencies.

# 3. Elicit Patient's Perspective: Ideas, Concerns, and Expectations ("ICE")

## EXPLORE PATIENT IDEAS ABOUT THE MEANING OF THE ILLNESS

At times the patient's ideas about the meaning of the illness are quite clear. However, this may not always be the case. (See Chapter Four). For example, the patient with some rather obscure abdominal pain might be concerned that cancer could be causing the pain. Alternatively, the concern might be social embarrassment from the passing of flatus. Unless the clinician knows the patient's ideas about the meaning of the symptom (i.e., the patient's "explanatory model"), the clinician will be inefficient in his or her care and may not be able to meet the patient's needs.[6,7]

The clinician should directly ask the patient what he or she thinks could be causing the symptom. For example:

**PHYSICIAN:** *Could you tell me what you think might be causing this stomach pain?*

**PATIENT:** *I don't know, you're the doctor. That's why I came to you.*

**PHYSICIAN:** *Of course I am the doctor, and I will do what I can to help. But it will help me if you could tell me what thoughts have crossed your mind about what could be causing these problems.*

Some patients may be unwilling to discuss their own ideas about the meaning of the illness, even with encouragement. However, when given an opportunity, many patients will be able to talk about their fears and ideas directly with the clinician. This discussion can contribute to the efficiency of the doctor-patient interaction, as well as to the ability of the clinician to reassure the patient. It can also enhance patient satisfaction. For example:

**PATIENT:** *Well, I know it's probably nothing. But my father died of colon cancer, and I'm kind of worried that I might have the same problem.*

**PHYSICIAN:** *I'm glad you could tell me that. It will help me understand your problem. After we talk about your pain and perhaps do some tests, I will do what I can to reassure you about your concern about cancer.*

## EXPLORE PATIENT <u>CONCERNS</u> ABOUT THE ILLNESS

Patient's concerns about the illness may become apparent as the meaning of the illness is explored. If the concerns are not immediately apparent, the clinician should ask directly:

**PHYSICIAN:** *I wonder what concerns you most about your stomach pain and fatigue?*

**PATIENT:** *Well, I just want to feel better, but I am worried that this might be some kind of hepatitis. I've been reading about hepatitis and I know someone who just died from hepatitis.*

## EXPLORE PATIENT <u>EXPECTATIONS</u>

Sometimes the patient's expectations of the clinician are quite clear. In other cases, however, the patient's expectations are less clear. (See Chapter Four). The specific desires of the patient are even more important in cases in which the patient has a chronic illness with difficulty adapting or some other psychosocial problem.

For example, a patient who is impotent because of diabetes may only want to talk about how the impotence is affecting his marital relationship. To bring back his sexual abilities, the patient may simply want a pill or think he may be interested in a penile implant. Asking directly about the patient's expectations can increase rapport in the relationship, improve efficiency in the interview, and achieve a more satisfied patient in the long run. If the clinician knows what the patient wants, the clinician will have an easier time satisfying the patient.[8-10]

Patient expectations can be elicited directly:

**PHYSICIAN:** *Please tell me as specifically as you can how you think I might be able to help you with your back pain.*

# 4. Agenda Setting

Once the chief complaint and the complete problem list have been developed through a systematic survey of problems and the clinician also understands the patient's ideas, expectations, and concerns, the clinician and the patient together can negotiate an agenda for subsequent interactions, investigations, and interventions. This should be a collaborative effort guided by the clinician's medical understanding of which problems might be most imminently threatening to the patient's health and balanced by the patient's personal hierarchy of concerns. When there is conflict between the doctor's and the patient's list of priorities, the order in which problems will be addressed should be directly negotiated. In general, the clinician should let the patient determine the order of priority as much as possible. For example:

> **PHYSICIAN:** *Now that we have outlined all of your problems, I'd like to hear from you about which ones bother you most.*
>
> **PATIENT:** *I'd really like to know more about this prostate thing. I think that's what is causing my problem with sex and my wife.*
>
> **PHYSICIAN:** *I'm also concerned about your prostate and I see it's a problem for you. I'll make sure that we get to it, but if it's acceptable to you, I think we need to make sure that we've dealt appropriately with the chest discomfort first. This may be something we need to take care of right away.*
>
> **PATIENT:** *Okay.*

## Summary

This chapter describes elicitation of:
1. The chief complaint
2. The problem survey and
3. The patient's perspective (ICE = ideas, concerns, and expectations).
4. Agenda setting is then discussed.

## References

1. Jackson G: "Oh ... by the way ...": doorknob syndrome. *Int J Clin Pract* 59(8):869, 2005.
2. Olson KP: "Oh, by the way ...": agenda setting in office visits. *Fam Pract Manag* 9(10):63–64, 2002.
3. White J, Levinson W, Roter D: "Oh, by the way ...": the closing moments of the medical visit. *J Gen Intern Med* 9(1):24–28, 1994.
4. Baker LH, O'Connell D, Platt FW: "What else?" Setting the agenda for the clinical interview. *Ann Intern Med* 143(10):766–770, 2005.
5. Minton PR: Setting the agenda for the clinical interview. *Ann Intern Med* 144(4):306, 2006.
6. Kleinman A, Eisenberg L, Good B: Culture, illness, and care: clinical lessons from anthropologic and cross-cultural research. *Ann Intern Med* 88(2):251–258, 1978.
7. Johnson TM, Hardt EJ, Kleinman A: Cultural factors in the medical interview. In Lipkin M, Jr, Putnam SM, Lazare A, editors: *The medical interview: clinical care, education, and research*, New York, 1995, Springer.
8. Lazare A: The interview as a clinical negotiation. In Lipkin M, Jr, Putnam SM, Lazare A, editors: *The medical interview: clinical care, education, and research*, New York, 1995, Springer.
9. Eisenthal S, Koopman C, Lazare A: Process analysis of two dimensions of the negotiated approach in relation to satisfaction in the initial interview. *J Nerv Ment Dis* 171(1):49–54, 1983.
10. Eisenthal S, et al: "Adherence" and the negotiated approach to patienthood. *Arch Gen Psychiatry* 36(4):393–398, 1979.

# History of Present Illness

## OVERVIEW

Chapter 9 explains how to develop a coherent narrative thread in the history of the present illness, using Function Two skills to explore and integrate all eight key elements of the patient's illness experience: WW, QQ, AA, LC, and I:

W—Where

W—When

Q—Quality

Q—Quantity

A—Aggravating and alleviating factors

A—Associated factors

LC—Life context

I—Impact on quality of life

Patient emotions commonly emerge during the elicitation of these eight elements of the present illness, and clinicians should respond to these feelings whenever they appear.

The history of the present illness is an elaborated description of the patient's chief complaint and is the most important structural element of the medical history. Obtaining an accurate account of the patient's present illness in an efficient manner while also maintaining rapport is the key challenge of the medical interview.

Constructing the history of the present illness represents the physician's effort to understand the full story of the development and expression of the chief complaint in the context of the patient's life. The chief complaint could be a pain somewhere (e.g., chest pain), a symptom of discomfort (e.g., fatigue), a loss of usual function (e.g., inability to walk), or a troublesome body change (e.g., numbness in the fingertips). A psychiatric symptom or illness such as depression, anxiety, or hearing voices can also be the chief complaint.

The history of the present illness is different for every patient and provides essential information for optimal diagnosis and management. It also serves as a useful summary of the patient's problems for communication purposes with other caregivers.

## Narrative Thread and Open-to-Closed Questioning

The physician's goal in understanding the history of the present illness is to obtain a coherent, orderly portrait of the development of the patient's chief complaint. Lipkin[1] describes how the physician elicits the story of the patient's illness by developing a "narrative thread" linking the chronologic emergence of symptoms with the overall life circumstances of the patient. This requires considerably more skill than obtaining a recitation of relevant signs and symptoms; the physician must have the ability to understand the development and impact of an illness as one unified entity in the life of a unique patient. The physician cannot obtain this narrative thread from a patient as one can take a blood pressure. Rather, the physician must work in partnership with the patient to develop an accurate and useful understanding of the illness in the patient's life.

Understanding the difference between a disease and an illness may be useful at this point. As described by Kleinman et al,[2] "disease" refers to a measurable physiologic, biologic disorder. "Illness, on the other hand," refers to a pattern of symptoms experienced by an individual: pain, discomfort, disability, and dysfunction. An individual may suffer from a disease (e.g., hypertension or occult cancer) without experiencing any illness. Similarly, a person may suffer from an illness (e.g., abdominal pain and disability) without any diagnosable disease. The narrative thread, therefore, refers primarily to the experience of an illness and not, necessarily, to a disease. Insofar as the patient may have already received objective confirmation (such as echocardiography) of an underlying disease related to his or her illness experience, these disease-related data also become embedded in the narrative thread of the history of the present illness.

To make the story coherent, it is essential for the narrative thread to determine **when** the very first symptom of this illness appeared:

PHYSICIAN: *You mentioned that you noticed this sudden onset of chest pain just as you finished mowing the lawn on Sunday. Was this your very first episode of chest pain, or have you ever had chest pain before? If you've ever had this pain before, when was the very first time you had this pain?*

If the patient has not had any chest pain like this before,[A] the clinician continues the development of the narrative thread while retaining this focus on orderly chronology. In order to maintain a coherent story, the most important question throughout the history of the present illness is: *"What happened next?"*

PHYSICIAN: *After you first noticed the pain on Sunday, what happened next?*

PATIENT: *I went inside to tell my wife.*

PHYSICIAN: *After you went inside to tell your wife, what happened next?*

The physician may find it necessary to interrupt the patient's narrative to ask some clarifying questions. After the patient provides this clarification, the physician should generally return to the question, "What happened next?" in order to get back to the sequential narrative thread.

PATIENT: *My wife said she was taking me to the hospital.*

PHYSICIAN: *Before we go further, can you describe the pain in some more detail?*

PATIENT: *It kind of grabbed me—deep down, tight.*

PHYSICIAN: *Can you show me exactly where it hurt?*

PATIENT: *Right here in my chest, and then it went down my left arm and into my back.*

PHYSICIAN: *How bad was it?*

PATIENT: *Not too bad at first, but then I had trouble catching my breath.*

PHYSICIAN: *Did you notice anything else unusual?*

PATIENT: *No, that was about all I noticed that I can remember.*

PHYSICIAN: *Okay, so you noticed a dull, tight, hard pain in your chest that went down your arm. It wasn't too bad at first, but then it started to bother you a whole lot when you got short of breath.*

PATIENT: *That's right.*

PHYSICIAN: *What happened next?*

In terms of question format, the skilled interviewer generally starts with open-ended questions to establish the broad outlines of the story. As the patient recounts symptoms and patterns, the interviewer becomes more focused and uses progressively more specific and narrow questions to fill in specific details. Eventually, final details are usually elicited by using closed questions. Mini-summarization (or "checking") is used frequently to ensure that details have been understood correctly. This progressive narrowing of focus has been called an "open-to-closed-cone" style of questioning (see Chapter Four).[3]

The overall process of developing the present illness as a narrative thread establishes coherence and an order that helps make sense of the patient's experience, both to the doctor and to the patient. For the patient, it may represent the first time that he or she has actually articulated the pattern of symptom development in this logical manner. An orderly recounting of symptoms and the sense that the doctor understands this orderly progression can be quite reassuring.

## Problem Exploration: WW, QQ, AA, LC, I[B]

W—Where

W—When

Q—Quality

Q—Quantity

A—Aggravating and Alleviating Factors

A—Associated Signs and Symptoms

LC—Life Context

I—Impact on Patient's Quality of Life

These eight core dimensions of illness must be investigated in detail.[4] In general, they provide information necessary to generate diagnostic hypotheses and formulate management strategies. A common challenge for the interviewer in investigating each of these areas is to obtain specific information without prematurely closing off the open-ended phase of the interview.

In general, each of the eight content areas is investigated in detail after the open-ended phase of the interview. In reality, few interviews proceed in this linear fashion and follow an idealized open-to-closed cone. In practice, skilled interviewers usually interrupt or direct a patient in the early stages of an interview to prevent the physician from getting "lost" in a sea of seemingly unrelated details. When necessary, the physician interrupts briefly to gather needed details by using closed questions and then returns to an open-ended format. Care and discretion must be used to prevent such interruptions from terminating the open-ended nature of the overall interview process.

### WHERE (LOCATION)

The physician must have a precise understanding of the location of the problem. At times the patient may speak in generalities or use a vocabulary that is not familiar to the physician. When this occurs, the physician must ask the patient to clarify the words. For example, a patient may indicate that his or her stomach hurts. It is sometimes useful to ask the patient to show the doctor specifically where it hurts. If the open-ended portion of the history was interrupted, the patient can be redirected in a more open-ended manner after a specific detail has been clarified.

PHYSICIAN: *Can you take one finger and show me exactly where it hurts? (clarifying question)*

PATIENT: *Right here, doctor. (patient points to the location)*

PHYSICIAN: *Okay. Can you now describe the pain to me in more detail? (return to more open-ended questioning)*

## WHEN (TIMING)

As described previously, the timing of the symptoms and associated responses is essential to the development of a coherent narrative thread. The physician needs to know when each symptom or problem began and also needs to know the rough chronology of the development of the problem. The physician occasionally needs to briefly interrupt the patient's story to make sure the timing of events is clear. If the patient begins reciting an array of symptoms without providing the details of the timing, it is helpful, indeed necessary, to interrupt:

PHYSICIAN: *So what is it that brought you to the clinic today? (open-ended elicitation of the chief complaint)*

PATIENT: *It's these headaches. They're getting worse and worse. Now I've started to become nauseated, and I threw up yesterday.*

PHYSICIAN: *Can you say some more about the headaches?*

PATIENT: *Well, yesterday was just terrible. The pain started slowly just as I woke up, and it got worse and worse during the day. I had to leave work, and that's when I went home and threw up. I took some of my wife's pain medicine and was able to go to sleep.*

PHYSICIAN: *What medicine was that? (physician interrupts for clarification)*

PATIENT: *I think it was Tylenol Number Three.*

PHYSICIAN: *And can you tell me when this problem first started? (physician interrupts to establish the time frame)*

PATIENT: *I guess I had my first bad headache like this about 2 years ago.*

PHYSICIAN: *Okay, so can you tell me some more about what it was like when the headaches started about 2 years ago? (physician returns to more open-ended questioning)*

As new or associated symptoms develop that are related to the problem being discussed, the physician needs to know about the timing of these related symptoms:

PATIENT: *Then I began throwing up with the headaches.*

PHYSICIAN: *About when did you begin to throw up with the headaches?*

PATIENT: *I guess the first time I began to throw up was about 6 weeks ago.*

## QUALITY

It is important for the patient to attempt to describe the quality of the symptom, because different disease syndromes can produce specific recognizable patterns of complaints. For example, a pain may be stabbing, sharp, dull, throbbing, continuous, etc.

It is usually best for the doctor to ask this question in as open-ended a way as possible.

PHYSICIAN: *Could you describe the pain? What is it like?*

Patients usually know what the doctor wants in asking for such a description. However, if the patient seems to be at a loss for words, the physician can provide some useful guidance:

PATIENT: *What do you mean "describe the pain"? Doctor, it just hurts.*

PHYSICIAN: *Okay, I guess I mean I would like to hear a little bit more about what it actually felt like. Was it sharp or dull? Did it come and go or just stay there all the time?*

## QUANTITY (SEVERITY)

It is important for the physician to get some ideas about how severe the discomfort, sensation, or pain was or is to the patient. This can sometimes be ascertained by noting nonverbal signals of acute discomfort by the patient, but the question about severity should also be asked directly.

PHYSICIAN: *How bad was the pain?*

PATIENT: *It was terrible.*

PHYSICIAN: *Was it the worst pain you've ever experienced?*

PATIENT: *No, my kidney stone was actually worse.*

A crude analogue scale can be very useful in measuring subjective levels of discomfort.

PHYSICIAN: *Could you tell me how bad this headache pain has been?*

PATIENT: *Well, it's sort of achy and pressured.*

PHYSICIAN: *Well, on a scale of zero to ten, where zero represents no pain and ten represents the worst pain you've ever experienced, how bad was your last headache?*

PATIENT: *I guess about a five or a six.*

## AGGRAVATING AND ALLEVIATING FACTORS (MODIFYING FACTORS)

The physician needs to find out what the patient has done to try to help himself or herself feel better and what types of things may make the symptoms worse:

PHYSICIAN: *Could you tell me what tends to help this pain?*

PATIENT: *Well, if I lie down in a dark, quiet room, the pain calms down a little.*

PHYSICIAN: *Have you tried any medicines?*

PATIENT: *Aspirin or Tylenol used to help, but they don't work anymore. Yesterday I took that Tylenol Number Three. Sometimes I need to go to an emergency room for a shot to stop the pain.*

PHYSICIAN: *What kinds of things make the headaches worse?*

PATIENT: *If I cough, it hurts. Looking at bright light hurts. Trying to concentrate hurts. That's about it.*

## ASSOCIATED SIGNS AND SYMPTOMS

The physician should inquire about associated signs and symptoms. These can provide essential additional information for diagnosis or management of a patient's problem.

PHYSICIAN: *When you get these headaches, what other sensations or feelings do you get?*

PATIENT: *Well, sometimes I get nauseated. I feel weak and dizzy. If I try to walk, I feel unsteady on my feet.*

PHYSICIAN: *Any other symptoms you can think of?*

PATIENT: *No.*

Under the category of associated signs and symptoms, physicians ask patients directly about "pertinent positives and negatives." From their understanding of illness patterns, physicians inquire about specific symptoms and signs whose presence or absence can make a great deal of difference in clarifying the final diagnostic possibilities. However, beginning students will generally not know very much about what may or may not be "pertinent." This section of the interview will necessarily be much shorter for medical student interviews than for interviews of more experienced clinicians.

## LIFE CONTEXT

The context of the symptom development is essential to an understandable narrative thread and can give environmental or psychosocial clues for diagnosis and management:

> PHYSICIAN: *Can you tell me where you are or what you are doing when you tend to get these headaches?*
>
> PATIENT: *I guess they mostly start at work.*
>
> PHYSICIAN: *Can you say some more about that?*
>
> PATIENT: *I guess they mostly come in the afternoons, especially on days that are very busy and when I feel pressured.*
>
> PHYSICIAN: *Is there anything else that comes to mind about the situations in which these headaches seem to develop?*
>
> PATIENT: *Not really.*

## IMPACT ON PATIENT'S QUALITY OF LIFE

To understand a patient's illness and to facilitate coping, the clinician must also evaluate the impact of the illness on the patient's quality of life. This information forms part of the history of the present illness. The physician should explore the effect of the illness on the patient's general functioning. This includes the impact on (1) interpersonal relationships (especially spouse, significant other, and family), (2) work, (3) sexual relationships, and (4) emotional stability.

As the physician nears the completion of the history of the present illness, he or she will already have obtained a great deal of information indirectly about the effect of the illness on the patient's quality of life, just by listening to the chronological story of life events as they have unfolded. This is especially true if the physician has responded to the emotions the patient has manifested throughout the process. The physician should then complete the quality-of-life evaluation by direct questioning:

> PHYSICIAN: *I'm interested in hearing more about how this illness has affected your life in general.*
>
> PATIENT: *What do you mean?*
>
> PHYSICIAN: *I'd like to hear about the impact this illness has had on your life, your home situation, your work, and things like that.*

Chapter Four reviewed in detail how to evaluate the impact of illness on a patient's quality of life.

## Respond to Emotions Throughout

As patients recount the story of their illness, they invariably experience emotional reactions. And as they experience these reactions, physicians should respond to them as they appear (see Chapter Three, Rule # 1). Each time a patient experiences an emotion that is overlooked by the physician, a wedge develops in the doctor-patient relationship and the physician has lost an opportunity for the development of deepened rapport.[6]

A sensitive physician can respond to a patient's emotions in numerous ways. A nonverbal acknowledgment is often sufficient. For example, a patient who becomes tearful may respond to a soft touch on the arm or to the physician's moving his or her chair a little closer (for support) and talking in a softer voice.

A reflective verbal intervention is suggested for situations in which the physician is uncertain of how to proceed. For example:

> **PHYSICIAN:** *I can see that this is hard to talk about.*

If the patient becomes more emotional and more tearful, it is important to stop the general informational direction of the interview and continue exploring and supporting the patient's emotional responses. This can be accomplished by using more reflective comments, legitimation, support, partnership, and respect (see Chapter 3), as well as by other intuitive or higher-order skills of the physician for more complicated emotional reactions (see Chapters 16 and 17).

Some interviewers may wonder whether devoting time to the emotional domain may interfere with the other task of collecting data. To the contrary, research indicates that attention to patients' emotional responses seems to facilitate the task of gathering biomedical information, perhaps by improving overall doctor-patient rapport.[5]

## Complete the Narrative Thread

As the patient provides responses to these eight content areas, the physician should endeavor to weave the responses together into a coherent story within the patient's life experience. To accomplish this effectively often requires considerable skill. When the physician has completed the history of the present illness, he or she should have attained a good understanding of when the symptoms began; the quality, location, and severity of the symptoms; how the symptoms progressed; the timing of new symptoms; the context of the symptoms; modifying factors; associated signs and symptoms; life context; and impact on the patient's quality of life. Perhaps most important of all, in obtaining this coherent story, the physician will have communicated a sense of compassion and understanding that will, in itself, build rapport and impart an element of therapeutic healing.

## Complete This Process for Every Problem

The physician must obtain a history of the present illness for every current problem. If the patient has a problem with headaches, chest pain, back pain, and depression, each of these problems must be explored in the detail described previously. In practice, physicians may not have the time in the first meeting with a patient (particularly in an outpatient practice with patients having multiple nonacute problems) to obtain a complete history for every one of the problems. In this case, the physician and the patient should negotiate a priority problem list that can be addressed adequately in the time available. Other problems can usually wait for another appointment.

## Summary

Chapter 9 explains how to develop a coherent narrative thread in the history of the present illness, using Function Two skills to explore and integrate all eight key elements of the patient's illness experience: WW, QQ, AA, LC, and I:

W—Where

W—When

Q—Quality

Q—Quantity

A—Aggravating and alleviating factors

A—Associated factors

LC—Life context

I—Impact on quality of life

## References

1. Lipkin M, Jr: The medical interview and related skills. In Branch WT, editor: *The office practice of medicine*, ed 3, Philadelphia, 1994, Saunders.
2. Kleinman A, Eisenberg L, Good B: Culture, illness, and care: clinical lessons from anthropological and cross-cultural research. *Arch Intern Med* 88:251–258, 1978.
3. Goldberg D, et al: *Training family practice residents to recognize psychiatric disturbances*, Rockville, MD, 1983, National Institute of Mental Health.
4. Morgan WL, Engel GL: *The clinical approach to the patient*, Philadelphia, 1969, Saunders.
5. Roter DL, et al: Improving physician's interviewing skills and reducing patients' emotional distress: a randomized clinical trial. *Arch Intern Med* 155:1877–1884, 1995.
6. Suchman T, Beckman H, Frankel R: A model of empathic communication in the medical interview. *JAMA* 277:1680–1681, 1997.

## Endnotes

A. If this patient has had chest pain like this before, the clinician must obtain the full details of the patient's previous episodes of chest pain chronologically up to the present episode.

B. Adopted from acronym in Silverman J, Kurtz S, Draper J: *Skills for communicating with patients* (Second Edition), San Francisco, 2005, Radcliffe Publishing.

# Past Medical History

## OVERVIEW

Chapter 10 explains how to elicit the patient's past medical history, which includes the following elements:

1. Hospitalizations
2. Surgeries
3. Illnesses
4. Injuries
5. Medications
6. Allergies
7. Pregnancies (for women)
8. Exposures
9. Health maintenance

The past medical history records the patient's experiences with hospitalizations, surgeries, other illnesses, injuries, medications, allergies, pregnancies (for women), exposures, and health maintenance. Some of this information may have already emerged during the exploration of the history of the present illness and conversely, when the past medical history is being formally explored, it is not uncommon for the interviewer to uncover additional information that "belongs" in the "history of the present illness." When this occurs, the interviewer will reorganize the information obtained into its most relevant components of the medical history when it is eventually written up and presented (see Chapter 15).

The information in the past medical history is important to collect in a systematic and efficient manner for numerous reasons, including its relevance for subsequent patient management. Most physicians develop a set of routine, relatively closed-ended questions for this part of the interview to ensure that all important areas of inquiry are covered. When new problems are uncovered that need to be investigated, the style of questioning can change appropriately to a more open-ended form. In outpatient settings, because of time constraints and the lack of urgency of this information for immediate management, some physicians develop strategies for completing this database over several visits. However, whether this information is collected during the first visit or over several visits, it does need to be completed for every new patient.

The past medical history includes the following areas: (1) hospitalizations, (2) surgeries, (3) illnesses, (4) injuries, (5) medications, (6) allergies, (7) pregnancies (for women), (8) exposures, and (9) health maintenance. This chapter discusses each topic and provides sample questions.

It is usually helpful to introduce this part of the interview by letting the patient know that the investigation of the current problem has been completed and that a different format and style of questioning will be used in conducting the evaluation of the past medical history. This introduction can contribute to the efficiency of interviewing by letting the patient know the kind of information that is now desired. For example:

> PHYSICIAN: *I think I have a good understanding now of your problem with chest pain. I'd like to go on and ask a series of questions about other medical problems you may have had in the past.*
>
> PATIENT: *Okay, sure.*

## Hospitalizations

A relatively closed-ended question is usually sufficient to inquire about past hospitalizations and surgeries. For example:

> PHYSICIAN: *Please tell me about your previous hospitalizations.*

Some patients may become overly concerned about recounting exact details of previous hospitalizations, such as exact dates or exact symptoms. Similarly, some patients may think that the physician wants to hear the details of the symptoms that led to previous hospitalizations in the same way that the details of the present illness were discussed. Such patients need to be gently directed toward the kind of answers that are most appropriate for this phase of the interview. Consider the following example:

> PHYSICIAN: *Please tell me about your previous hospitalizations.*
>
> PATIENT: *Well, let's see. I had this stomach problem a while back. I think it was 10 years ago … no, it may have been 11 … no. It was ten. They eventually decided it was a gallbladder problem. The pain was terrible, but it came and went. It took them a long time to figure things out, but they eventually decided to take out the gallbladder, and the pain went away. It started with a sharp pain right here, and then it went around.…*
>
> PHYSICIAN: *Excuse me a moment, I'm sorry to interrupt. I appreciate your efforts to be very specific. But since we are a little short of time, I want to make sure you know that I only need a very rough idea of each time you have been in a hospital before and for what problem. For example, for your gallbladder operation, I only need to know about when it was taken out. I don't really need to know the symptoms that led up to the operation, and whether it was 10 or 11 years ago is not really that important for what we need to accomplish now.*

## Surgeries

Many significant surgeries will already have been mentioned in the patient's review of hospitalizations. However, since more and more surgery is now being performed on an outpatient basis, it is important to ask about surgeries as a separate category to make sure the area has been completely covered:

> PHYSICIAN: *Besides the operations you've already mentioned in hospitals, have you had any other surgeries as an outpatient?*

## Illnesses

The physician can investigate previous illnesses by using the same strategies discussed above. For example:

> PHYSICIAN: *Now that we have discussed hospitalizations, can you tell me about any serious or troubling illnesses you have had in the past?*

As the patient brings up past experiences with illness, the physician should find out general information concerning the severity of the illnesses, treatments, and outcomes. Experienced physicians, at this point in the interview, usually check with patients about other common illnesses:

> PHYSICIAN: *Has anyone ever told you that you've had high blood pressure, diabetes, lung disease, thyroid disease, anemia, cancer, arthritis, coronary artery disease, (etc).?*

## Injuries

> PHYSICIAN: *Have you ever had any serious accidents or injuries? (What happened? Did you break any bones? Were you hospitalized?)*

## Medications

If not already covered, a complete and systematic review of the patient's experience with medications is essential. This must include over-the-counter medicines as well.

> PHYSICIAN: *What medicines are you taking now? (What strength? How often do you take it? How often do you miss a dose?)*

> or

> PHYSICIAN: *Are you taking any over-the-counter medications? (Anything for sleep or bowels? Vitamins or pain pills?)*

The patient's past experience with medications is also essential.

> PHYSICIAN: *What medications have you taken in the past?*

## Allergies

Because patients may not routinely inform the physician of allergies, this information must be elicited directly.

> PHYSICIAN: *Do you have any allergies? (What kind of allergic reactions have you had? Have you had any allergic reaction to penicillin or injections used for x-ray studies?)*

## Pregnancies

> PHYSICIAN: *Have you ever been pregnant? (How many times? Any problems or complications?)*

## Exposures

> PHYSICIAN: *In your work or other activities, have you been exposed to chemicals, dusts, or fumes that might be dangerous? (Are your work conditions safe? Are you exposed to any other dangerous situations that you are aware of?)*

## Health Maintenance Practices

The past medical history includes inquiries regarding health maintenance practices concerning immunizations, screening tests (mammography, colonoscopy, lipids, etc), and lifestyle issues (exercise, nutrition).[1]

## Summary

Chapter 10 explains how to elicit the patient's past medical history, which includes the following elements:

1. Hospitalizations
2. Surgeries
3. Illnesses
4. Injuries
5. Medications
6. Allergies
7. Pregnancies (for women)
8. Exposures
9. Health maintenance

### Reference

1. Bickley L: *Bates' guide to physical exam and history taking*, ed 11, Philadelphia, 2013, Lippincott, Williams and Wilkins.

# CHAPTER 11

# Family History

## OVERVIEW

The family history is important because it identifies risks of potentially heritable illnesses or risk factors. In addition, the process itself of obtaining a family history often uncovers core fears driving some illness behaviors; uncovering these fears and responding empathically to this anxiety builds rapport and is broadly "therapeutic." Furthermore, this understanding contributes to the development of more effective collaborative management strategies.

The family history focuses on the health problems of the patient's closest relatives. This information can be especially important in investigating the possibility or implications of genetically related or transmitted diseases.

As the physician inquires about family illnesses or causes of death, many of the patient's concerns about his or her own condition may emerge. The patient may also experience significant emotional reactions when discussing family illnesses. In both of these cases the physician should notice these concerns and reactions and respond to them. For example:

PHYSICIAN: *I'd like to ask a few questions about illnesses in your family. Please tell me about your parents' health.*

PATIENT: *My mother has high blood pressure, and my father is dead. He died of a heart attack 5 years ago.*

PHYSICIAN: *I'm sorry. How old was he at the time?*

PATIENT: *Fifty-eight. My grandfather also died of a heart attack.*

PHYSICIAN: *How old was your grandfather when he died?*

PATIENT: *I don't know for sure. Probably about 65 or so. Do you think I have heart disease too?*

PHYSICIAN: *I can see why you might be concerned about your chest pains with this family history. That's understandable. I don't know yet whether there is a problem there or not. We still need to do the physical examination and a few tests. If you do have a heart problem, I want you to know there's a lot we can do for you to help prevent any major problems. We'll discuss your options in detail if we need to do anything.*

The physician needs to inquire in detail about health problems and treatment of all first-degree relatives (parents, siblings, and children). In addition, the physician needs to especially look for general health problems that might run in a large family:

PHYSICIAN: *Are there any other illnesses that run in your family, in your cousins or aunts and uncles?*

After specific information has been elicited, the physician will usually also ask whether anyone else in the family has ever had problems similar to the ones the patient is currently experiencing:

PHYSICIAN: *Has anyone else in the family ever had problems like yours?*

After eliciting this information, the clinician will usually also go back and check for major diseases categories in the family, for example:

PHYSICIAN: *Has anyone in the family ever had trouble with high blood pressure? Coronary artery disease? High cholesterol? Stroke? Diabetes? Thyroid or renal disease? Arthritis? Asthma or lung disease? Mental illness, substance abuse, or suicide?*[1]

## Summary

The family history is important because it identifies risks of potentially heritable illnesses or risk factors, and it is also important because the process itself of obtaining a family history often uncovers core fears driving the illness behavior and thus may contribute to the development of more effective collaborative management strategies.

### Reference

1. Bickley L: *Bates' guide to physical exam and history taking*, ed 11, Philadelphia, 2013, Lippincott, Williams and Wilkins.

# CHAPTER 12

# Patient Profile and Social History

## OVERVIEW

The patient profile/social history is an essential part of the medical history because understanding your patient as a person will help you develop more efficient and effective collaborative management strategies. The social history includes:

1. The patient profile
2. Lifestyle risk factors
3. Stresses and supports

The patient profile and social history are important parts of the database. The information elicited in this part of the interview helps with both assessment and collaborative management. For example, a patient's lifestyle, family and cultural history, social environment, and employment situation significantly influence the expression of symptoms, decisions to seek treatment, levels of functional disability, and willingness to adhere to collaborative management strategies.

Similarly, family structure profoundly influences patient care and outcome. For example, cohesive families help patients cope and adapt to functional limitations. Alternatively, significant family conflict may be predictive of problematic outcome in a physical illness. Family stability is further associated with adherence to medical regimens. Unfortunately, because the psychosocial aspects of a patient's life are so complex, trainees often have difficulty deciding how much of this information to pursue. Hours could be spent on this part of the interview alone. Students may be reassured to realize that this is also a significant challenge for experienced physicians.

There is often a difference between what experts recommend and what many physicians actually do. Medical textbooks routinely propose an extensive list of psychosocial areas that should be addressed (e.g., sibling relationships, developmental milestones, early work experiences, and relationships to parents when growing up).[1] In practice, however, most medical charts do not mention these topics,[2] and most clinicians find it impractical to address all these topics routinely.

Clinical discretion plays a key role in the determination of the balance between psychosocial exploration and more routine biologic assessment. Different patients and different medical problems clearly influence the pattern and balance of evaluation. When psychosocial variables seem to play a significant role in the etiology, exacerbation, or management of a medical problem, more thorough assessment of the social history becomes key.

This chapter reviews what can be considered a basic but adequate evaluation of the patient profile and social history. More extensive investigation is necessary for more complex cases. It is also worth noting that the evaluation of the social history is often different for inpatient and outpatient settings. For outpatients, physicians often use several visits to develop an adequate understanding of the patient profile and social history.

The basic patient profile and social history comprise the following components: (1) patient profile, (2) lifestyle risk factors, (3) stresses, and (4) supports. Each of these dimensions will be considered separately.

# Patient Profile

The patient profile represents the physician's understanding of a patient's uniqueness as a person. This generally includes three domains:

1. **Interpersonal relationships:** Ask about the patient's primary social (e.g., married, single, divorced, children, extended family, and friends) and sexual (activity, sexual orientation, and use of protection) relationships.

2. **Daily activities:** Evaluate how the patient spends his or her time (e.g., work, leisure, spiritual, other organized groups).

3. **Other factors:** Note other factors the patient considers important to mention. Many physicians obtain some of this information at the beginning of an interview, whereas others elicit it throughout the interview or wait to investigate social history in detail after the physical evaluation is complete.

Regardless of when the physician chooses to evaluate the patient profile, he or she can introduce the topic by saying something like the following:

> PHYSICIAN: *Can you tell me a little about yourself as a person? I'd like to know something about your family and the people who are important to you.*

This type of open-ended question usually elicits a great deal of information about a patient's family and social relationships. The physician can follow the patient's leads as appropriate.

Given the prevalence of sexually transmitted diseases, the physician's inquiry into patterns of sexual behavior has become a requisite part of the general medical evaluation. Although many medical students and practicing physicians may be uncomfortable with this line of questioning, these basic questions should be incorporated into every complete medical history. An orienting statement can be helpful before asking the questions about sexual activity, orientation, and protection. For example:

> PHYSICIAN: *I now need to ask you some questions about your sexual life. I ask these questions of all my patients. Are you currently sexually active? Are you active with men, with women, or with both? Do you ever have unprotected sexual relations?*

Because medical students and physicians find it so difficult to discuss sexual issues with their patients, Chapter 21 provides further guidance on this challenging topic.

After the physician learns something about the patient's social and sexual relationships, finding out more about how the patient spends his or her time (e.g., working, watching TV, keeping house, raising children, fishing, going to church) is usually helpful.

> PHYSICIAN: *Can you tell me a little about how you spend your time?*

The question about how a patient spends his or her time yields valuable information about the ability to function and cope with physical problems. It helps the physician learn about a patient's ability to work and function in the home with an illness. The question about time also yields information about the use of leisure time and activities such as church attendance that may be central to the lives of some patients.

After the physician has elicited information about social relationships and time, it is usually helpful to ask the patient at least one more open-ended question about himself or herself:

> PHYSICIAN: *What else would you like to tell me about yourself that you think might help me understand you better?*

An open-ended question like this prompts the patient to select aspects of his or her life that may be central to future patient management.

# High-Risk Health Behaviors

Negative health habits are important risk factors for the development of future illnesses and need to be evaluated. Patients need to be asked about their smoking habits and their use of alcohol and nonprescription drugs. These include over-the-counter medicines as well as substances of abuse (e.g., street drugs).

Because alcoholism is so common (about 20% of men have clinically significant alcoholism at some time in their lives) and denial is so common among alcoholics, special interviewing techniques are usually required to elicit a history of alcoholism.[3] Most patients who have problems with alcohol do not openly admit to this difficulty, and when asked to specify amounts of alcohol consumed, they tend to minimize the amount.

The CAGE interview, which inquires about the effects of drinking rather than drinking itself, can be helpful in eliciting information suggestive of alcohol abuse.[4] The four letters in CAGE are used as an acronym to remember the four important questions that should be asked of all patients to explore the possibility of alcohol abuse.

**C** Have you ever felt the need to **cut** down on your drinking?

**A** Do you ever get **annoyed** when people tell you to cut down on your drinking?

**G** Do you ever feel **guilty** about drinking too much?

**E** Have you ever needed an **"eye-opener"** in the mornings?

If the patient answers yes to any of the four questions of the CAGE model, the possibility of alcohol abuse or risky drinking is present and must be explored in more detail. Interviewing patients about their drinking behavior is complex and difficult (see Chapter 29).[5]

Patients should also be asked about their use of illicit drugs. Some physicians ask these questions after they have inquired about prescription and nonprescription drugs. For example:

PHYSICIAN: *You've mentioned some medications prescribed by the doctor and some you've bought in drug stores. Have you ever used drugs for recreation? Have you ever used uppers or downers? Have you ever tried a drug like cocaine?*

Physicians also need to inquire about smoking. For example:

PHYSICIAN: *Do you smoke? How much do you smoke? About how many packs do you smoke a day? For how many years have you smoked this much?*

Total years of experience smoking are conventionally expressed in pack-years. One year of smoking one pack of cigarettes a day equals one pack-year. Thus, 10 years of smoking three packs of cigarettes a day is counted as 30 pack-years.

# High-Risk Life Situations (High Stress and Low Support)

Social stress and social support are significant risk factors for most physical and psychiatric illnesses. For example, among patients experiencing their first heart attacks, those patients with low support and high stress were four times more likely to die of a repeat heart attack in the subsequent year.[6] This was true even after controlling for factors such as underlying cardiac condition, smoking and other negative health habits, visits to the doctor, and the prior state of health. The magnitude of this effect on outcome was as large as any physical risk factor (e.g., arrhythmias and congestive failure).

Because of the wealth of evidence that points to the important health consequences of life stress and social support, a brief consideration of both of these factors should be included in every new patient evaluation. This need not consume a great deal of time; two specific questions may be sufficient. However, more extensive evaluation may be necessary for patients who indicate problems in either of these areas.

**PHYSICIAN:** *Can you tell me a little about the kinds of stress you are under?*

It is generally preferable to ask the question in this open-ended form rather than a closed-ended one, for example, like asking the patient, "Are you under stress?" The suggested format helps decrease patient defensiveness when reporting psychosocial difficulties.

Domestic violence as well as previous physical or sexual abuse has become increasingly apparent as a hidden cause of visits to emergency rooms as well a factor in underlying chronic illnesses. Therefore screening for domestic violence and/or present or previous abuse is mandatory. This can be delicate and difficult but should be addressed with open-ended questions such as the following:

**PHYSICIAN:** *Have you ever felt unsafe at home? Or in your relationships? Has your partner ever hurt/threatened/abused you or your children? Growing up, were you ever afraid or hurt by any grown-ups around you?*

After inquiring about stresses, the physician should investigate sources of social support as well. For example:

**PHYSICIAN:** *To whom can you turn for support?*

## Summary

The patient profile and social history is an important part of the medical history because understanding your patient as a person will help you develop more efficient and effective collaborative management strategies. The patient profile and social history includes:

1. The patient profile
2. Life style risk factors
3. Stresses and supports

### References

1. Bickley L: *Bates' guide to physical exam and history taking*, ed 11, Philadelphia, 2013, Lippincott, Williams and Wilkins.
2. Cohen-Cole SA, et al: Psychiatric education for internists: a randomized controlled comparison of two teaching models. *Psychosom Med* 44:122, 1982.
3. Saitz R. Unhealthy alcohol use. *N Engl J Med* 352:596–607, 2005.
4. Ewing JA: Detecting alcoholism: the CAGE questionnaire. *JAMA* 252:1905, 1984.
5. NIAAA: *Helping patients who drink too much: a clinician's guide*, Washington, D.C., 2005, Government Printing Office (updated, January, 2007). http://pubs.niaaa.nih.gov/publications/Practitioner/Clinicians Guide2005/clinicians_guide.htm; accessed 12/4/2012.
6. Rozanski A, et al: The epidemiology, pathophysiology, and management of psychosocial risk factors in cardiac practice: the emerging field of behavioral cardiology. *J Am Coll Cardiol* 45(5):637–651, 2005.

# CHAPTER 13

# Review of Systems

## OVERVIEW

The review of systems is an essential part of the medical history to ensure that significant problems have not been overlooked. Clinicians typically develop an individualized systematic approach to gather this information in an efficient manner. Care should be taken to include screening for hidden psychiatric issues or domestic violence, both of which contribute to excessive health care use.

The review of systems is an important part of the medical history that allows the physician to survey the various bodily systems and uncover significant symptoms that may not have already been revealed in the history of the present illness or the elaboration of the past medical history.

Because the review of systems is designed to screen an enormous array of possible problems, interviewing skill is required to gather data systematically and efficiently without missing important details. Most patients understand the point of this part of the interview and cooperate with the physician in completing it rapidly and efficiently. Because most information relevant to the patient's current problems will already have been elicited in the discussion of the present illness and the past medical history, the review of systems should be possible to complete in 5 to 10 minutes for most patients. Some patients who demonstrate a positive review of systems, however, find some way to report symptoms in virtually every organ system. Such patients have also been said to present a laundry list of complaints and can be frustrating to interview. In general, these patients need to be directed toward the goal of reporting common, recurrent, or troubling symptoms and omitting infrequent or mild symptoms.

Experienced physicians often complete the review of systems while performing the physical examination. Screening questions can be asked of the patient while the physician is examining the relevant body part. Although this method is efficient, the physician must ensure that the patient knows the physician is asking general screening questions. Some patients become anxious because they imagine that questions are being asked about some physical abnormality that has appeared on the physical examination.

Because of the complexity of the review of systems, however, beginning students generally need to complete this part of the interview before they examine the patient. To remember important topics, most students also find it helpful to consult a list of relevant questions while they are interviewing patients. Students may write key questions on a sheet of paper, a clipboard, or an index card to refer to while they interview patients. Students are soon able to develop their own systems for remembering relevant questions and will no longer need reminders.

In general, an efficient review of systems is organized around body systems. These are the systems that must be evaluated:[1]

1. General
2. Skin
3. Head, eyes, ears, nose, throat (HEENT)
4. Neck
5. Breasts

6. Respiratory system
7. Cardiovascular system
8. Gastrointestinal system
9. Peripheral vascular system
10. Urinary organs
11. Genital organs
12. Musculoskeletal system
13. Neurologic system
14. Hematologic system
15. Endocrine system
16. Psychiatric state

The patient should be told that a separate part of the evaluation process is about to begin and that the clinician will screen a wide variety of organs, organ systems, and physical problems to see whether anything important was omitted in the interview so far.

> **PHYSICIAN:** *The next part of the interview is different. I'm going to ask you a series of standard questions about common medical problems that you may or may not have experienced. This is our way of making sure we don't miss something that might be important.*

A few selected questions are listed as examples for each of the organ systems. As students gain experience, they will develop skill in evaluating the significance of symptoms uncovered in the review of systems and they will learn to recognize patterns of patient responses that require more detailed follow-up. Several general questions are asked for each organ system. Clinicians can also give patients a short list of symptoms and ask them whether they have ever experienced any of the symptoms. Positive responses by patients then need to be followed by more focused questions inquiring about the details of the complaint. The following list of questions represents an acceptable approach for beginning students:

1. **General:** Have you ever had any problems with weight change, clothing that fits more tightly or loosely than usual, weakness, fatigue, or fever?
2. **Skin:** Have you ever had rashes, lumps, sores, itching, dryness, changes in color, changes in nails or hair, changes in size or color of moles?
3. **Head, eyes, ears, nose, throat (HEENT):** Have you ever had headaches, head injury, dizziness, or lightheadedness,? What about vision problems, glasses or contacts, eye pain, redness, excessive tearing, double or blurred vision, spots, specks, or flashing lights? Have you ever had ringing in the ears, earaches, discharge, decreased hearing, frequent colds, nasal stuffiness, discharge, itching, nosebleeds, sinus trouble, gum trouble, teeth trouble, sore tongue, dry mouth, frequent sore throats, or hoarseness? When did you last see the dentist? Do you wear dentures?
4. **Neck:** Have you ever had "swollen glands," lumps, pain, or stiffness in the neck?
5. **Breasts:** Have you ever had lumps, pain, discomfort, nipple discharge? Do you do self-examinations?
6. **Respiratory system:** Have you had a cough? Have you coughed up sputum or blood? Have you had chest pain, shortness of breath, or wheezing? When was your last chest x-ray?
7. **Cardiovascular system:** Have you had chest pain, palpitations, shortness of breath, swelling? What were the results of previous EKGs, other cardiac tests, stress tests?
8. **Gastrointestinal system:** Have you had trouble swallowing, heartburn, reflux, trouble with appetite, nausea, bowel movements, change in stool habits or color, stomach pain, rectal bleeding, constipation, food intolerance, passing of gas?
9. **Peripheral vascular system:** Have you had pain in your calves, cramps, swelling, color changes in fingers or toes in cold weather, swelling or tenderness?

10. **Urinary system:** Have you had urinary frequency, urination at night, urgency, burning or pain on urination, hesitation, blood in the urine, flank pain, suprapubic pain, decreased stream or dribbling?

11. **Genital organs:** (male)—Have you had hernias, discharge, sores on penis, testicular pain or masses, STDs or treatments? What about your sexual habits, interests or function, birth control methods, concerns?; (female)—age of menarche, regularity, frequency and duration of periods, amount of bleeding, bleeding between periods or after intercourse, last menstrual period, dysmenorrhea, premenstrual tension, age of menopause, menopausal symptoms, postmenopausal symptoms, vaginal discharge, itching, lumps, sores, STDs, number of pregnancies, number and types of deliveries, number of abortions, complications of pregnancy, birth control methods, sexual preferences, concerns, dyspareunia, concerns about HIV?

12. **Musculoskeletal system:** Have you had muscle or joint pain, stiffness, arthritis, gout, backache, joint tenderness, weakness, limitation of movement, neck or low back pain, joint pain with systemic features such as fever, chills, rash?

13. **Neurologic system:** Have you had changes in attention or speech, orientation or memory, headache, dizziness, vertigo, blackouts, weakness, paralysis, numbness, "pins and needles," tremors or other involuntary movements, seizures?

14. **Hematologic system:** Have you had easy bruising, anemia, transfusions, transfusion reactions?

15. **Endocrine system:** Have you had "thyroid trouble," heat or cold intolerance, excessive sweating, excessive thirst or hunger, polyuria, change in glove or shoe size.

16. **Psychiatric state:** Have you felt nervous or tense? Have you had mood changes, depression, or anxiety; memory changes, suicidal thoughts or attempts? Were you ever afraid of being hurt at home when you were growing up? What about now?

It is important to highlight the special importance of the psychiatric review of systems. Many patients in the general medical system, especially those with unexplained physical complaints, suffer from unrecognized depression or anxiety or are victims of current or previous physical or sexual abuse.[2,3] These patients typically use excessive health care resources before their underlying psychiatric disorders or abuse history is recognized and appropriately treated. Sadly, sometimes the psychiatric problems or abuse are never recognized, or even worse, sometimes patients with unrecognized mental disorders in the general medical sector ultimately go on to make suicide attempts or complete suicidal acts. Therefore, special efforts should be made to make sure to include the psychiatric screening questions in every complete medical evaluation.

## Summary

The review of systems is an essential part of the medical history to ensure that significant problems have not been overlooked. Clinicians typically develop an individualized systematic approach to gather this information in an efficient manner. Care should be taken to include screening for hidden psychiatric issues or domestic violence, both of which contribute to excessive health care utilization.

### References

1. Bickley L: *Bates' guide to physical exam and history taking*, ed 11, Philadelphia, 2013, Lippincott, Williams and Wilkins.
2. Warshaw C, Alpert E: Integrating routine inquiry about domestic violence into daily practice (editorial). *Ann Intern Med* 131(8):619–620, 1999.
3. Kroenke K, Jackson JL, Chamberlin S: Depressive and anxiety disorders in patients presenting with physical complaints: clinical predictors and outcome. *Am J Med* 103(5):339–357, 1997.

# CHAPTER 14

# Mental Status

## OVERVIEW

This chapter discusses the importance of the brief mental status examination in every general medical workup and presents an outline for a six-point assessment, most of which can be elicited without any specific questioning:
1. General appearance/behavior
2. Speech/language
3. Mood/affect
4. Thought/perception
5. Cognition/sensorium
6. Insight/judgment

An evaluation of mental status belongs in every complete medical workup. As with the patient profile and social history, the recommendations in medical texts for the mental status examination are sometimes far different from what is actually incorporated into routine medical practice. Most medical texts present a complex discussion of the mental status evaluation. However, few physicians routinely incorporate a "formal" mental status examination into their interviews, and most written evaluations of mental status in patients' charts refer to "orientation" only with statements such as "oriented × 3," "confused," or "disoriented."

This chapter presents the rationale for including a brief mental status evaluation in every medical workup and presents a succinct version of the mental status evaluation that can be easily and efficiently adapted for routine office practice.[1] Because some patients (especially elderly patients or those with possible delirium or dementia) require more extensive cognitive testing, physicians can develop further competencies in this area by consulting other references.[2]

### Why Every Medical Workup Should Include a Mental Status Evaluation

The mental status of every patient should be assessed for multiple reasons. Physicians need to be aware of cognitive abnormalities that can lead to unreliability in the data collection process and are important for further workup. Clinicians also need to be aware of early signs of affective and anxiety disorders.

As pointed out in Chapter 2, mental illness is common in the general population (about 20% of the population over any 6-month period of time) and among patients seeking general medical care.[4]

Carefully conducted studies have revealed that 25% to 33% of primary care patients suffer from a mental disorder and another 20% have significant emotional problems or symptoms complicating their physical illnesses. One third to one half of these problems are not recognized by primary care physicians.[3]

Some students may wonder about the importance of recognizing mental disorders in their patients. They may believe that mentally ill patients really "belong" in the mental health sector of the health care system, and that it may not be appropriate for primary providers to explore such problems in their patients. However, there are several reasons that general medical physicians need skills in the recognition and management of mental disorders. First, 50% to 60% of the mentally ill patients in the United States obtain their only mental health care from primary care providers.[4] Second, many mentally ill patients seek general medical attention because physical complaints are more "legitimate" avenues for the expression of psychiatric problems. Most psychiatric conditions are psychobiologic conditions in which physical complaints are common (e.g., sleep disorder in depression and palpitations or shortness of breath in panic disorder). Many patients focus on these physical symptoms when seeking medical attention rather than face the stigma of psychiatric care. Primary care patients with mental illness use twice as much nonpsychiatric medical care as patients without mental illness.[5] Furthermore, most patients who eventually commit suicide seek some type of medical help in the weeks before their suicide.[6]

For general humanitarian reasons, then, as well as for public health and efficiency, physicians should have the skills to recognize and manage psychiatric disorders that occur in their clinical and hospital practices. Developing proficiency in the use of a brief mental status examination is one important part of learning to recognize mental disorders.

In addition to missing affective and anxiety disorders in medical patients, cognitive impairment in hospitalized patients is also commonly overlooked. One study in an inner-city hospital found that 33% of the medically ill patients had significant cognitive impairment and that with 50% of these patients the condition was unrecognized by their physicians.[7] It is important for physicians to recognize cognitive impairment because limited cognitive capacity can lead to inaccurate data collection by the physician and poor compliance. In addition, many cognitive problems are associated with treatable and sometimes reversible disorders.

# Brief Mental Status Examination

Most parts of the brief mental status evaluation can be completed without asking the patient specific questions. Significant information about mental status is obtained throughout the interview process through careful observation: note the patient's general appearance, motor activity and behavior, speech, thought process, judgment, recounting of medical history, and affect. The physician may need to ask the patient only three or four screening questions to complete the entire mental status examination as presented here. Thus the mental status examination is an ongoing process throughout the interview and may require only 3 or 4 minutes of additional directed questioning.

The brief mental status evaluation includes six basic categories. By convention, the oral presentation or written description of the mental status evaluation are usually included as the first part of the neurologic examination (which is part of the overall physical examination).

## 1. GENERAL APPEARANCE/BEHAVIOR

The physician can complete the general description of the patient without asking any specific questions. The general description is a short statement about how the patient appears overall to the examiner, and can include motor activity and general behavior if particularly remarkable. The general description should give the listener or reader a "snapshot" of the patient's presentation and can provide a great deal of information about the patient's general condition, if notable. Areas of concern are the patient's attention to or ability for self-care (neat? disheveled?) and rapport with the physician (cooperative? suspicious?). For the purposes of oral presentation or written documentation, the following description might be appropriate:

> **Mr. Barnes was lying quietly in bed and appeared somewhat disheveled. He answered questions slowly and somewhat hesitantly.**

## 2. SPEECH/LANGUAGE

The quality and quantity of speech and language should be described. For example, speech can be rapid or slow, coherent or disorganized and rambling, or clear or slurred. The description of a patient's speech gives a great deal of information concerning emotional and neurologic functioning. Again, the quality and quantity of speech can be observed without asking any specific questions:

>  **Mrs. Fander's speech was clear and coherent.**
>
>    or
>
>  **Mr. Spike's speech was slurred and rambling.**

When there are inconsistencies and incoherence in speech or language, more careful psychiatric evaluation for psychosis or neurologic examination for aphasia may be necessary.

## 3. MOOD/AFFECT

"Mood" generally refers to an underlying emotional state, or alternatively in some systems of mental status, how the patient describes his or her own mood. "Affect" describes more momentary modulation of feeling in the course of an interview, or in some systems of mental status, what the physician observes during the examination. For the purposes of the brief mental status evaluation, it is not always necessary to separate the two categories. In this section the physician should describe the predominant feeling tone communicated by the patient (e.g., sadness, anger, or anxiety) and what the physician observes. The patient occasionally demonstrates more than one significant feeling. When this occurs, the physician should record it. If the physician observes an inappropriate or flat affect, this also should be described. For example:

>  **Mr. Kline said he has not been depressed or anxious and demonstrated appropriate affect throughout the interview but seemed very anxious when we discussed his test results.**
>
>    or
>
>  **Mr. Blanc said he's been depressed and he appeared sad throughout the interview and cried several times as he discussed his difficulty in working.**

One or two screening questions can be productive for the evaluation of mood and affect. For example:

>  **PHYSICIAN:** *How have you reacted to all these problems? How much stress or tension have you been feeling lately? How often do you feel sad or "blue"?*

When the clinician inquires about mood or stress, the patient often expresses some distress (e.g. crying, anxiety). The clinician should respond empathetically to those expressed feelings with the skills of Function One. (Rule #1, Respond to the patient's feelings as soon as they appear, Chapter Three).

## 4. THOUGHT/PERCEPTION

The evaluation of thought refers to the patient's main concerns, the presence of psychotic phenomena such as delusions and hallucinations, and the presence of suicidal or homicidal ideation.

Some systems of mental status create a separate category of perception for psychotic processes such as hallucinations. But I do not think that is necessary for the purposes of a brief mental status in a general medical setting. Under the category of thought/perception, the clinician can include the patient's thought content and concerns, the presence or absence of hallucinations/delusions, and the presence or absence of suicidal or homicidal ideation. For the purposes of most medical interviews, the patient's main concern is the chief complaint and present illness, and there is no need to ask further questions about the patient's main concern. Here is an example of a possible chart notation on thought.

**THOUGHT:** *Patient is concerned about heart disease because his father died of an MI at age 60; no evidence of psychosis; no suicidal or homicidal ideation.*

Patients demonstrating emotional distress should be asked about suicidal ideation. Physicians should be reassured that this type of inquiry can be lifesaving and does not "put ideas" into patients' heads. Of course, concern and sensitivity to the patient's emotional concerns must be shown, and then the physician can sensitively ask a question such as the following:

**PHYSICIAN:** *With all these problems you've been having, I wonder—do you ever think that life is not worth living?*

With this type of introduction the physician can begin exploring the patient's specific thoughts and plans about suicidal intent.

## 5. COGNITION/SENSORIUM

The physician should describe patients' orientation and general cognitive functioning. The patient's sensorium is a rough proxy for "attention" and the ability to interact with the environment. It is important as a separate category because of the frequency of delirium, which is a disorder of attention. Orientation to person, place, date, and situation (four separate dimensions) can be a rough test for intact sensorium. If a patient were fully oriented in all four spheres, it would be unusual for him or her to have an impairment in sensorium such that he or she could not interact meaningfully with the environment. Evaluating the cognitive status of every patient is essential. To minimize patient discomfort, this can be introduced as another part of the routine evaluation. For example:

**PHYSICIAN:** *Mrs. Smith, I need to ask you a few questions about your memory and thinking. These are routine. Some are quite easy, and some may be more difficult. Where are you right now? What is today's date?*

After the physician has asked the orientation questions, he or she should complete at least a brief cognitive screening. A short-term memory task and at least one other complex cognitive task is adequate for screening purposes. Patients can be asked to remember three objects after 3 minutes and to complete one more cognitive challenge that may be appropriate to their educational level. The physician can complete this test of short-term memory by asking the patient to repeat three specific words after the examiner has said them and then to remember them when asked, a few minutes later. For example:

**PHYSICIAN:** *Now, Mr. Brown, I'm going to say three words, and I would like you to say them after me. Then I would like you to try to remember them for a few minutes. I will ask you for them again. The words are "apple," "table," and "penny."*

After the patient has registered the words, one complex cognitive task appropriate to educational level should be administered. For example, college-educated patients can be asked to subtract 7 from 100 and keep going for about 1 minute (or typically five subtractions). If the patient is less well educated, suitable alternatives could be to spell "world" backward, subtract serial 3s from 100, recite the months of the year or days of the week backward, or recite seven numbers forward or four numbers backward, for example. Alternately, patients can be asked to draw the face of a clock, put in the numbers, and place the long and short arms of the clock at the appropriate place to indicate a specific time (e.g., 10 minutes before 2). After this task is complete, the patient can be asked to recall the three words. This final screening cognitive task is useful, especially in elderly patients, because impairment in short-term memory can be a subtle sign of early dementia. If performance on the screen is equivocal, physicians can perform a more complete bedside screening cognitive assessment (e.g., the Mini-Mental State Examination).[8]

## 6. INSIGHT/JUDGMENT

Assessment of insight concerns the extent to which the patient understands his or her own illness and assessment of judgment refers to his or her ability to make appropriate and adaptive decisions about his or her situation or condition. In the general medical setting, the insight and judgment of most patients without dementia will generally be adequate. On the other hand, insight and judgment can be considered impaired in those patients who do not accept their chronic illnesses, who are grossly non-adherent with lifesaving medical recommendations, and who repeatedly demonstrate poor judgment in life or medical situations. Such patients will usually be suffering from some form of delirium or dementia. Thus, evaluation of insight and judgment can usually be inferred from the interview, personal behavior, and recent medical history; it rarely requires a specialized set of questions.

## Conclusion

In general, the brief mental status evaluation will take no more than 3 or 4 minutes for patients who do not have a significant mental disorder or significant cognitive impairment but will detect many patients with mental disorders whose impairments are often missed in general medical settings.

## Summary

This chapter discusses the importance of the brief mental status examination in every general medical workup and presents an outline for a six-point assessment, most of which can be elicited without any specific questioning:

1. General appearance/behavior
2. Speech/language
3. Mood/affect
4. Thought/perception
5. Cognition/sensorium
6. Insight/judgment

### References

1. The model for mental status presented in this chapter is very similar to the discussion of mental status in Bickley L., *Bates' guide to physical exams and history taking*, 11th Edition, Lippincott, Williams and Wilkins, Philadelphia, 2013.
2. Snyderman D, Rovner B: Mental status exam in primary care: a review. *A Fam Physician* 80(8):809–814, 2009.
3. Kessler RC, et al: Prevalence and treatment of mental disorders, 1990-2003. *N Engl J Med* 352(24):25, 15–23, 2005.
4. Regier DA, et al: The de facto U.S. mental and addictive disorders service system. Epidemiologic catchment area prospective 1-year prevalence rates of disorders and services. *Arch Gen Psych* 50:85–94, 1993.
5. Unetzer J, et al: Depressive symptoms and the cost of health services in HMO patients aged 65 years and older. A 4-year prospective study. *JAMA* 277(28):618–623, 1997.
6. Barraclough B, et al: A hundred cases of suicide: clinical aspects. *Br J Psychiatry* 125:355–373, 1974.
7. Gehi M, et al: Is there a need for admission and discharge cognitive screening for the medically ill? *Gen Hosp Psychiatry* 3:186–191, 1980.
8. Folstein MF, Folstein SE, McHugh PR: 'Mini-mental state.' A practical method for grading the cognitive state of patients for the clinician. *J Psychiatr Res* 12(3):189–198, 1975.

# Presentation and Documentation

# CHAPTER 15

# Presentation and Documentation

Susan Lane

## OVERVIEW

Learning the verbal and written case presentation stands as one of the foundation tasks of medical education. This chapter reviews the basic elements of the medical write-up and provides suggestions for effective presentations.

The medical write-up has three purposes. The write-up is an accounting of the medical care of the patient and provides essential information to other health care providers who will also be caring for the patient. It also serves as the permanent legal record of the medical care provided to the patient and may be referenced for future care as well as for medicolegal purposes. Last, it forces the clinician to carefully consider the patient's health state, to distill and organize the information gathered so as to formulate a coherent assessment of the illness to plan for collaborative management.

An excellent written or oral case presentation facilitates the give-and-take learning that occurs between teacher and student in the clinical setting. With an excellent presentation you demonstrate the thoroughness of your investigation, your understanding of the case, and the research you have done to develop your differential and your management plan. The medical note you generate is the product of your hard work. Take pride in your written documentation.

The comprehensive health history (for inpatient admissions or new outpatient visits) and the focused health history (for follow-up care in both settings) share many commonalities but also have some important differences, both of which are discussed below.

Before even getting started, students often find the following general guidelines helpful.

1. Take care to recognize and avoid one common pitfall of beginners: a tendency to editorialize. This obfuscates rather than clarifies and decreases efficiency. For example, the word "I" should not appear in your written note and, in general, should not be included in your oral presentations. For example, rather than saying, "I think I heard a mitral stenosis murmur but I'm not sure," simply describe what you hear: "There is a 2/6 diastolic rumble heard best over the 5th intercostal space, midclavicular line."
2. In the history of present illness, choose simple language over flowery and choose direct language rather than elaborate. For example, it is better to say, "the patient reported increased chest pain during stress at work," as opposed to, "the patient manifested increased severity of substernal discomfort during periods when his judgment was challenged by his supervisor at work."
3. Describe what you personally observe in your physical exam rather than stating a diagnosis ("scattered vesicles on pink base" rather than "shingles").

## Chief Complaint

Every write-up and presentation should include a chief complaint (CC). By convention, this is a very short description, using the *patient's* words, about why the patient has come to the office or has been admitted to the hospital. Some examples include "cough for 3 days," "follow-up of type 2 diabetes mellitus," and "severe pain in the abdomen." During the course of a hospitalization, the CC becomes a brief statement as to why the patient is admitted and evolves over the course of the admission. The patient may have been admitted for "cough and fever for 5 days" but has subsequently been diagnosed with right lower lobe pneumonia. In this instance, the CC becomes "cough and fever for 5 days, diagnosed as RLL pneumonia."

## History

The write-up and presentation centers around the history, which presents the greatest challenge to the developing physician for good reason. For example, it is sometimes difficult to know if a piece of information belongs in the history section, or in the past medical history (PMH), or the review of systems (ROS). The choice is sometimes ambiguous, but more often than not this difficulty resolves as you gain more clinical experience. You will begin to recognize patterns of disease and will be able to determine that which is relevant to the history of the present illness and that which may be of only peripheral importance, and therefore, more appropriately placed into another part of the write-up or presentation. If you understand and adhere to the following guideline, you will generally make the right decisions:

> *The history is the patient's own chronological story, or narrative, of his or her present condition.*

The history of present illness (HPI) is part of the comprehensive health assessment for a new admission to the hospital or when a patient is establishing care with a new provider. Here you describe the story of the present illness as told to you by the patient and as experienced by the patient. Do not overly quote, but do not alter the patient's representation of the story by imposing your own interpretation over the patient's or introducing unfamiliar medical jargon that may change the patient's meaning. On the other hand, it is acceptable, and even preferable, to rephrase some of the patient's words using common medical terminology (e.g., "sputum" rather than "spit") as long as this does not lead to misinterpretation or alteration of the patient's actual experience. When a patient uses a diagnosis to describe his/her symptoms (e.g., "I have sciatica"), be sure to ask the patient specifically what is meant by "sciatica," in terms of their own subjective experience of symptoms (e.g., pain).

When you are a beginner eliciting patient histories, you likely will not have had enough clinical experience to form an early impression (or problem representation) of the clinical situation. As your experience grows, you will begin to recognize patterns of disease and your questioning will become more focused as you seek to identify the defining and discriminating features of the case. Both the initial and follow-up histories should contain pertinent positives and negatives with regard to symptoms and history. Your listener is formulating a differential diagnosis while you are presenting and is listening for clues to narrow the diagnosis.

All of the active medical problems that are pertinent to the history (medical, surgical, psychological, social, family) are to be included in the history section. Often, particularly in the outpatient setting, a patient may have a number of issues to be discussed. It is helpful to number these problems in the HPI.

The student must investigate eight essential dimensions for every patient problem, as described in more detail in Chapter 9. The following acronym can be a helpful memory aid for these eight dimensions: *WW, QQ, AA, LC,* and *I.*

1. Where
2. When
3. Quality
4. Quantity

5. Aggravating and alleviating factors
6. Associated factors
7. Life context
8. Impact on quality of life

Objective information related to the narrative should also be included in the history; for example, the last visit to the ophthalmologist for the diabetic patient or a recent visit to the cardiologist, in which a medication was adjusted for a patient with congestive heart failure. The patient's ideas, concerns, and expectations about the illness ("ICE," see Chapter 8) are part of the medical interview with the patient, and relevant "ICE" information obtained should be judiciously and efficiently integrated into the written and oral presentations. As discussed above, these decisions about what is relevant for the HPI will become more facile and efficient as you gain more clinical experience and clinical judgment throughout your training.

The history should be presented in chronologic order, starting with the current episode and adding background information as needed.

The focused health history is used for the follow-up progress note during a hospital admission or an outpatient visit. Traditionally the SOAP note format is followed, in which S represents the subjective portion of the note (the history), O is the objective (the examination) and data, and A and P represent assessment and plan, respectively.

Some medical centers or physicians prefer to structure the follow-up note as History, Examination, Data, Assessment, and Plan. If a chronic disease is being discussed as opposed to an acute problem, it is important to document the following points in the history: how long the patient has had the disease, manifestations and complications from the disease, adherence to therapy, changes in therapy, and present status. In the inpatient setting, it is important to avoid restating the initial, detailed HPI in the history section of your daily progress notes. It is far better to *briefly* summarize the HPI and then detail the recent events during the hospitalization, overnight events, and symptoms the patient is currently feeling.

## Medications

The medication list should be reviewed in its entirety with the patient. It is good practice to use the generic names of the medications. You should know the indication for every medication that you are recording. Document the dose, route, and frequency of each medication. Include non-prescription medications and supplements. If you are using an electronic medical record, be sure to reconcile the medication list and remove outdated information. Drug, food, and environmental allergies should be noted along with the reaction for each.

## Past Medical History

The past medical history (PMH) should list all medical problems, indicating parenthetically whether active or resolved. The items should be subcategorized as medical, surgical, obstetric/gynecologic, and psychiatric. Some of these medical problems may already have been mentioned in the HPI/history sections. (See Chapter 10)

## Family History

The family history details important aspects of the patient's family's medical history. In addition to case-specific inquiries you may have, you should routinely ask about cardiovascular disease, diabetes, hypertension, colon cancer, and breast cancer. Note the relationship of the individual to the patient (e.g., first-degree relative or paternal grandfather) and the age of onset. The answers may have implications for disease screening for your patient as well as your assessment of the possible diagnosis. (See Chapter 11)

## Social History

The social history helps us understand the social context of the patient's life. This should include information on the living situation (safety, caregiver support, type of residence such as apartment with one flight of stairs, assisted living facility), exercise, occupation, tobacco and alcohol use, use of illicit substances, sexual activity, activities of daily living (dressing, eating, ambulating, toileting, transferring, bathing), and instrumental activities of daily living (shopping, housekeeping, accounting, food preparation, taking medications, transportation). Consider the elderly patient who becomes debilitated after a prolonged hospitalization for pneumonia who lives in a second-floor walk-up apartment. She is evaluated by physical therapy and although she is able to transfer, she is unable to climb stairs and thus cannot be discharged to home. It is essential to know the patient's social context as this frequently impacts illness and medical care. (See Chapter 12)

## Review of Systems

Explore the review of systems (ROS) in detail for a new patient. Include any items that are pertinent to the present illness in the HPI/history. Important items that are not relevant to the HPI/history but are identified in the review are recorded in the ROS section. A less extensive and more focused ROS is appropriate for a follow-up visit. (See Chapter 13)

## Examination

Begin the physical examination section with the vital signs, including heart rate, blood pressure, temperature, respiratory rate, height, weight, and body mass index (BMI). Level of pain may be included if relevant. There may be additional data that are relevant in this section, particularly in the inpatient setting, including oxygen saturation (indicate whether obtained on room air or with oxygen, quantifying the amount), I/O (fluids in and out), blood sugar readings, or ventilator settings and pressures. You may want to indicate the Tmax (maximum temperature) or the range of blood pressures, if relevant to the case.

A brief description of the general appearance is helpful and alerts your listener to the acuity of the presentation ("seated comfortably on the exam table" vs. "breathing rapidly and not able to speak in full sentences"). A new patient requires a thorough examination, whereas a follow-up patient will have a more focused examination. You will need to carefully consider the pertinent positives and negatives to include in your focused examination.

> *Limit your reporting in the examination section to the physical findings that you have observed.*

Do not let subjective phrases find their way into your examination section! Rather than stating that something is "normal," it is more instructive to give relevant findings. For example, an examination of the lungs would be documented as follows: "clear to auscultation, no rales, wheezes, or rhonchi" as opposed to "normal lung exam." Remember that you are learning and you should always take the opportunity to ask your supervisor to help you confirm findings that you feel unsure about. This is best done at the end of the presentation.

## Data

In this section you should list recent and important test results with dates and trends noted. Tables are useful when displaying data trends over time.

## Assessment

Often you are so exhausted from documenting the previous sections that this section is not given sufficient attention. Be sure to give the assessment section your full attention and effort!

This is where you demonstrate your understanding of the case, and where you will learn the most in your preparation. There are several ways to approach this section. If you are performing an initial assessment of a new hospital admission, your assessment will be a summary of the pertinent findings in the history, exam, and data sections. Be sure to include the discriminating features you noted in the history and physical examination. You will then suggest possible etiologies of the problem, thus generating a differential diagnosis. Your differential should contain your reasoning strategy—why you do or do not think the patient has a particular disorder. You should consult a textbook or online resource to broaden and define your differential.

As you compose your assessment, use what are known as opposing discriminators (or abstract semantic qualifiers) to transform the patient-specific details into a defined problem.[1] For example, for the patient who describes pain in his right knee that began yesterday, you would summarize "*acute* onset of *mono*articular pain" as opposed to "*chronic poly*articular pain." Using opposing discriminators in your assessments will foster the development of disease pattern recognition and you will be on the road to becoming an expert clinician!

Although a patient who presents with new signs and symptoms may have many diseases, try to follow the law of diagnostic parsimony (Occam's razor) and seek to find a unifying diagnosis that ties the subjective and objective findings together. Keep your differential broad, do not ignore or omit information that does not seem to fit your diagnosis, and apply common sense as you develop your assessment.

In a follow-up visit, if there are no new problems, the assessment may be more of a summary of the visit, noting pertinent history, exam findings, and data. When there are multiple, distinct problems, it may be easier to provide an assessment (and plan) for each problem individually.

## Plan

Spend time organizing this section, with items listed from your determination of highest to lowest priority, and avoid redundancy. A problem-focused plan works well and is easy to organize. A problem may be a symptom, a diagnosis, or a condition (e.g., cough, pneumonia, or homelessness). Each problem is numbered and is followed by an assessment or a brief summary (e.g., hypertension stage I: at goal with blood pressure <130/80).

Avoid generating a problem/solution list—this will curtail your ability to demonstrate your true understanding of the patient's issues. The problem list for an admitted patient in the hospital should evolve over time as the disease process becomes better understood (e.g., from "cough" to "pneumonia"). Make sure your problem list accurately represents the complexity of the patient's illness (e.g., "UTI with hypotension" rather than "UTI"). Bulleted action items under each problem make the plan easy to read and track. The plan should address diagnosis, therapy, and patient education for each problem.

Your well-organized note enables other health care providers involved in the patient's care to understand the patient's health issues and the plan of therapy. Your note is also a tool for you, the clinician, to monitor your patient's health status over time. It is helpful to include contingency plans because they facilitate subsequent care (e.g., "If the chest x-ray is normal, would pursue CT scan of lungs").

If the patient is obese, it is wise to include this in the problem list to ensure that it is properly addressed at the visit because obesity has major implications for health status. Tobacco and other substance dependencies are often listed as separate problems as well.

On the inpatient service, a section labeled Disposition helps you keep track of plans necessary to help the patient transition from the hospital to home or to rehabilitation.

Finally, it is good practice to include health care maintenance on the problem list, particularly for outpatient visits. This will help you to remember to address gender- and age-appropriate care, including disease screening, immunizations, and anticipatory guidance.

Before you sign your note, read it over, check for internal consistency, and look for discordance. Are all of the issues raised in the HPI/history, exam, and data sections addressed in the Assessment and Plan? Finally, indicate that you have discussed the case with your supervising physician (indicate that doctor's name) and then sign your name and year of medical school training. Record the time and date that your note was written.

The information you gather in your patient interview does not necessarily flow to you in an organized form—HPI, then PMH, then ROS, and so on. You must take the information you have gathered from the patient and then organize it into a logical and effective document or presentation. This takes time and practice. You should take a few moments after you have completed your history and physical to gather your thoughts and develop an assessment with a differential and a plan, rather than rushing straight to the preceptor to present. It is perfectly reasonable to request some time for this from your supervisor by saying, "May I have a few minutes to organize my presentation?"

## Some Pearls for the Presentation

You will have many opportunities to present your patients on inpatient units and outpatient clinics as new and follow-up cases. Your presentations should be *concise* and *organized*. You want to engage your listeners with an interesting story. The following pearls for presentation have proved helpful for many students:

- Be concise and do not use flowery language when simpler words will do.
- Do not editorialize ("I think I heard a heart murmur."). Speak decisively.
- Always give the chief complaint!
- Always start your physical section with a report of the vital signs.
- Summarize appropriately and quantify when possible (post-op day #3 from appendectomy, day #7/10 of levofloxacin for pneumonia).
- Clearly state your assessment using opposing descriptors and include your differential and your clinical reasoning.

## Guideline for the New Patient Presentation

You will give a focused summary of all of the details of the patient's history and illness. You should include pertinent positives and negatives in the history, exam, and data sections. Generally speaking, a typical new patient should take approximately 10 minutes to present. Be sure to include your assessment with your differential diagnosis, your reasoning, and your plans for the case.

(In your introductory workshops in which you will first learn these presentation skills you may be allowed, or even encouraged for training purposes, to take longer than this "target" 10 minutes. At the point of care, however, once you are members of a functioning team, you will be expected to communicate a new patient presentation in about 10 minutes.)

## Guideline for the Follow-Up Presentation

This is a more focused presentation based on the current issues at hand. Only relevant details of the history, examination, and data may be included. Generally speaking, a follow-up patient should take approximately 5 minutes to present.

## Summary and Conclusion

Mastering the interview leads directly to the write-up and the presentation. All three provide the foundation for clinical medicine. This chapter provides an overview of how to move from the medical interview to the medical write-up and clinical presentation.

### Reference

1. Bordage G: Why did I miss the diagnosis? Some cognitive explanations and educational implications. *Acad Med* 74(10):S138–S143, 1998.

# Understanding Patients' Emotional Responses to Chronic Illness

# CHAPTER 16

# Understanding Chronic Illness: Normal Reactions

## OVERVIEW

This chapter reviews seven common stresses of chronic illness:
1. Threat to efficacy
2. Threat of separation
3. Threat of loss of love
4. Threat of loss of body function
5. Threat of loss of body parts
6. Threat of loss of rationality
7. Threat of pain

To manage these common threats and maintain psychological balance, patients with chronic illness face seven specific adaptive challenges:
1. Coping with symptoms, pain, and disability
2. Coping with treatment
3. Adapting to a variety of health care providers
4. Managing emotions
5. Relating to family members and friends
6. Preserving a positive self-image
7. Coping with the unknown

Finally, the chapter reviews common mechanisms of defense used by patients with chronic illness (regression, repression, suppression, denial), as well as common emotional reactions (anxiety, anger, sadness). Physicians who better understand these common stresses, adaptive tasks, mechanisms of defense, and emotions will be better able to help their patients weather the emotional storms and challenges of chronic illness.

With few exceptions, illness generates emotional distress. In particular, chronic illness leads to a wide variety of negative emotional reactions as patients endure the many stresses of illness and struggle to meet the adaptive challenges posed by their illness. This chapter reviews the common stresses and related adaptive tasks of chronic illness. Physicians who understand these stresses and challenges will be better able to help patients cope with the emotions that often result. Chapter 17 presents strategies to help patients who present maladaptive emotional reactions to chronic illness. Chapter 19, on the other hand, discusses communication approaches suitable for long-term relationships with your chronically ill patients over time.

## Common Stresses of Illness

Strain and Grossman[1] have described numerous stresses of illness. The list that follows represents a modification of their contributions, describing seven significant stresses:

## 1. THREAT TO EFFICACY

Patients who are sick usually become less effective in the world. Self-esteem and a sense of value in the world derive in part from what a person is able to do. Illness interferes with this ability to perform effectively at a job, at home, or in leisure activities. If patients had been working, they often must cope with the loss of a job or the threat of the loss of a job. For patients who are homemakers, illness may compromise the ability to work in the home. Sickness may make it impossible for fathers to "roughhouse" with their children or take them fishing. Mothers may be unable to function in the ways that bring them pleasure or recognition from those around them.

## 2. THREAT OF SEPARATION

Especially when the possibility of hospitalization is involved, illness can generate the fear of separation from people who are loved and who are perceived as needed for comfort and support. The enforced dependency of illness or hospitalization can reawaken early childhood separation fears.

## 3. THREAT OF LOSS OF LOVE

Many patients fear that illness will make them unattractive or unlovable to the people around them.

## 4. THREAT OF LOSS OF BODY FUNCTION

Illness often leads to urinary or fecal incontinence. This is usually embarrassing to patients and sometimes terrifying. It makes a person feel like a baby, with all the associated and complex meanings that being baby-like signifies to different individuals.

## 5. THREAT OF LOSS OF BODY PARTS

Sometimes patients are afraid (many times with good reason) that they might lose an important part of their body.

## 6. THREAT OF LOSS OF RATIONALITY

Illness often compromises mental and cognitive functioning. Patients who are ill or who take medications may become more forgetful, may have trouble concentrating, or, in general, may lose some of their previous levels of mental control. The idea of "going crazy" terrifies many patients who do not realize that this cognitive loss is commonly associated with many physical illnesses and treatments, especially for any patient hospitalized with any new illness causing a delirium.

Physicians can be quite helpful to patients by educating them with a simple statement such as the following:

> PHYSICIAN: *Many patients feel that they are losing their ability to think well when they get sick ... sometimes that they even are losing their minds. This is really very common ... and the mental confusion you may be experiencing now can be expected to clear in a few days.*

## 7. THREAT OF PAIN

In general, patients are afraid of pain and do not want to suffer.

# Adaptive Tasks of Illness

The stresses of illness described previously confront the patient with a host of challenges to which he or she must adapt. The consequences of good or poor adaptation have significant implications for the quality of life of the patient and for the type of care the physician attempts to administer. There are seven common challenges, three directly related to the illness itself (coping with the symptoms, coping with the treatment, and coping with the health care team) and four associated challenges (managing emotions, preserving relationships with family members and friends, maintaining a positive self-image, and preparing for an uncertain future).[2]

## 1. COPING WITH SYMPTOMS, PAIN, AND DISABILITY

Illnesses have diverse symptoms, many of which are uncomfortable, unpleasant, embarrassing, humiliating, evolving, disabling, or frightening. Pain is often the worst. And severe pain may be present or anticipation of severe pain may be in the future. Patients must learn to live with this pain in a way that enables them to continue functioning in as productive a manner as possible.

Illness is often associated with physical impairments that render some type of disability. Among the possible impairments are difficulty ambulating, trouble using one's hands, difficulty seeing or hearing, trouble sleeping, inability to carry out activities of daily living, and inability to drive. Adapting to the physical impairments causing the disability is a continuing and sometimes overwhelming task for patients.

## 2. COPING WITH TREATMENT

Treatment itself for many, or most, illnesses is challenging and complex, and is associated with disruptions of life schedules, side effects, and impairment to quality of life. Hospitalizations, dialysis, radiation therapy, surgeries, and so on all take a toll on individuals and their families.

## 3. ADAPTING TO A VARIETY OF HEALTH CARE PROVIDERS

Chronic illness requires patients to come into contact with a great variety of health care professionals. Patients must try to deal with many different physicians representing different specialties and with different individual temperaments as well. For example, nurses, secretaries, nutritionists, and physical therapists represent specialties and personalities to which the patient must try to adapt. This can be a manageable task for some and an impossible one for others.

## 4. MANAGING EMOTIONS

The stresses of illness lead to a variety of patients' emotional reactions that are described later in the chapter in more detail. Patients are faced with the challenge of experiencing these emotional dislocations and trying to weather them and continue with their lives. This is difficult and sometimes impossible to accomplish.

## 5. RELATING TO FAMILY MEMBERS AND FRIENDS

Because illness creates so many complicated difficulties in many patients' lives, normal social relationships often become strained. The ability to sustain relationships in spite of illness is a core task for patients, especially those with chronic illness.

Preserving family relationships can be even more difficult and important than maintaining social relationships in general. Sickness often alters relationships in the family; breadwinner and homemaker roles may switch. Patterns of intimacy, role responsibility, sexuality, and parenting can all be altered by chronic illness. A favorable outcome is usually associated with patients who are able to preserve their core relationships despite necessary alterations in social role functioning.

## 6. PRESERVING A POSITIVE SELF-IMAGE

Good outcome requires that the patient preserve a positive self-image in spite of any changes in physical appearance or functional abilities that result from the illness. This may require some changes in short- or long-term goals, changes in values, or changes in cognitive sets. Patients who have greater flexibility in thinking about one's self and one's role in life will generally fare better in comparison to those who are more rigid.

## 7. COPING WITH THE UNKNOWN

Many illnesses have an unpredictable course. Some patients may get better, some worse, and some stay about the same. Patients have to cope with this enormous uncertainty when predicting the future level of their physical impairment. Some patients do not know whether they will die from their current illness.

## "Normal" Emotional Reactions to Illness and Mechanisms of Defense

As described, most patients experience a variety of emotional reactions to illness. In general, patients often experience anxiety, anger, or sadness, each of which is discussed in the following section. From a psychological point of view, individuals use mechanisms of defense as a protection from experiencing emotions that are too strong.

The common mechanisms of defense that we all use to defend ourselves against the anxiety of illness are regression, repression, suppression, and denial. Each of these emotions and defense mechanisms is discussed briefly in the following.

### REGRESSION

Regression refers to the psychic phenomenon of reliance on more childlike stages of emotional functioning in response to illness. This universal response to illness encourages increased physical and emotional dependence during illness. For the most part, limited regression can be adaptive, to permit rest and recovery from acute illnesses or during exacerbations of chronic illness. Indeed, our health care system values this dependency to some extent because being a "good" patient is often perceived as doing what the doctor says without question.

Chronic illness demands severe limitations on this regression and dependency. Functioning in the face of chronic illness often requires considerable effort on both the physician's and patient's parts to overcome the regressive tendencies of illness. Patients respond differently to this dependency; some patients find it hard to assume and/or to relinquish dependency once it is assumed, and others find any dependency at all to be extremely threatening.

### DENIAL, SUPPRESSION, AND REPRESSION

One of the initial emotional reactions to news about an illness is the absence of an observable emotion. The consequences and emotional impact of an illness may be so great that many patients deny the news.

Denial can take many forms. When the patient simply pushes the idea of the illness out of his or her mind and manages to avoid thinking about it, this coping mechanism can actually contribute to better functioning. Technically, this is called *suppression*, which is considered a relatively healthy type of defense mechanism. The thoughts are still on the borders of consciousness, but the patient is able to divert his or her attention from the problem for short periods.

Repression refers to the unintentional movement of a thought from consciousness to unconsciousness. This can also be adaptive in some circumstances, but it can lead to negative consequences, such as forgetting to keep appointments and forgetting medicine.

Denial is potentially the most deleterious of this group of defenses, in which the information received from physicians is turned into its opposite. If a patient is told he or she has cancer, the patient who denies this information insists that the physician is wrong.

Typical problems related to denial appear in patients with coronary artery disease who insist that their chest pain symptoms are "heartburn" and not heart disease because they cannot face the implications of having a heart attack. Unfortunately, this type of denial can be life threatening when it leads to a delay in the time it takes for patients to receive treatment.

## ANXIETY

Anxiety is, of course, another common and expected part of almost all illnesses, and almost every ill patient experiences at least some degree of anxiety. For the purposes of this text, anxiety and fear are not distinguished. Anxiety refers to the subjective experience of fear, dread, and foreboding. This can take many forms and vary in intensity throughout the course of any illness. Each of the stresses and threats described previously is usually associated with some fearful reactions on the part of the patient.

Patients can experience anxiety as an internal state of fearfulness, but the anxiety can also have somatic manifestations and influence the course of the primary physical illness. For example, anxiety can cause autonomic nervous system activation such as palpitations, gastrointestinal hypermotility, sweating, and sleeplessness. When anxiety is unrelieved, it can exert a negative influence on the disease process. At times, anxiety becomes so intense and pervasive that it actually becomes an independent psychiatric condition. (This situation is reviewed in Chapter 17.)

## ANGER

Anger, too, is a common concomitant of chronic illness. Patients wonder, "Why me?" They are often angry with their God or feel spiritual uncertainty as they try to understand the ultimate meaning of the illness. This commonly leads to anxiety as well as anger.

Many patients feel a generalized anger that cannot be focused on any one particular idea or person. When this occurs, they often lash out unexpectedly and seemingly without good reason at everyone around them. Physicians and other medical providers are typical targets, as are valued friends and family. This is unfortunate because some angry patients alienate the people they most need for support during physical and emotional crises. However, when made aware of these reactions, medical providers and family can often deal with them better with fewer maladaptive consequences for the patient.

## SADNESS

Sadness is a common reaction to any illness. In fact, physicians would suspect the "normalcy" of anyone who becomes chronically ill and does not experience sadness. Chronic illness usually leads to many losses—such as loss of work function, leisure pleasures, physical pleasures, and relationships. Sadness is the most common and expected emotional reaction to loss, although other reactions such as anger and anxiety also play a role in loss.

However, sadness is not the same as persistent, clinically significant major depression. This distinction is highlighted in more detail in Chapter 17. In brief, a normal sad reaction to illness will not color every aspect of a person's relationship with those around him or her. "Normal" sadness still allows the anticipation and experience of pleasurable activities over time, even if they are more limited when compared with life before illness. Clinical depression, on the other hand, pervades every aspect of life, to the extent that the patient no longer experience any interest or pleasure in living.

## Summary

This chapter reviews seven common stresses of chronic illness:
1. Threat to efficacy
2. Threat of separation
3. Threat of loss of love
4. Threat of loss of body function
5. Threat of loss of body parts
6. Threat of loss of rationality
7. Threat of pain

To manage these common threats and maintain psychological balance, patients with chronic illness face seven specific adaptive challenges:
1. Coping with symptoms, pain, and disability
2. Coping with treatment
3. Adapting to a variety of health care providers
4. Managing emotions
5. Relating to family members and friends
6. Preserving a positive self-image
7. Coping with the unknown

Finally, the chapter reviews common mechanisms of defense used by patients with chronic illness (regression, repression, suppression, denial), as well as common emotional reactions (anxiety, anger, sadness). Physicians who better understand these common stresses, adaptive tasks, mechanisms of defense, and emotions will be better able to help their patients weather the emotional storms and challenges of chronic illness.

## References

1. Strain JJ, Grossman S: Psychological reactions to medical illness and hospitalization. In Strain JJ, Grossman S, editors: *Psychological care of the medically ill: a primer in liaison psychiatry*, New York, 1975, Appleton.
2. Moos RH, Holahan CJ: Adaptive tasks and methods of coping with illness and disability, In Martz E, Liveneh H, editors: *Coping with chronic illness and disability*, Memphis, 2007, Springer.

# CHAPTER 17

# Understanding Chronic Illness: Maladaptive Reactions

## OVERVIEW

This chapter discusses three prototypical maladaptive emotional reactions to chronic illness:
1. Persistent anger
2. Depression
3. Persistent anxiety
Communication strategies are suggested for each.

The various emotional responses to illness that were discussed in Chapter 16 should be considered "normal" in the sense that most individuals facing chronic or serious illness experience them to some degree. Sometimes these emotions, by themselves (i.e., independent of the illness that caused them) do not disrupt a patient's quality of life. On the other hand, for some patients these emotional responses can start interfering with functioning, independent of the physical illnesses that may have precipitated their initial expression. In such cases these reactions can be considered maladaptive.

In general, the concept of maladaptive responses to illness is more useful to patients and physicians than is the concept of "abnormality." The idea of an abnormal emotional reaction conveys such a pejorative tone that physicians and patients shrink from accepting such a label. This text therefore urges the use of functional terms such as "adaptive" and "maladaptive" to describe emotional reactions to illness.

Emotions can be considered maladaptive when they interfere with a patient's quality of life or overall functioning. There are many types of maladaptive emotional responses, and sometimes these take the form of mixed emotional reactions. This chapter focuses on three basic types of responses that can develop into relatively fixed patterns of maladaptive emotional response sets: anger, depression, and anxiety.

## Persistent Anger

As was discussed in the previous chapter, most patients with a chronic illness become angry at some point in the coping process. Patients often ask bitterly, "Why me? What did I do to deserve this sickness?" The anger can take the form of lashing out at family members, at physicians, or at anyone who happens to be around. It is often helpful for physicians to remember that this inappropriate anger, at times directed at them, may be a displacement of the anger that the patient feels about the illness itself.

Anger can become seriously maladaptive when it is so persistent and offensive that the patient alienates the people he or she most needs for physical and emotional support. The patient can be so unpleasant that nurses and physicians stay away. This can lead to more angry demands for attention and to further isolation. Thus the angry response may lead to a self-defeating circle of angry demands and withdrawal of staff. It is worth noting that this anger often functions to mask underlying fear.

The angry patient often alienates friends and family. For example, when receiving visitors, an angry patient may demand to know why they came and may insinuate ulterior motives rather than graciously accepting whatever sympathy and concern the visitors may sincerely feel and offer. Such attitudes can lead to even more isolation and loneliness than the physical illness itself might cause. In addition, this apparent social rejection may feed an already low sense of self-esteem.

## Adjustment Disorder with Depressed Mood and Major Depression

Most serious or chronic illnesses also lead to sadness. This is certainly an expected response. However, some patients develop persistent despondent feelings that interfere with their ability to work, to function in social roles, or to relate to the important people in their lives. When sadness becomes this severe, current psychiatric nomenclature would probably describe this sadness as meeting the first diagnostic criterion either for an adjustment disorder with depressed mood or for a major depression ("persistent sadness").[1]

An adjustment disorder with depressed mood is defined as an emotional response (i.e., a sad response) to a stressful life event that is stronger and more persistent than would be expected in most individuals. Major depression, on the other hand, describes a particular set of syndromal signs and symptoms that include at least 2 weeks of persistent sadness or anhedonia (pervasive loss of interest or pleasure). A characteristic set of physical signs (poor sleep, loss of appetite, fatigue, and psychomotor agitation or retardation) and psychologic symptoms (poor concentration, low self-esteem or guilt, and hopelessness) constitutes the syndrome of major depression. In general, major depression is best conceptualized as a psychobiologic illness. It tends to occur in genetically predisposed individuals and may also develop in response to significant life stressors.[2] Depending on the individual and the biologic substrate, these stressors may be extraordinarily potent or in some cases may be rather minor. In fact, with sufficient biologic loading, major depression may appear in the absence of any discernible stressor.

Some physicians and patients tend to explain away a major depression by saying things like, "Anyone with this condition would be depressed." Although this statement might be true in the sense that anyone with the condition would be sad, it is not true that everyone with a serious illness develops major depression. Studies of terminally ill cancer patients, for example, as well as studies of patients with other serious illnesses, indicate that fewer than half of such patients demonstrate the signs and symptoms of major depression.[2]

Patients who develop major depression in the context of a significant and chronic physical illness develop levels of functional impairment that far exceed the impairment expected from the physical illness itself. Relationships are damaged, the ability to function is impaired, and the overall quality of life is grossly damaged. This maladaptive response to illness is important to recognize because in many instances it can be effectively treated. Therefore, major depression occurring in the context of a physical illness should always be considered a "dread complication" of the illness that needs immediate and aggressive treatment rather than an expected reaction that warrants no special treatment in and of itself. (Ned Cassem, verbal communication, circa 1995).

# Adjustment Disorder with Anxious Mood/Anxiety Disorders

Anxiety represents the third type of maladaptive response to illness discussed in this chapter. As pointed out in Chapter 16, most patients with a new or significant illness will also experience and manifest some degree of anxiety. Patients usually feel anxious about the meaning of the illness in their lives and about how the illness will affect their lives as it unfolds. This is universal.

Persistent anxiety, on the other hand, can be disabling, interfere with the coping process, and in fact, impair physical recovery. Patients with this type of persistent anxiety cannot separate themselves from their fears. They cling to doctors, friends, and family with repetitive, sometimes superficial questions that seem to spring from a deep thirst that cannot be sated. Such "questions" cannot be "answered" because the questions may mask deeper real fears that remain tacit and unexpressed. Alternatively, anxious patients at times present unrealistic, seemingly preposterous demands for attention or care. Many anxious patients also suffer from autonomic system arousal with tachycardia, sweating, diarrhea, cramps, shortness of breath, hyperventilation, and trouble sleeping—all of which can become independent problems themselves. When patients suffer from persistent anxiety in the face of chronic illness, physicians should recognize this anxious state and manage it thoughtfully and directly. Persistent anxiety that is co-morbid with chronic general medical illness may meet criteria for psychiatric disorders such as adjustment disorder with anxious mood, panic disorder, or generalized anxiety disorder.[1]

An adjustment disorder with anxious mood is nosologically similar to an adjustment disorder with depressed mood. The name of this condition refers to a situation in which the patient reacts to a stressor with an emotional reaction that exceeds what might be expected in most individuals. On the other hand, panic disorder is a severe psychiatric condition marked by unpredictable attacks of sudden panic that are often characterized by a sense of impending doom, hyperventilation, chest pain, sweating, and other signs of autonomic activation. Panic attacks are often associated with agoraphobia (a fear of going outside).

A generalized anxiety disorder, on the other hand, is a severe anxiety disorder marked by 6 months or more of significant anxiety symptoms, including autonomic arousal (e.g., hyperventilation and palpitations) and fearful behavior toward the environment (e.g., vigilance and scanning).

# Interviewing Strategies for Patients with Maladaptive Emotional Responses

In general, communicating effectively with patients who demonstrate maladaptive emotional responses requires skills that are more advanced than the ones described so far in this text. Despite the need for more advanced skills, the interventions presented in Chapter 3 provide a solid foundation for responding to patients with intense emotional, or maladaptive, reactions to illness, that is, patients who are persistently angry, depressed, or anxious. Some principles and examples are presented below (see Chapter 18 for further discussion of advanced emotional response skills, some of which may also be useful to the kinds of reactions discussed in this chapter).

## PERSISTENTLY ANGRY PATIENTS

Most angry patients will respond to reflection and legitimation, as discussed in Chapter 3. Consider the following case:

> Mr. Bailes is a 56-year-old construction worker in the intensive care unit with arrhythmias after an acute myocardial infarction. He is enraged because the nurses will not allow him

to get out of bed to use the bedside commode. His anger seems to be leading to autonomic arousal, which itself can exacerbate potentially dangerous, lethal arrhythmias.

The physician might try to initiate a dialogue with a statement along the lines of the following:

PHYSICIAN: *Mr. Bailes, I can see that you're pretty upset.* (reflection)

PATIENT: *You bet I am! Wouldn't you be upset too if they wouldn't let you out of bed to take a crap? I don't mind pissing into a jug, but this bedpan thing is just too much. The toilet is 10 feet from my bed ... but they won't even let me out to use it!*

PHYSICIAN: *I see this is really making you miserable* (reflection) ... *I understand. I would probably feel frustrated too.* (legitimation) *Can you say some more about what's been going on?* (exploration)

By expressing empathy through reflecting and legitimating the patient's feelings, followed by a request for further exploration (see "Empathic Communication to Deepen Understanding [ECDU]" in Chapter 3), the physician can rebuild or establish a new therapeutic alliance. The patient can express frustration and the physician can listen and hear the story from the patient's point of view. Expressed empathy and shared understanding will help the patient calm down.

With improved rapport, a physician and an angry patient will usually be able to negotiate a solution that facilitates better outcomes. Sometimes a negotiated solution may, of necessity, include some concessions by the health care team to achieve an adequate level of patient cooperation. The intensive care unit patient discussed above felt so humiliated by enforced dependency on a bedpan that the staff decided to let him use a bedside commode (vs. walking all the way to the bathroom). This was clearly the best "biopsychosocial" solution, even though it may not have been the most desirable solution from an immediate and narrow physiologic point of view.

## PATIENTS WHO HAVE AN ADJUSTMENT DISORDER WITH DEPRESSED MOOD OR MAJOR DEPRESSION

The sad or depressed patient can also be approached by starting with reflection and legitimation.

Mr. Gaines is a 62-year-old businessman with worsening chronic obstructive pulmonary disease and feels despondent about returning to work. When asked about the impact of the illness on his life, he weeps.

The physician might say something like this:

PHYSICIAN: *I see you feel overwhelmed.* (reflection)

PATIENT: *I'm just so upset, I don't know what to do. I can't sleep and I don't have any appetite. Nothing seems important.* (patient begins to cry)

PHYSICIAN: (attentive silence)

PATIENT: *I think I'm going to have to give up my business.* (patient continues to cry)

PHYSICIAN: *That sounds like it's going to be very hard* (reflection) ... *I can understand* (legitimation). *I want to assure you that I'm going to stand by you through this.* (personal support). *There's a lot we do to help you get physically stronger and feel better and there's also a lot we can do to help you with those sad and depressed feelings you're having.* (support)

Expressed empathy and support from a physician clearly helps many patients with persistent depressed moods. On the other hand, some patients' depressive state remains refractory to these interventions and more formal psychotherapy, antidepressant medication, or psychiatric consultation may be needed to achieve relief.

## PATIENTS WHO HAVE AN ADJUSTMENT DISORDER WITH ANXIOUS MOOD OR AN ANXIETY DISORDER

The following patient suffered from persistent, or maladaptive, anxiety:

> Ms. James is a 21-year-old married female with a congenital liver problem who needs a liver transplant. She has always been anxious, but now her anxiety has become disabling. In fact, she is so afraid of the surgery that she may not be able to undergo the operation.

The physician may pursue the interview in the following way:

PHYSICIAN: *I'd like to know more about how you've been feeling lately.*

PATIENT: *Doctor, I'm just so scared about the surgery. My palms are sweaty, I can't sleep, and I've got butterflies in my stomach all the time.*

PHYSICIAN: *I see you're very anxious.* (reflection) *First of all, I hope you realize that anxiety is understandable and common in these circumstances.* (legitimation) *Can tell me some more about your specific worries?* (exploration) (See "Empathic Communication to Deepen Understanding [ECDU]" in Chapter 3)

PATIENT: *I'm worried about what the operation will be like. I don't know who will take care of my kids. I'm afraid I won't do well after the surgery. And I've been getting more panic attacks. I thought they were gone ... but now they're back.*

PHYSICIAN: *Okay. Thank you. Now I understand your concerns a little better. We (that is, the whole medical team) can help you understand more about the details of the surgery and help you make specific plans for your recovery. More specifically, we can also help you think through how to best take care of your kids during your recovery.* (support) *By the way, I should also tell you that I'm impressed with your thoughtfulness and concern to plan ahead so constructively and in such detail.* (respect, affirmation)

Targeted use of reflection, legitimation, exploration, support, and respect (affirmation) can all help reassure patients with persistent (maladaptive) anxiety. Some patients, however, may need more extensive interventions, for example, by clinicians with advanced communication skills to provide appropriate therapeutic support, psychotherapy, or appropriate antianxiety medication. Psychiatric referral may also be indicated.

## Summary

This chapter discusses three prototypical maladaptive emotional reactions to chronic illness:
1. Persistent anger
2. Depression
3. Persistent anxiety
Communication strategies are suggested for each.

### References

1. American Psychiatric Association: *Diagnostic and statistical manual of mental disorders, V*, Washington, D.C., 2013, American Psychiatric Association Press.
2. Belmaker RH, Agam G: Major depressive disorder. *N Engl J Med* 358:55–68, 2008.

# Advanced Applications

# CHAPTER 18

# Stepped-Care Advanced Skills for Action Planning

Steven Cole ■ Damara Gutnick ■ Joseph Weiner

## OVERVIEW

Stepped-care advanced skills for action planning (SAAP) focus on eliciting, recognizing, and responding to change talk by:
1. Responding to discord or distress
2. Understanding personal benefits or obstacles to change
3. Using higher-order Motivational Interviewing (MI) skills

Stepped-care advanced skills for action planning (SAAP) involve the application of 13 specific advanced skills to elicit, recognize, and respond to change talk. As the amount and strength of change talk increases, the clinician gains confidence that the patient will become more likely to respond positively to Question One of Brief Action Planning (BAP). Use of SAAP requires thorough working knowledge and clinical mastery of the eight core competencies of BAP (see Chapter 5).

Because of the complexity of the skills themselves as well as their stepped-care application, this chapter is divided into seven sections to facilitate presentation, understanding, and mastery.
A. Why Are Advanced Skills Necessary?
B. Overview: The SAAP Model
C. What Is Change Talk? Why Is It Important?
D. SAAP and Change Talk: How Elicitation, Recognition, and Response to Change Talk Drive the Model
E. Skills and Case Study of SAAP Step One: Responding to Discord or Distress
F. Skills and Case Studies of SAAP Step Two: Understanding Benefits or Obstacles to Change
G. Skills and Case Study of SAAP Step Three: Using Higher-Order Motivational Interviewing Skills

## A: Why Are Advanced Skill Necessary?

Brief Action Planning (BAP), a straightforward set of eight Function Three skills described in Chapter 5, provides the foundation for collaborative management, allowing clinicians to help patients set and accomplish their own personal health goals. In general, about 50% of all medical patients can make at least some concrete action plans for health in 5- to 10-minute interactions; and patients follow through (at least partially) on these action plans about 70% to 80% of the time.[1,2]

Other patients, however, may be unwilling or unable to make brief action plans or follow through successfully. This chapter presents a three-step model of 13 advanced skills, which clinicians can use to help motivate such patients to move forward with realistic action planning for health.

Expressed in another way, this chapter focuses on what clinicians can do to help motivate patients who are not willing or not able to respond positively to Question One of BAP:

*Is there anything you would like to do for your health in the next week or two?*

Consider the following clinical examples:

Ms. Johnson, a 54-year-old obese woman with type II diabetes, binge eats and drinks five glasses of wine three to four days each week. At the end of your initial meeting, you educate her about the unhealthy impact of binge eating and problem drinking. You ask her to repeat her understanding of this information and she summarizes it very well. You then ask her:

*Is there anything you would like to do for your health in the next week or two?*

Her response is:

*No. I'm fine just the way I am.*

Mr. Gilson, a 70-year-old man with coronary heart disease, hypertension, peripheral vascular disease, and type II diabetes takes more than 20 medications each day. He does not adhere to this complex regimen in a reliable and consistent manner. You ask:

*Is there anything you would like to do for your health in the next week or two?*

His response is:

*You bet there is! Pills, pills, pills. So many pills! I'm sick of them. I hate them. I'd like to flush all these pills down the toilet! That's what I'd like to do for my health!*

How do physicians tend to respond to patients like Ms. Johnson and Mr. Gibson and what happens to the physician-patient-family relationship as a result of these reactions? The following are common reactions and outcomes.

- Some physicians simply give up, thinking, "Okay, I'll just back off. If he wants to kill himself by not taking his medication, that's his business."
- Patients may mislead physicians or leave treatment. One of the authors' patients told her rheumatologist that she was taking her anti-inflammatory medication for years, when she actually was not. This led to the patient's apparent failure to respond to "prescribed" medications and the subsequent prescription of additional, unnecessarily complex medication regimens. Another patient left treatment with a physician because he kept pressuring her to change, clearly not accepting her right to lead her life as she chose. (See Chapter 5 on the "spirit of MI" and respecting the patient's autonomous decision to change or not to change.)
- Loved ones may become frustrated with the patient. A patient who becomes "stuck" with persistently unhealthy behaviors often introduces enormous stress into family relationships. The deleterious impact of alcoholism or other substance abuse upon a family represents just one example; but other or less obvious situations, such as nonadherence with a healthy diet, can also lead to intense conflict between spouses or within an extended family. One of the authors is treating a patient who is contemplating divorce because her husband cannot control his eating.
- The clinician may resort to lecturing the patient about why he or she needs to change persistent unhealthy behaviors.[3] Smoking cessation, exercise, and weight reduction are common topics for such physician-driven lectures. How useful are these lectures? In fact, most patients with persistent unhealthy behaviors already understand what they need to do, so clinician pressure typically leads to shame and humiliation and, ultimately,

resentment, all of which increase patient reluctance to change. Such discord between patient and physician threatens their relationship, thus rendering further attempts at collaborative action planning worthless until a working alliance can be established or restored.

Because of these complexities, the clinician's use of the eight core competencies of BAP may prove insufficient to help motivate patients like Ms. Johnson and Mr. Gilson to move forward with meaningful action planning for health. Therefore, those clinicians who would like to help patients with persistent unhealthy behaviors will generally need to use more advanced, more robust and powerful skills to support action planning for change. The SAAP model presents advanced skills which can help motivate such patients towards meaningful action planning for health.

## B. Overview: The SAAP Model

This chapter introduces a three-tiered step-care communication model that conceptualizes increasing levels of challenge and complexity that clinicians (and their patients) encounter when addressing behavioral change for persistent unhealthy behavior. If the patient does not develop an action plan with the application of skills from the first step, then skills from the second step can be used. If Step Two skills do not prove sufficient, then skills from Step Three can be recruited. Brief summaries of the three steps follow. Later sections in the chapter discusses each of the steps in more detail.

### STEP ONE: RESPOND TO DISTRESS OR DISCORD TO MEET RELATIONAL CHALLENGES

*Relational challenges* manifest themselves when Function One (Chapter 3) skills have not been adequately used, either to address the emotional suffering inherent in difficult behavioral change or to repair a disruption in the patient-physician relationship. Therefore, to implement Step One of SAAP, this chapter discusses the adaptation of previously described Function One skills to situations of increasingly complex distress or discord. Once the relationship has been repaired and rapport established/reestablished or patient distress has been soothed, the patient often can feel freer emotionally to take on the challenge of behavior change.

### STEP TWO: UNDERSTAND BENEFITS OR OBSTACLES TO CHANGE TO MEET EXPLORATORY CHALLENGES

*Exploratory challenges* can be addressed, in Step Two, when and if relational challenges have been met and patients still remain unable or unwilling to engage in action planning. Physicians can adapt previously described Function Two skills for assessment/understanding (Chapter 4) to help patients explore personal benefits of change, or conversely, to better understand underlying reasons for the persistence of maladaptive behaviors. Such exploration increases self-awareness, facilitating action planning for change.

### STEP THREE: USE HIGHER-ORDER MOTIVATIONAL INTERVIEWING SKILLS TO MEET COMPLEX MOTIVATIONAL CHALLENGES

*Motivational challenges* are often marked by complex and/or deep ambivalence about change. Such challenges can be addressed if use of Step One and Step Two skills has not led to adaptive action planning for health. This chapter describes two higher-order motivational interviewing[4] skills to address these challenges in the service of action planning: (1) elicit and resolve ambivalence about

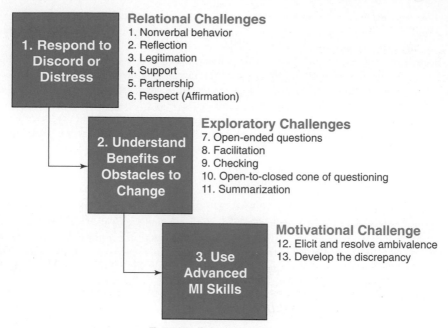

**Figure 18.1** The three-tiered model.

a persistent unhealthy behavior; and (2) develop potential discrepancies between the patient's current health behaviors and longer-term life goals.

This three-tiered model presents a highly structured and logically progressive approach to the use of advanced skills for action planning. Figure 18.1 illustrates these three steps, along with the skills associated with each step.

Students and practicing clinicians should realize, of course, that there will always be some patients with very persistent unhealthy behaviors who will not be able to generate meaningful action plans in a single or even multiple encounters regardless of how skillfully the advanced skills have been used. Such patients should not be pressured into making action plans before they are ready, because such pressure becomes counterproductive, leading to discord and sustained reluctance to change. Patients with refractory behaviors may need several visits to discuss these behaviors before they are ready for action planning; they may need or want referral to behavioral specialists; or they simply may never decide to change, regardless of whom they talk with and whatever skills are used.[A]

## C. What Is Change Talk? Why Is It Important?

Miller and Rollnick define change talk as "any client speech that favors movement toward a particular change goal." Numerous studies document a relationship between patient change talk and subsequent patient behavior change. That is, increased change talk predicts increased likelihood of positive behavior change. Furthermore, clinicians can systematically and strategically increase patient change talk by using skills described in this text (or others described in the Motivational Interviewing literature).[4]

Change talk has two broad components: (1) preparatory or (2) mobilizing; each has its own subtypes of change talk. The acronym DARN CATs (Desire, Ability, Reason, Need, Commitment, Activation, and Taking Steps about change) captures these concepts and subtypes. Using the example of weight loss, Table 18.1 illustrates these various forms of change talk.

TABLE 18.1 ■ Change Talk

| **Preparatory Change Talk (DARN)** | |
| --- | --- |
| Desire: | *"I'd really like to lose some weight."* |
| Ability: | *"I think I really could lose weight if I put my mind to it."* |
| Reasons: | *"I know it's important for me to lose weight or I'll need to go on insulin soon."* |
| Need: | *"I really need to lose weight for my family. I owe it to them."* |
| ***Mobilizing Change Talk (CATS)*** | |
| Commitment: | *"I've made up my mind to join Weight Watchers."* |
| Activation: | *"I'm going to go online and look for meetings I can go to."* |
| Taking Steps: | *"I found a meeting I'll go to next Saturday night."* |

When BAP doesn't lead to concrete action plans for health, clinicians using SAAP start listening for change talk in each statement made by the patient about the problem at hand, asking themselves, for example: *"Is there change talk here? Did the patient's response to my intervention (i.e., advanced skill) demonstrate any change talk?"*

The clinician's focus on action planning can effectively respond to any change talk that emerges in a manner that promotes and further strengthens it. As change talk increases and strengthens, the physician can make decisions about the most opportune moment to rechallenge the patient with Question One of BAP. In many patient-care circumstances, the introduction of advanced skills elicits change talk quickly; and once it emerges, patients are more likely to respond adaptively to Question One.

# D. SAAP and Change Talk: How Elicitation, Recognition, and Response to Change Talk Drive the Model

As discussed, the stepped-care approach to action planning suggests a natural hierarchy to the use of advanced skills. This hierarchy should be considered a rough roadmap or guide pointing the way to efficient and effective care in most situations, although clinical judgment at the point of care may indicate a different direction for special or unusual presentations. *Clinical judgment always take precedence over any roadmap.*

This section of the chapter discusses how elicitation, recognition, and response to change talk drive the implementation of each unique step of the model as well as progression through consecutive steps.

## 1. RESPOND TO DISTRESS OR DISCORD TO MEET RELATIONAL CHALLENGES (ADVANCED APPLICATION OF FUNCTION ONE SKILLS)

As pointed out, the first set of advanced skills to use involves those that rely on ensuring that the working alliance is still working. No meaningful collaborative action planning can occur if the working alliance between the clinician and patient is broken or if patient distress exists. The clinician must think, "Is mutual respect, rapport, and trust present?" "Is the patient feeling upset, sad, frustrated, or demoralized?" If this is the case, advanced skills can be used to help clinicians reengage the patient or address patient distress before proceeding with further action planning for health.

If the clinician begins to address discord or distress, especially as it relates to problem behavior(s), patients often begin to make statements about willingness to change their behavior

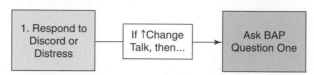

**Figure 18.2** The sequence of Step One leading to change talk.

(i.e., "change talk"). When this change talk is then recognized and cultivated as part of the process of the response to discord or distress, the clinician can then return to Question One of BAP soon after emotional equilibrium has returned. Figure 18.2 demonstrates the sequence of Step One leading to change talk that then, in turn, makes it possible for the clinician to rechallenge the patient with Question One.

Section E presents the skills and an extended case study illustrating the clinical implementation of Step One.

## 2. UNDERSTAND BENEFITS OR OBSTACLES TO CHANGE TO MEET EXPLORATORY CHALLENGES (ADVANCED APPLICATION OF FUNCTION TWO SKILLS)

The second step of advanced skills becomes important at any point when it is clear that engagement and emotional equilibrium are present and yet the patient is *still* not able or willing to enter into action planning for health. At that point, the model suggests using skills of assessment and exploration (Function Two, Chapter 4) to understand the patient's perception of personal benefits or obstacles to change.

With respect to understanding benefits, the physician might ask the patient a question like,

> *How might your life be different if you were able to change ... (the behavior under consideration)?*

Patients often respond to this question with remarkably strong change talk, which can lead rather quickly to an effective return to Question One.

If the exploration of personal benefits of change does not lead to sufficient change talk to move forward with action planning, it is at this point that SAAP suggests that clinicians look more deeply into the narrative history of the maladaptive behavior itself, seeking to understand the meaning of the behavior in the patient's life and the specific obstacles to change. As the patient recounts the history of the unhealthy behavior (to an empathic, supportive listener), it is likely that substantial change talk will emerge, which the clinician can continue to cultivate until such time as it becomes appropriate to "test the waters" again with Question One of BAP.

Figure 18.3 illustrates how the clinician might proceed through Step One, then Step Two, and back to Question One of BAP.

Section F presents the skills and extended case studies illustrating the clinical implementation of understanding benefits or obstacles to change in Step Two.

## 3. USE OF HIGHER-ORDER MOTIVATIONAL INTERVIEWING SKILLS TO MEET COMPLEX MOTIVATIONAL CHALLENGES (ADVANCED APPLICATION OF FUNCTION THREE SKILLS)

Finally, the last step of the advanced skills for action planning becomes important only when skills for responding to discord or distress and understanding personal benefits or obstacles to change do not lead to adaptive action planning for health. Complex and deep ambivalence to change present motivational challenges that block action planning and behavioral change

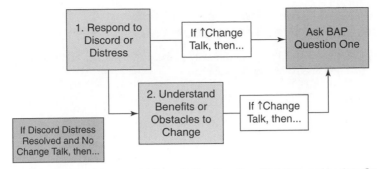

**Figure 18.3** How the clinician might proceed through Step One, then Step Two, and back to Question One of BAP.

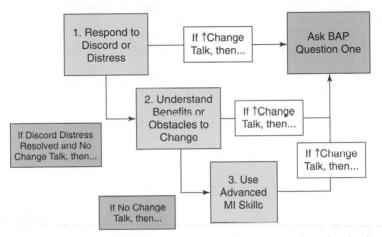

**Figure 18.4** The complete stepped-care approach to advanced skills for action planning.

at this point. Clinicians' use of two higher-order, very powerful competencies from the field of motivational interviewing (MI)—eliciting and resolving ambivalence and developing the discrepancy—can help patients move forward with action planning for health.

Ambivalence about change rests at the core of many patients' difficulties in making change. Motivational interviewing recognizes the central role that ambivalence plays in blocking behavior change and has developed methods to help clinicians elicit and resolve ambivalence. Change talk emerges as ambivalence is explored, thus providing opportunities for promotion of more change talk and, ultimately, to action planning for health.

The most complex skill addressed in this text revolves around "developing the discrepancy." Motivational interviewing suggests that patients with persistent unhealthy behaviors often maintain their maladaptive behaviors in the face of beliefs and values that would otherwise be inconsistent with these behaviors. By highlighting the contrast between these beliefs and values and the patient's current behavior, clinicians can elicit and cultivate change talk that can lead, ultimately, to action planning for health.

Figure 18.4 illustrates the complete stepped-care approach to advanced skills for action planning, demonstrating the key roles that elicitation, recognition, and response to change talk play at each step.

Section G presents the skills and an extended case study illustrating the clinical implementation of these two higher-order MI skills in Step Three.

## E. Skills and Case Study of SAAP Step One: Responding to Discord or Distress

Chapter 3 presented six basic Function One skills to assist physicians in building the relationship/ responding to emotions. To review, the skills are:

- Nonverbal behavior
- Reflection
- Legitimation
- Support
- Partnership and
- Respect (affirmation)

All of these skills are basic in the sense that they can be readily described, demonstrated, practiced by trainees, and learned (given sufficient coaching and feedback).

Of particular interest for this chapter on advanced skills, however, is the understanding that an enriched application of these core skills provides the foundation for subtler, more finely tuned approaches to empathic communication. Many situations in general medical settings arise in which these advanced skills for reengagement or responding to distress become essential, especially when discord emerges, threatening a working alliance. Sometimes, as tension emerges, the patient may get labeled and blamed as a "difficult" patient, rather than viewing the relationship, itself, as disrupted. What needs repair at that point is the relationship, not the patient. And the skills needed are relationship skills.

This section of the chapter describes and illustrates how basic relationship skills can be adapted to complex clinical situations through an actual case example from Dr. Cole's practice.[B] Specific skills are identified in parentheses. Comments on the use of particular skills are also in parentheses. Three specific types of "complex" reflections (see Chapter 3) are introduced by example in this dialogue and then defined. The three types of complex reflections include: reflection with a twist, double-sided reflection, and amplified negative reflection.

> Mr. V. is a heavy cigarette smoker with diabetes, heart disease, high blood pressure, depression, and grief over loss of a child several years ago. Toward the end of a recent check-up, at a point in the meeting of good rapport and engagement, the physician asks Question One of Brief Action Planning (BAP):

> *I wonder if there is anything you might like to do for your health in the next week or two?*

> **PATIENT:** *Are you kidding!* (very angry) *Why don't you just ask my wife and kids ... they'll tell you what I need to do ... they told me I HAVE to stop smoking.* (pause) *... I know I have to stop.* (quiet and thoughtful) *But do you hear me? THEY told ME that I have to stop smoking.* (loud again) *Can you believe that? I mean since when do kids tell parents what they're going to do! Well, no one's going to boss ME around. No way, no how.* (still angry)

> **PHYSICIAN:** (pauses and nods his head) (attentive silence is facilitative)

> **PATIENT:** *What I'm trying to tell you is that I'm in charge of my own home. No one told my father what he was going to do, and no one is going to tell me what to do! Not them and not you!* (challenges physician)

> **PHYSICIAN:** *Well, I can see that this makes you angry.* (simple reflection)

> **PATIENT:** *You bet it does. I know I have to stop smoking,* (calms down a little) *and I know they're only trying to help me, but I'm going to do it my own way and when I'm good and ready.*

> **PHYSICIAN:** *Okay. When your wife and kids tell you what to do, even if it's really just about your health, you somehow feel like you're not the head of the family anymore, even though deep down you know it's really because they care.* (complex reflection)

PATIENT: *That's right.*

PHYSICIAN: *Okay. I think I understand why you're feeling this way. It sounds like you know you need to stop smoking and I heard you say that you're going to do that. You just don't want someone else to tell you what to do and when. Especially not your wife and kids. And when they do tell you what to do, it makes you angry, and it makes you feel like you're really not in charge anymore. So I certainly understand why that would bother you. You just want to be the one who decides what you're going to do and when you're going to do it.* (reflection, legitimation, empathy; reflection with a twist)

PATIENT: *You got it doc, you got it.*

PHYSICIAN: (silence)

In this dialogue so far, the clinician introduced Question One of BAP, as recommended, at a point in the interview when there was reasonably good clinician-patient engagement and rapport. Unfortunately, the question itself unleashed a firestorm of anger toward the family (and potentially toward the doctor) because they have been pressuring him to stop smoking before he is ready. Because his smoking is such a high-risk behavior in a diabetic with heart disease, it would not be hard for the clinician to fall into the trap of joining the family with a "righting reflex" by trying to force the patient into a more adaptive or healthy lifestyle through forceful persuasion or coercion. Unfortunately, these approaches are rarely successful in patients with persistent unhealthy behaviors and often generate more discord, which happened here.

It is worth noting how, in this complex situation, the use of enriched basic skills facilitated better outcomes. The clinician's initial response to the patient's anger was *silence*. This silence is a very powerful nonverbal signal of acceptance and allows the patient to continue talking and express himself further. Rather than trying to cut off the dialogue or redirect it, silence gives the patient permission to keep talking and sends the message that the clinician is willing to keep listening. As the patient keeps talking, the patient often provides further information, which is very useful clinically. It is also hard to stay angry very long at someone who is willing to listen without defensiveness. So, *attentive silence* also serves the function of diffusion of anger.

As the patient continues talking for another sentence or two, we learn that he comes from a family with an autocratic father who ran the household with an unchallenged iron hand and that when his wife or children challenge him, he feels his authority is undermined. When the clinician makes a simple, empathic reflection ("you feel angry"), the patient is relieved that someone understands, and accepts, him and he calms down.

Of even greater interest, his defensiveness about smoking cessation dissolves momentarily and he admits, as if in a passing thought, "I know I need to stop smoking." Here we have spontaneous change talk, emerging as the working alliance is reestablished. The physician picked up on the patient's change talk as he ended his summary with a statement about the patient wanting to stop but not knowing exactly when he was going to do it. This has been called "reflection with a twist" because the physician reflected the feeling of the patient but added something that was not entirely present, though implied, in the patient's presentation about not knowing when he was planning to stop.[4]

PATIENT: *It's just so hard.* (mood changes) *I just don't know how I'm going to do it.*

PHYSICIAN: *It is hard. But it sounds like this is something that you do want to do.*

PATIENT: *I do want to stop. But I don't know … I don't know. Maybe this just isn't the time.*

PHYSICIAN: *Okay. I hear you. It sounds like you're just not going to stop smoking now … this isn't the time … you're just not ready to try anything at all right now.* (complex reflection, amplified negative reflection)

PATIENT: *Well, I'm not ready to just stop cold turkey; but I didn't say I wasn't ready to try anything at all. Maybe I can start to cut down a little. What do you think?*

**PHYSICIAN:** *I think this really is your decision. If you decide you're going to keep smoking, I will support your right to do that ... but if you decide you want to start cutting down a little, I'm here to help you with that.* **(partnership, spirit of MI: acceptance—support for autonomy)**

**PATIENT:** *Really! You're behind me even if I decide to keep smoking?*

**PHYSICIAN:** *Absolutely. I care about you* **(support—statement of caring)** *and your health, so, of course, I would like to see you cut down or stop, but if you decide to keep smoking, I really think that is your decision and I will back you up on that.* **(acceptance—support for autonomy)**

**PATIENT:** *You know, I do think I could start thinking about how to cut down. What should I do?*

**PHYSICIAN:** *It takes a lot of strength and determination to make any change at all in a habit as strong as smoking, especially for someone like you who has smoked so long and has a family who's gotten him irritated by making demands. So you have a lot of courage to even start thinking about how you might want to start cutting back.* **(affirmation)**

*This is the kind of thing you and I can work on together,* **(partnership)** *but it occurs to me that you're the kind of person who has probably already given this a lot of thought already* **(affirmation),** *which is a good thing. I wonder if you'd share some of the ideas you've had about what you might start doing to help you cut down. Then we can talk about them and I can share any other ideas that I might have.* **(partnership)**

In this short dialogue, the physician continues to use enriched adaptations of all six basic relationship-building skills in this complex clinical situation of persistent unhealthy behavior. As already noted, he used the nonverbal skill of *attentive silence* very effectively. Attentive silence is always facilitative; that is, silence encourages the patient to keep talking. In situations of high emotional intensity, however, attentive silence may be one of the most powerful and nonintrusive facilitation techniques available. Deliberate use of *attentive silence* often helps diffuse intense emotions more effectively than selected verbal exchanges might accomplish. In the preceding example, two instances of attentive silence facilitated communication and helped to diffuse angry feelings.

Reflection of patient feelings facilitates empathic communication, which builds understanding and trust between the patient and physician. In the preceding example, the physician reflected his awareness that the patient was angry *(simple reflection)* and also used *complex reflections* to communicate his emotional understanding that the patient was unhappy about the symbolic loss of power in the family (see Chapter 3). Use of complex reflections to enhance empathic communication deepens the relationship and builds trust. With a better working alliance built on deeper empathic understanding, patients are more likely to be ready to make action plans for health or, in general, work in partnership with physicians toward more adaptive health behaviors.

The dialogue also includes another higher-order skill, a special type of complex reflection called an "amplified negative reflection." Note that as soon as the physician suggested that the patient seemed "ready" to make some changes in smoking behavior (after the patient had said he "knows" he needs to stop smoking), the patient backtracked and expressed ambivalence about being ready for change. This ambivalent dance commonly marks situations of persistent unhealthy behaviors.

Many clinicians might attempt to take on the role of cheerleader with a patient with persistent unhealthy behavior, asking permission to make suggestions for change (e.g., behavioral menu) or trying to directly influence the patient in the direction of the desired change, even after he or she has expressed ambivalence. This rarely works with the ambivalent patient, especially one with persistent unhealthy behavior.

Therefore, in the preceding example, as soon as the patient expressed ambivalence, the physician recognized the ambivalence but chose to "amplify" the negative (i.e., "no change") side of the ambivalence a bit more negatively than the patient himself expressed it.

**PHYSICIAN:** *Okay. I hear you. It sounds like you're just not going to stop smoking, or even cut down a little.* **(complex reflection, amplified negative reflection)**

This type of reflection often functions as a powerful motivator for change. By amplifying the negative side of the ambivalence more than the patient actually stated, the clinician encourages the patient to make a correction by clarifying the ways in which the clinician has overstated the negative. Through this clarification, however, the patient will be making statements about change that he is interested or willing to make (i.e., change talk), and when patients hear themselves voice reasons for change, they feel more motivated to change.

When a clinician uses an amplified negative reflection, however, care must be taken to always continue to communicate respect for the patient's autonomy (MI spirit; see Chapter 5) as well as avoiding any tone of sarcasm.

Let's look at this specific interaction more closely because at least two other kinds of reflections besides the amplified negative reflection might have been chosen in response to the patient's statement:

*I just don't know. Maybe this isn't the time.*

Miller and Rollnick call this sustain talk, which is the opposite of change talk, and define it as "any client speech that favors status quo rather than movement toward a change goal."[1]

A simple reflection would have been acceptable.

**PHYSICIAN:** *It sounds like you just don't know if you're ready for a change now.* **(simple reflection)**

or

**PHYSICIAN:** *It sounds like you're of two minds now: Part of you doesn't feel ready for change, but part of you does feel ready.* **(double-sided reflection)**

Either of these reflections would have been acceptable or adequate. The first was a simple reflection and the second was another type of complex reflection, termed "double-sided reflection." Double-sided reflections are useful for bringing ambivalence to the surface in a non-confrontational, nonjudgmental manner, facilitating direct discussion of the ambivalence itself. Each side of the ambivalence has merit, and double-sided reflections can help the patient and physician begin a dialogue about the relative benefits of each side of the ambivalence and the patient's decision to change or not to change.

From a technical point of view, in the preceding example of the double-sided reflection, it is worth noting that the clinician ended with the positive side of the ambivalence, weighting the dialogue a bit toward the direction of change.[c]

The legitimating comment about how the demanding behavior of his wife and children makes him feel out of control with respect to his family is another example of a complex reflection. And the case presentation also demonstrates multiple examples of enriched applications of legitimation, support, partnership, and affirmation.

To summarize, use of advanced skills to respond to discord in the relationship, or distress, is an essential first step of SAAP when BAP doesn't work. As rapport becomes reestablished or distress resolves, change talk usually emerges and the clinician can judiciously revisit the earlier probe for change (Question One of BAP). Many patients will be able to make action plans at that time and the clinician will not need to move on to higher steps of advanced skills.

In virtually all cases, the advanced skills for rebuilding relationships remain qualitatively the same as the core relationship skills presented in Chapter 3 (nonverbal skills, reflection, legitimation, support, partnership, and respect), although the clinical context and emotional intensity present higher degrees of challenge than more routine medical encounters.

The challenge for the clinician in using advanced skills for responding to discord or distress in the service of action planning for change becomes how to mobilize these skills effectively and efficiently in the context of the unique clinical issue at hand. Practice and clinical experience are, of course, essential, but the following general principles can be helpful.

1. *Attentive silence* has particular usefulness in situations of emotional complexity. It invariably facilitates patient expression of feeling.
2. Starting with simple reflection and moving toward more complex reflections can help the clinician communicate empathy. Strategic use of complex reflections, including double-sided reflections and amplified negative reflections, can be particularly effective in helping patients with persistent unhealthy behaviors move toward expression of change talk and into a frame of mind to respond positively to a challenge or rechallenge with Question One of Brief Action Planning.
3. Other relationship skills including support for autonomy, respect (affirmation), and partnership all have enduring value in situations of high emotional complexity.

## F. Skills and Case Studies of SAAP Step Two: Understanding Benefits or Obstacles to Change

Clinicians face situations in which there may be no discord or distress and yet the patient still has no interest in change. The next logical step, then, in SAAP centers around understanding personal benefits or obstacles to change.

By asking the patient to think about the personal benefits of change, the clinician seeks to motivate the patient to envision a life without the problematic behavior. Table 18.2 proposes a structured question that clinicians can use to ask patients about the personal benefits of change.

If the patient begins to sincerely talk about how life might be different, this discussion generates change talk, often sufficient rather quickly to allow the clinician to successfully reintroduce Question One.

Other patients, however, do not generate sufficient change talk to move forward to action planning. For these patients, the stepped-care approach suggests moving forward to the strategic use of data-gathering skills to explore and understand the personal meaning of the problematic behavior and the obstacles to change; for example, "What is the history of this behavior? What function does it serve? What attempts have been made to change in the past?"[D] As the patient recounts the narrative story of the problematic behaviors along with the history of obstacles to change to an empathic listener, change talk almost always emerges. If the clinician recognizes the change talk and responds to it strategically, the strength and intensity of the change talk will increase, leading to a point, eventually, at which Question One may be successfully reintroduced.

The specific advanced skills of Understanding Benefits or Obstacles to Change include enriched applications of the basic skills of assessment and understanding presented in Chapter 4:

- Open-ended questions
- Facilitation
- Checking

---

TABLE 18.2 ▪ **Understanding Personal Benefits of Change**

| | |
|---|---|
| Aim: | *To evoke personal benefits of change* |
| Ask: | *"How might your life be different if you were able to change … ?"* (the behavior under consideration) |

- Open-to-closed cone of questioning
- Summarizing

Similar to Step One of SAAP, which had two components (discord and distress), this second step of the advanced skills also has two components: (1) understanding benefits of change and (2) understanding obstacles to change. The components are placed in the same strategic SAAP step because they both involve the concept of clinician understanding and both rely on the same strategic data-gathering skills, beginning with open-ended questions.

We suggest that clinicians start Step Two with exploration of the *benefits* of change because it is conceptually easier and clinically more time efficient than exploration of *obstacles*. If the patient is able to talk about the benefits of change with sufficient emotional investment in the change talk that emerges, the clinician can often introduce Question One soon afterward with good results.

Consider Dr. Gutnick's approach to one of her actual patients, Mr. Smith, which illustrates exploring the benefits of change in Step Two of SAAP.[E]

> Mr. Smith, a 68-year-old man with a heavy smoking history, had an excellent relationship with Dr. Gutnick, his primary care physician for more than 15 years. He respected his physician and understood that she always had his best interest in mind but was frustrated that she brought up his smoking at every visit since he enjoyed smoking and was not interested in quitting. Over the years Dr. Gutnick tried various strategies to encourage and support Mr. Smith to quit smoking, including educating him about the health consequences of smoking.

> **DR. GUTNICK:** *Mr. Smith, if you quit smoking your breathing would be better.*

> **MR. SMITH:** *Doc, I am not complaining, my breathing is fine now.*

> **DR. GUTNICK:** *Mr. Smith, you mentioned that you are stressed about finances. Think about how much money you could save if you gave up the cigarettes.* (Tries to pressure patient by bringing up the financial cost of cigarettes.)

> **MR. SMITH:** *Doc, my wife's family brings me my smokes from Ecuador when they visit so that's really not a problem. Cigarettes are cheap there.*

> **DR. GUTNICK:** *Mr. Smith, if you keep smoking, you can get cancer and die.* (uses scare tactics)

> **MR. SMITH:** *Doc, when it is my time, that will be my time. Anyway my dad smoked all his life and lived till 100, longevity runs in my family.*

> **DR. GUTNICK:** *Mr. Smith, as a doctor it is my responsibility to speak to you about your smoking. But I must not be a good doctor since I cannot get you to stop.* (And even resorting to guilt)

> **MR. SMITH:** *Doc, you are not a bad doctor, I am just a bad patient. Why don't you just write down in your notes that we discussed it, but let's not!!*

The preceding dialogues, which are near-verbatim excerpts from real conversations that Dr. Gutnick had with Mr. Smith over the years, illustrate Mr. Smith's resistance to engage in smoking discussion no matter which strategy Dr. Gutnick attempted to employ. None of these strategies were successful, and Mr. Smith got so frustrated with the redundancy of his physicians' efforts to bring up the smoking conversation that eventually he would walk into his physician's office with his hand in front of his face, exclaiming:

> *Doc, let's not go there today, Okay? Let's not go there.*

After attending a Motivational Interviewing workshop, Dr. Gutnick tried a new strategy to explore the benefits of change:

> **DR. GUTNICK:** *Mr. Smith I respect the fact that you are not ready to quit smoking.*

> **MR. SMITH:** (sigh of relief and nonverbal cue that the patient is more relaxed)

**DR. GUTNICK:** *But can I ask you one question?* **(asking permission, see Chapter 5)**

**MR. SMITH:** *Sure doc, anything.*

**DR. GUTNICK:** *I know you don't want to stop smoking, but if you did, how might your life be different?*

**MR. SMITH:** *Oh, I see where you are going doc, I see where you are going.* (But Mr. Smith went on to answer the question.) *Well if I did stop smoking, my breathing would be better* **(change talk: reason)**, *my wife wouldn't be on my case all the time* **(change talk: reason)**, *and I would have some extra cash in my pocket.* **(change talk: reason)**

Then Mr. Smith went on:

**MR. SMITH:** *You know I really could cut down just a bit. It wouldn't be so hard.* **(change talk: ability)** *I don't want to end up needing to breathe through a straw in my neck.* **(change talk: reason)**

**DR. GUTNICK:** *You recognize that there are many benefits of stopping that would improve the quality of your life, and it sounds like cutting down a bit is something you feel confident that you could do. Would you like to make a specific plan around this for the next week or two?*

Dr. Gutnick used the emergence of change talk as a queue to ask Question One of BAP. She first reflected back the personal benefits of change that Mr. Smith alluded to, emphasizing the personal confidence she heard in his change talk. Question One of BAP then flowed naturally and logically into the conversation.

Mr. Smith represents an example of a patient who responded well to questions about the benefits of change.

As pointed out, however, for other patients clinicians need to explore and understand the personal meaning of the problem behavior and the personal obstacles to change.

Consider the following case example: a 55 year-old cigarette smoker, with diabetes, heart disease, high blood pressure, depression, and grief over loss of a child. Toward the end of a recent checkup, at a point in the meeting at which there had been, up to that point, good rapport and engagement, the physician wonders if the patient is ready to make an action plan for health and asks him Question One of Brief Action Planning (BAP):

**PHYSICIAN:** *I wonder if there is anything you might like to do for your health in the next week or two?*

**PATIENT:** *You bet there is! I'd like to flush all these pills down the toilet! Pills, pills, pills. So many pills! I'm sick of them. There's just too many. I hate them. That's what I'd like to do for my health!* **(very angry)**

**PHYSICIAN:** *Wow. You're pretty angry and upset. There are just too many pills.* **(simple reflection)**

**PATIENT:** *I'm sick of it. And I can't do it. Every time I go to the doctor, there's another pill. I just can't keep them straight. I guess I need them and I guess I should take them, but sometimes I really wonder if I really wouldn't be better off flushing them all down the toilet. It's hard to remember to take them the way I should. I do forget sometimes. And then when I forget for a whole day, sometimes I actually feel better.*

**PHYSICIAN:** *Well this sounds important. I can understand why you wouldn't want to take the pills if you're not really sure you need them.* **(legitimation; empathy)**

**PATIENT:** *No, I know I need them. We've gone over the reasons lots of times. I know I need to take them all, just the way you've prescribed them. It's just hard to keep my mind on it day in and day out. I'm just not sure what to do next.*

Up to this point in the conversation, it is clear that BAP has not worked and Step One of SAAP did not elicit sufficient change talk to launch action planning for change. The physician realizes that the next step of advanced skills must be introduced in the effort to elicit action planning for change with respect to this patient's focus of change: medication nonadherence.

Consider the following dialogue from the point at which the preceding conversation stopped:

PHYSICIAN: *Well, Mr. James first of all, you should feel good about yourself that you understand why the medications are important and that you think it is important to take them. That's a really important first step and something that lots of people have trouble with. You've made a lot of progress if you've already made it through that step and come to that resolution for yourself.* (**respect; affirmation**)

PATIENT: *Well, you're right I have. It's just been hard to follow through.*

PHYSICIAN: *Okay, and second, I'd like to reassure you that many patients who are taking a lot of different medications find it hard to take them regularly, as prescribed.* (**legitimation**)

*So, I'd like to take a few minutes to understand your particular situation, and then maybe together we can come up with some solutions. Does that sound okay to you?* (**asking permission, see Chapter 5**)

PATIENT: *Sure.*

PHYSICIAN: *Great. So, can we start with you giving me a little background about what's been making this so difficult for you?* (**open-ended question**)

PATIENT: *Well, I used to be very strong and athletic. I worked all day and then I would come home and run at least 3 to 5 miles most nights. Now I can't work anymore and I'm still young, only 55, but I can't work and I can't run anymore.*

PHYSICIAN: *Okay. Go on.* (**facilitation**)

PATIENT: *So I know it doesn't make sense, but taking all these pills make me feel even older and sicker than I really am. And I stare all day at all those bottles on the kitchen table and I hate them. They remind me of my aunts and uncles ... when I was growing up ... old and sick.*

PHYSICIAN: *So, you used to be so active, strong, and athletic. Taking pills now makes you feel old and sick, and looking at the bottles on the table gives you uncomfortable memories of family members who've been old and sick.* (**checking**)

PATIENT: *That's right.*

PHYSICIAN: *Okay. Please go on.* (**facilitation**)

PATIENT: *And then my wife keeps reminding me to take the pills and I get mad, so I refuse to take them, just to make a point that I don't want to do what she says. I tell her I'll take them later. And I do think I really will take them later, but then I sometimes forget.*

PHYSICIAN: *Okay. I'd like to bring up one other thing. I know you've been struggling with depression too. You've been recovering from the tragic death of your son in that car accident 2 years ago. Has that affected this medication issue?*

(Open-to-closed cone of questioning. As questions become more focused, open questions are more directed and closed questions eventually are important for clarification and accuracy.)

PATIENT: *Well, maybe a little, I guess. Sometimes I get really down and out and think, "What's the point? I really don't want to go on like this." Maybe the funk lasts a day or two and I'll miss some more pills, but I realize that I don't want to kill myself that way ... so I get back on the pills because I realize I still do have a lot to live for. I know I need to take them if I want to go on living to enjoy life and be with my wife and grandkids.* (**patient ends this paragraph with change talk of need to change nonadherent behavior**)

PHYSICIAN: *Thanks for that background. It's very helpful. I can certainly understand better now why taking the pills regularly has been such a problem for you. As I said before, taking pills regularly is generally difficult for everyone. But this has been especially difficult for you because just taking the pills and especially having them on your kitchen table day in and day out, and having your wife on your case regularly, reminds you of illness, disability, and frailty in your own family and brings up feelings of loss of your independence, your work life, and your athletic activities, all of which have also been really hard for you. At times, you've even wondered whether going on living makes sense, but you've decided that you still have a lot to live for.* (**summarization**)

PATIENT: *That's right.*

PHYSICIAN: *And it sounds like you understand all the reasons why it's important to take the medications regularly. You just haven't been able to find a method to do that yet.*

PATIENT: *That's it.*

PHYSICIAN: *Would it be alright with you if I suggested some medication-taking methods that have worked for some of my other patients that might interest and help you?*

PATIENT: *Sure, that'd be great.*

In this situation, after using advanced skills to rebuild the relationship and other advanced skills to understand roadblocks to change, the physician now uses summarization skills to re-state and emphasize some of the patients' own change talk statements. The physician then asks for and receives permission to present this patient with a behavioral menu for medication nonadherence (see Chapter 5). The patient goes on and makes a personal action plan around one of the methods in the behavioral menu for medication nonadherence, specifically buying a weekly medication pillbox in a local pharmacy, putting his pills in the box, and keeping the pills near his toothbrush in the bathroom (not on the kitchen table) to help remind him to take the medications regularly when he brushes his teeth.

It is worth noting that the skills of "checking" and "summarization" are essentially the same; the term "checking" is used to refer to the skill earlier in the interview and the term "summarization" is used for the longer form when it used near the conclusion of the interview.

## G. Skills and Case Study of SAAP Step Three: Using Higher-Order Motivational Interviewing Skills

When neither Step One nor Step Two of SAAP lead to effective action planning, clinicians can turn to Step Three, the final step of the 13 advanced skills. This step includes two higher-order Motivational Interviewing (MI) competencies:

1. Elicit and resolve ambivalence.
2. Develop the discrepancy.

Use of either of these skills requires special training, practice, coaching, and re-practice. Nevertheless, the general concepts are presented in this chapter and a case is provided to demonstrate how the skills are used in practice. Links are provided for interested readers to pursue this specialized, advanced training.[F]

## Elicit and Resolve Ambivalence

Most patients with persistent unhealthy behavior harbor some significant ambivalence about that behavior. Higher-order MI skills aim to draw attention to this ambivalence and elicit change talk around the healthy side of the ambivalence, which can then lead to action planning for change.

One way to do this has been to help patients look at both valences of a particular unhealthy behavior, not just what is "bad" about the behavior but also what is "good." This has sometimes been called the decisional balance. There is clearly quite a lot that is good about the unhealthy behavior for the patient, or he or she would not have been engaging in the behavior in the first place. So, in exploring the ambivalence, the clinician seeks to clarify all that is good about the behavior, often before the clinician seeks to clarify what is not so good (or bad) about the behavior.

This approach usually comes as a surprise to patients, who usually expect the physician to tell them directly to stop the unhealthy behavior or "lecture" the patient about what is bad. Once the discussion turns to what is "good" about problematic behaviors, it is interesting to note that in actual practice, it turns out to be the patient himself or herself who usually spontaneously starts to come up with a list of things that are bad or "not so good" about the behavior. These "not so good" aspects of the behavior quite naturally soon become the basis of the argument or plan for change. With the emergence of change talk, the patient may be ready soon to consider action planning for change.

## Develop the Discrepancy

To "develop the discrepancy" refers to the clinician's effort to elicit and make explicit a patient's long-term goals, values, or life objectives and place those consciously alongside his or her current behaviors to discuss with the patient the extent to which there seems to be a conflict or discrepancy between the two. For the patient with persistent unhealthy behavior, of course, this underlying discrepancy will virtually always be present. Because people feel uncomfortable with this cognitive discrepancy,[5] once it is drawn to their attention, without shame or humiliation, they often begin making change statements, to which the clinician can respond and ask for elaboration. As the patient elaborates on the discrepancy and the wish to resolve it, sufficient change talk may emerge to allow a probe for action planning; that is, Question One, "Is there anything you'd like to do about (this behavior of focus) in the next week or two?"

Consider the following example of an actual emergency room visit from Dr. Cole's clinical experience, which illustrates the use of advanced MI skills, eliciting and resolving ambivalence, and developing the discrepancy.

> A 42-year-old married woman with a long history of alcoholism was brought by the police to the ER at 2 AM after a neighbor's call about a family disturbance. The police told the ER physicians that she was inebriated and threatening to kill her husband. The police report quoted her as saying, "I'm going to kill him. I'm going to pull him apart limb by limb and love every minute of it!"
>
> The patient had a history of three previous ER admissions in the last 5 years but no criminal record of actual violence. Her alcohol blood level was 1.6. She was seen by the ER resident and held overnight to sleep off the inebriation to be reevaluated when sober.

Dr. Cole was the attending physician the next morning and heard the following report from the ER resident:

> "This is another chronic alcoholic who's ready for discharge. She is a 42-year-old married woman with a long history of abuse and dependence. She was brought in by the police for making violent threats against her husband, but she was drunk at the time. She has no history of actual violence and she's clear now and denies any suicidal or homicidal intent. She has no depression, anxiety, or psychosis. Her husband denies any history of real threats, attempts, or risks and is comfortable with her returning home. I gave her the usual list of referrals for alcohol treatment, but it's no use. She has no interest in getting any help or changing. She's just a chronic alcoholic. She's ready to go."

As the attending, Dr. Cole needed to "eyeball" the patient anyway, so he asked the resident if he minded if he asked the patient a few questions. The resident reminded Dr. Cole that they were "very busy" and needed the bed opened up, sending nonverbal signals of reluctance (eyes roll up). Unfortunately, medical professionals, frustrated by the tenacity of maladaptive chronic addictions, often feel and express negative attitudes when caring for patients with persistent unhealthy behaviors.

Dr. Cole's conversation with the patient went like this:

> **DR. COLE:** *Hello, Mrs. Henry. I'm Dr. Cole, the attending physician. I understand you're ready to go home and Dr. Jones has already reviewed the case with me in detail. I need to complete the evaluation and then you can go.*
>
> **PATIENT:** *I don't understand what else you need to know, doctor. I'm an alcoholic and I love to drink. That's not going to change. I'm not going to hurt anyone, so you can let me go now. You can't keep me.* **(It is clear that any attempt at immediate BAP will not work.)**
>
> **DR. COLE:** *Well, you're right. You're anxious to go. I understand that and I am going to let you go in just a few more minutes.* **(simple reflection, legitimation, attempt at building a relationship)**
>
> *I just need to ask you one or two more questions. And then we can call your husband and he can come and get you. Is that Okay?* **(Attempt to understand obstacles to change; asking permission, although the context is not exactly one of equal power in that the patient is locked up and doesn't really have power to refuse absolutely.)**
>
> **PATIENT:** *Okay, please make it quick.*
>
> **DR. COLE:** *I will. I want to start by recognizing that you enjoy drinking, that it adds a lot to your life, and that you are not going to stop. I do understand that.*
>
> **PATIENT:** *You got it. I love drinking. It's everything to me. I've been drinking for 25 years. That's what I do and that's who I am.*
>
> **DR. COLE:** *My main question is this one. Is there anything at all in your life that is not going so well? Is there anything in your life or your drinking that is on the negative side, that is not going the way you might want it to go?*
>
> (This is a question strategically aimed at understanding the complexity of the drinking behavior in its full impact on her life; seeking information related to potential *ambivalence* or *discrepancies*.)
>
> **PATIENT:** *Well, my doctor did tell me that I have a bad liver, that it's actually very bad. It could fail.*
>
> **DR. COLE:** *I'm not sure I understand. Could you say some more about that?* **(understanding obstacles to change: facilitation)**
>
> **PATIENT:** *Well, he said my tests, chemicals … enzymes. I think that's what they're called … that's right … they've been going up … and are now so high that my liver could fail all together.*
>
> **DR. COLE:** *And is that related to the alcohol?* **(understanding obstacles, open-to-closed cone of questions)**
>
> **PATIENT:** *That's what the doctor said. The alcohol is killing the liver.*
>
> **DR. COLE:** *And is that a big problem or a little problem?* **(understanding obstacles, closed question)**
>
> **PATIENT:** *It's a big one. You need your liver to stay alive.*

**DR. COLE:** *Okay. Let me see if I understand what you're telling me. I know that you love drinking, that you're an alcoholic and that you're not going to stop, but now you're also telling me that if you keep drinking, your liver is going to fail and you're going to die. So, I guess what I'm hearing you say is that compared to your drinking, you don't care that much whether you live or die.* **(summarization to develop the discrepancy; not sarcastic)**

**PATIENT:** *No! That's not true, not at all! I love life! I'm not ready to die. I know I have to stop drinking. I'm just not ready to stop.* **(emergence of change talk)**

**DR. COLE:** *Okay, I understand better now. You know you have to stop drinking because you love life. You're just not ready. You're probably going to stop sometime in the very distant future, say 5 or 10 years.* **(reflection with a twist)**

**PATIENT:** *No way. I'll be long dead by then. I've got to stop in the next year. I don't know how I'm going to do it, but I know I'll just have to do it.*

**DR. COLE:** *Okay, I see. It sounds like this is actually a real problem for you. You love drinking and have no real interest at all in stopping. But if you keep drinking, even for a year or more, your liver will fail and you're going to die. So, you realize you're going to have to stop sometime in the next year, but don't know how you're going to do it. Is that right?* (Elicit and resolve ambivalence)

**PATIENT:** *Yeah, that's about it.*

**DR. COLE:** *Would you have any interest in getting some help with stopping? We can point you in the direction of programs that are there to help you.*

**PATIENT:** *Yes, I would like that kind of help. I need it.*

**DR. COLE:** *We actually already gave you a list of programs. You have it there in your hand. Would you like to look it over with me and make a plan with me about which one you might like to call and when you might do this?*

**PATIENT:** *Yes, I would.*

This patient went on to make a concrete action plan for her health. She chose a center and made a commitment to call that center the next day for an appointment.

This one interaction demonstrates the use of the full compliment of advanced skills for action planning: responding to discord and distress, understanding benefits and obstacles to change, eliciting ambivalence, and developing the discrepancy. It demonstrates how they can be used to elicit change talk that can lead directly to action planning for change.

## Conclusion

This chapter describes and demonstrates three steps and 13 stepped-care advanced skills for action planning when BAP is not sufficient. The three steps require eliciting, recognizing, and responding to change talk as the 13 specific skills themselves are used to: respond to discord and distress, understand benefits and obstacles to change, and implement higher-order MI skills.

As described and demonstrated in this chapter, the advanced skills for action planning may appear deceptively simple to use. In reality, they are complex and higher order. They take time and effort to master conceptually and even more work to integrate smoothly into actual practice. However, practitioners who do not plan to attend formal workshops or learning programs to master the skills themselves can benefit from taking time to understand the concepts and the way they are clinically applied.

Furthermore, this understanding may help practitioners begin to implement some of these concepts into their own clinical work and also help them better understand how their colleagues or other members of their interdisciplinary care teams may be use these skills to help motivate patients for self-care. Interested learners can enroll in targeted training programs to learn these skills for application in their own patient practices.[F]

## Summary

Stepped-care advanced skills for action planning focus on eliciting, recognizing, and responding to change talk by:
- Responding to discord or distress
- Understanding personal benefits or obstacles to change
- Using advanced motivational interviewing skills

### References

1. Cole S, Blader J: UB-PAP (Ultra-Brief Personal Action Planning): an innovative tool to support patient self-management, motivate healthy behavior change and improve adherence. Poster Presented at Annual Meeting of the Institute of Psychiatric Services, York, 2009.
2. Cole S, Waxenberg F, McCarthy D, McClure T, Lee R: Ultra-Brief Personal Action Planning (UB-PAP) and motivational interviewing: a prospective, pilot efficacy study. Paper presented at First International Conference on Motivational Interviewing, Interlaken, Switzerland, 2008.
3. Miller and Rollnick call this the "righting reflex". In Miller Wm, Rollnick S, editors: *Motivational interviewing*, ed 3, Helping People Change. 2012, Guilford Press.
4. Miller Wm, Rollnick S: *Motivational interviewing*, ed 3, Helping People Change. 2012, Guilford Press.
5. Cialdini R: *Influence: the psychology of persuasion*. New York 2010, Collins.

### Endnotes

A. Some physicians may want to pursue specific training in Brief Action Planning (BAP) or Stepped-Care Advanced Action Planning Skills (SAAP) to develop competencies and/or certification. Information is available at www.ComprehensiveMI.com or www.CentreCMI.ca Information on training in Motivational Interviewing itself is available through the website of the Motivational Interviewing Network of Trainers (MINT) at www.motivationalingerviewing.org.

B. This case, and other similar ones, can be practiced in classroom settings (with opportunities for practice and repractice) to help develop competencies in advanced applications. Teachers and learners, however, should appreciate that mastery of these higher order skills usually requires dedicated and specialized learning efforts or specialized learning programs that include simulations as well as live cases. www.ComprehensiveMI.com; www.CentreCMI.ca.

C. Ambivalence, of course, plays a role in virtually all situations of persistent unhealthy behavior. Section G, however, focuses more specifically on those higher-order methods that concentrate directly on patient ambivalence in the effort to motivate healthy behavior change.

D. It is worth noting that the stepped-care approach to basic and advanced action planning, places the step of understanding (or assessment) a long way down the path of interventions, in fact making understanding the next to last overall step. The SAAP approach might be considered unorthodox or anti-paradigmatic by standing the typical medical or psychological approach on its head by leaving assessment out of some interventions entirely and placing it towards the end, not the beginning of others. BAP and SAAP start with the assumption that the patient is the expert on himself/herself and may be able, if given the opportunity, to produce the "best" action plan that he/she is most likely to actually follow. Therefore, a lengthy "assessment" phase can sometimes be omitted or significantly truncated for the purposes of efficient action planning.

E. A dramatization of this dialogue can be seen in a YouTube video at the URL (Mr. Smith's Smoking Evolution).

F. www.ComprehensiveMI.com; www.CentreCMI.ca; www.motivationalinterviewing.org.

# CHAPTER 19

# Communicating with Patients with Chronic Illness

Connie Davis ▪ Steven Cole

## OVERVIEW

This chapter focuses on the special longitudinal and evolving challenges of caring and communicating with patients with chronic medical conditions who clinicians follow over extended periods of time.

Chronic illness affects more than 80% of people over the age of 65. Of more striking relevance, about 70% of people over 65 have more than one chronic condition. Although medical professionals tend to focus on physiologic parameters, patients worry about how chronic conditions affect their lives. In one recent poll of Medicare recipients, these concerns were:[1,A]

- Loss of independence
- Being a burden to family or friends
- Not being able to afford medical care

Chapter 16 also discusses chronic illness but focuses on understanding common stresses and adaptive tasks of illness, mechanisms of defense, and three common emotional reactions (anger, sadness, and anxiety) to chronic illness. Chapter 17 covers three common maladaptive reactions (anger, sadness, and anxiety) to chronic illness. This chapter, on the other hand, deals more specifically with the relationship and communication strategies that clinicians can rely on to help their patients cope better with the longitudinal and unfolding problems of chronic illness over time.

Clinicians may find it helpful to organize their thinking and conversations about chronic illness care by considering the broad tasks described by Corbin and Strauss (1988)[2,B] and Moos and Holahan.[3,C] They discovered that basic adjustment to chronic illness seemed to require attention to three new life tasks, similar to those reviewed in Chapter 16.

1. Straightforward caring for the illness itself became the first task, including taking medications, administering treatments, and interacting with health care professionals.
2. The second task concerned making adjustments in daily life, such as activity levels, diet, and work schedules.
3. The third task involved handling the emotions that come with chronic illness. The most typical emotions are anger, fear, sadness, and frustration.

Anticipating these broad tasks can help clinicians build trust and deepen the relationship (Function One); understand the personal experiences and assess the unfolding needs of their patients over time (Function Two); and educate and collaboratively build self-management skills to meet the specific needs of specific patients with specific conditions (Function Three).

It is worth noting that some patients experience profound alterations in their views of the future once the diagnosis of a chronic illness is made, which can lead to debilitating depression

145

(see Chapters 16 and 17). This depression adversely affects treatment care and outcome. For example, patients may find it difficult to focus on daily self-care of a physical condition when they feel hopeless and have little motivation for action. Therefore clinicians should, in general, make efforts to treat any depression that is present very early, or at least concurrently, to maximize potential for as much patient assumption of self-care of the chronic illness as possible.

Throughout the trajectory of chronic illness, these three challenges ebb and flow to various different levels and intensities. The clinician caring for the patient with chronic illness can help the patient cope with all of these challenges by strategic and caring use of the communication skills of the three function model discussed in the following.

Although all 30 skills of the Three Function Model are important, building patient self-management (or self-management support) comes to the fore as the core, primary, guiding principle in longitudinal chronic illness care.

Improved self-management leads to better outcomes. Self-management is defined (see Chapter 5) as "The individual's ability to manage the symptoms, treatment, physical and social consequences and lifestyle changes inherent in living with a chronic condition."[4] Self-management is what patients do. The term is neutral. Some patients are seen as "good" self-managers (often meaning compliant) and others are labeled as "bad" self-managers. In actuality, every decision made by a person with chronic illness is self-managing.

Self-management support is defined as the activities of the health care system that facilitate patient self-management. This occurs at many levels, including patient-provider, patient-health care team, patient-health care system, and patient-community. Self-management support is what others do to aid the person with chronic illness. The professional's role is to instill hope that a person can have a long and satisfying life with chronic illness, help him or her understand the possible consequences of daily choices, elicit the goals of the person with chronic illness, and assist the person in adopting behaviors that will help him or her meet goals.

Clinicians contribute to the patient's self-management ability. Messages given throughout the diagnostic process can influence the patient's understanding of his or her role in his or her care. The formation of a working partnership with the patient will affect the person's success in daily self-management. This partnership should not be solely with the primary clinician. Primary clinicians may discover that others may have more time and different skills that are ideally suited to provide self-management support. Studies have shown that other patients, as peers, in addition to health care professionals, can also provide self-management support.[5]

# Application of the Three Function Model to Chronic Illness

## FUNCTION ONE: BUILD (AND MAINTAIN) THE RELATIONSHIP

For patients with chronic illness, the relationship with the clinician often evolves into an important part of his or her life. Built on trust, respect, and mutual caring, the doctor-patient relationship in chronic illness care offers the patient a reliable source of comfort and care (technical and emotional) over time, while also offering the clinician a gratifying context within which to provide this comfort and care.

The patient's emotional reactions (as discussed) start very early in the chronic illness experience, and often include anger, fear, depression, or frustration. In general, these should be addressed right away using varying combinations of reflection, legitimation, support, partnership, or respect (Rule #1, see Chapter 3). For example:

*I can see the diagnosis of diabetes is upsetting for you.* (**reflection**)

*I understand why this would be hard.* (**legitimation**)

*I want you to know I'm going to be here to help you with this.* (**support**)

*I'm going to work with you. Together we can work out ways to deal with this.* (**partnership**)

*You know, I'm impressed with how you've been dealing with this so far.* (**respect**)

Once the initial diagnosis of chronic illness has been made and the patient has made his or her early adjustment, the clinician often continues working with the same patient over many years. The clinician has already built the initial relationship, which must be maintained. The basic skills for maintaining the relationship are exactly the same: empathy (reflection and legitimation), support, partnership, and respect. Effort taken to maintain the relationship will improve the outcomes for the patient and the satisfaction for the physician. Acknowledgment of the work of caring for a chronic illness will build rapport. Here the physician uses **legitimation**:

> **PATIENT WITH DIABETES:** *Every moment I have to be thinking about what I can eat, if I need more insulin or less because I'm trying to get some exercise.*

> **PHYSICIAN:** *I understand that's hard. Having a chronic illness can be a lot of effort.*

Here the physician formally describes the **partnership** and expresses **support**.

> **PHYSICIAN:** *Diabetes is an ongoing condition. You and I are going to work together to manage your diabetes so that you have a long and satisfying life.*

**Reflection** can be useful.

> **PATIENT:** *I just hate having this lung disease. I can't go fishing like I used to. I get winded just walking from my car to the river.*

> **PHYSICIAN:** *You are finding you get short of breath when walking.*

> **PATIENT:** *Yeah, that's it, doc. I wish I had more energy.*

> **PHYSICIAN:** *Let's look again at your inhalers. Tell me how you are using them.* (moving on to collaborate for management)

Patients appreciate knowing that their efforts are recognized. When a patient takes the time to complete a monitoring log, it is important for the physician to acknowledge these efforts.

> **PHYSICIAN:** *I am very impressed by your blood pressure log. You have certainly taken this seriously.*

The physician has conveyed **respect** through this interchange.

## FUNCTION TWO: ASSESS AND UNDERSTAND THE PATIENT

Sometimes physicians may find themselves puzzled by the actions or health behaviors of their patients with chronic illness. When the physician understands the patient's unique explanatory model of the illness, his or her expectations from the physicians, and the impact of the illness on his or her life, the physician will be in a much better position to provide meaningful emotional support and effective medical intervention, leading to better outcomes. In fact, just the process of elicitation of these data also tends to improve trust and rapport.

Open-ended questions allow the patient to express his or her personal understanding of the illness.

> **PHYSICIAN:** *What do you think caused your heart disease?*

> **PATIENT:** *It was going to happen no matter what I did. You see, my dad died at age 45 of a heart attack. My mom made it to age 60, same thing. My brother's already had one of those surgeries. Four-way bypass I think it was. I figure I'm doomed.*

The physician now has an understanding of the patient's **explanatory model** and his or her **expectations**. The physician can now work to impart hope and encourage the patient to accept treatment.

If the physician is assuming the care of a person with chronic illness, it is useful to allow the patient to tell his or her story **(develop the narrative)**. Notice the open-ended **questioning style**.

PHYSICIAN: *Tell me about how you came to find out you have lupus.*

PATIENT: *Well, it's been a hard road. I had all these odd things happening for many years and my former doctor just couldn't put his finger on it. Then one day he ordered some more tests and I started to get this funny mark on my face and—there it was. I had lupus. It changed everything. I had to cut back to part-time work. I have to admit I've been depressed.*

PHYSICIAN: *You have had some troubles with depression. What other troubles have you had with your lupus?* (The physician is beginning the survey of problems.)

PATIENT: *Well, I get real tired from the littlest thing. And I have to watch out for infections. I seem to catch every cold that comes along. I have a lot of aches, too. I think there is something going on with my joints. I just don't seem to be able to move about very well.*

PHYSICIAN SUMMARIZING AND NOTING THE IMPACT OF ILLNESS: *So there's the depression, fatigue, worry about infections, pain, and some joint problems. This has led to changes in your ability to work full time. What did I miss?*

PATIENT: *That about covers it.*

PHYSICIAN NEGOTIATING PRIORITIES: *Which of these concerns should we deal with today?*

PATIENT: *The fatigue is really getting me down. Is there something we can do about that?*

PHYSICIAN ELICITING EXPECTATIONS: *What would you like your energy level to be like?*

PATIENT: *I'd really like to be able to attend one of my son's basketball games. Right now I just get too tired and I have to leave at halftime.*

Through the course of a chronic illness, patients experience change on many levels: They age, their illnesses progress, the people or circumstances around them change, or other change occurs. Any or all of these changes have an impact on the illness, the chronic illness care, and the relationship. Function Two skills to assess and understand are essential for monitoring these changes over time. In managing the patient with chronic illness, the physician must always communicate a sense of being open to learning from the patient about these new developments with a question like:

*Tell me what's new in your life since I saw you last?*

An open-ended question like this, a Function Two skill, can cover both physical and emotional domains for the patient, allowing the physician the opportunity to get updated on the key new elements about chronic illness care so as to offer the best care for the patient until the next visit.

Depending on how the patient responds to this question, the physician may need to follow up with many more Function Two skills, such as facilitation and checking (if more details of new physical problems or new emotional events need exploration). If the patient demonstrates strong emotions in response to the open-ended question (perhaps there was a death, significant life stress, or other negative event), the physician must respond with Function One skills like reflection and legitimation (empathy) before learning more specific details about the event. In general, the physician needs to continue "in Function One" until the patient reaches sufficient emotional equilibrium to return to the narrative of the emotionally charged event. And the new event, itself, needs sufficient exploration (Function Two) for the physician to understand its potential impact on the patient's primary illness process. In a busy clinic, these tasks can usually be covered in 3-5 minutes, though in very troublesome situations or with troubled patients, more time may be required. The clinician may need to schedule new appointments or refer these patients to other providers (e.g., social workers or psychologists/psychiatrists) if indicated.

## FUNCTION THREE: COLLABORATE FOR MANAGEMENT

For the patient to live successfully with chronic illness, the physician can help by focusing on three key techniques of self-management: goal setting, action planning, and problem solving. These activities are natural for some patients, and others apply them successfully in some realms of their life (such as managing their job or their finances) but have difficulty applying them to self-managing a chronic condition. Nonphysician members of the team may also perform these tasks. Brief Action Planning (BAP), as a separate stand-alone complex skill, is discussed in Chapter 5. Action planning is presented here as part of a continuum with *broader* goal setting, which is more appropriately reasonable for longer-term planning in chronic illness care.

*Eliciting a Goal:*

PHYSICIAN: *Where would you like to be in 6 months with your arthritis?*

or

PHYSICIAN: *What would your life to be like in 6 months or so?*

If the patient says something vague, like "I would like to feel better," the physician can attempt to get more clarification:

PHYSICIAN: *How would I know you were better? What would be different?*

or

PHYSICIAN: *What would another person be able to see that was better?*

Prompts may be necessary, such as:

PHYSICIAN: *What is your pain preventing you from doing that you would like to do?*

Some patients may defer to the physician about goal setting. If this is truly a well-considered choice, the physician who focuses on function over clinical goals will be most likely to contribute to improved quality of life for the patient. Alternately, patients may be so overwhelmed with their condition(s) or demoralized by prior unsuccessful attempts at lifestyle changes that they will have difficulty thinking of a goal. A trusting relationship with the physician and other members of the health care team form the foundation for assisting patients to set goals in future interactions. The physician can also assist patients by encouraging interaction with other patients who have successfully managed by recommending self-management education programs, peer support, and peer mentors. Group medical visits can be a powerful motivator for self-management as patients see other people modeling self-management behaviors.

*Action Planning:*

Goals are global expressions of an aspiration. To reach a goal, new behaviors are undertaken in daily life. One tool to help patients learn new behaviors is to help the patient make an action plan. This process is described more fully in Chapter 5, and the following are examples of BAP in the care of people with chronic conditions.

PHYSICIAN: *Is there anything you'd like to do for your health in the next week or two?*

PATIENT: *I've been thinking a lot about my poor sleep. My daughter keeps telling me that I should cut back on the caffeine. I think I should try that.*

PHYSICIAN: *Is this something you really want to do? Or would you just be doing it to please your daughter?*

PATIENT: *No, I think I should, too. Those espressos are expensive.*

PHYSICIAN: *What is something specific you will do in the next week to cut back on your caffeine?*

PATIENT: *I will stop having coffee in the afternoon. Just one last latte on my afternoon break. You know, I don't drink so much coffee on weekends, just weekdays.*

PHYSICIAN: *That sounds like a good plan. Could you say it back to one more time so I make sure we're on the same page?*

PATIENT: *Yeah. I'm going to stop drinking coffee after my afternoon break when I'm at work.*

PHYSICIAN: *Great. Now another question: How confident are you that you can do this? Let's say confidence is something you could measure on a scale of 0 to 10, with 0 being not confident at all that you can stop having coffee after afternoon break and 10 being you are absolutely certain. What number would you give your confidence?*

PATIENT: *I'd say it's about a 7. I really like my coffee, but I am tired of sleeping so poorly.*

PHYSICIAN: *Seven is great. If it's okay with you, I'd like Marcia, my medical assistant, to give you a quick call next week just to see how it's going. Would that be okay with you?*

PATIENT: *Well, sure. I guess you're really interested in seeing how I do.*

If the patient says his or her confidence is less than 7, the physician will need to help the patient rework the plan until the patient's confidence is higher. The physician wants the patient to be successful in the plan so that confidence in making changes to his or her life will grow and he or she can work on more challenging aspects of life. If the patient persists in choosing an action plan that seems unrealistic to the patient or unrelated to the chronic condition, it is important to not insist on reworking the plan. The physician will then be ready to help the patient recover if the plan was too difficult for an initial effort and guide the patient to topics that will influence his or her chronic condition when the patient is ready. Remember that goal setting, action planning, and problem solving are techniques that can be used by any member of the health care team, and some patients prefer working with other members of the team. The tasks can also be split up among the team members.

If the physician is working with someone with depression, it is often helpful to create an action plan around scheduling pleasurable events. If a person with depression can succeed in having one small fun activity in his or her daily life, he or she may begin to create hope that life could be different.

Physicians are often natural problem solvers; it is part of the attraction of practicing medicine. **Problem solving** is a skill that can be taught. Problem solving related to Brief Action Planning (BAP) was covered in Chapter 5. Additional details about problem solving, a key skill for people with chronic conditions, are included here. The outline for this approach was developed by Kate Lorig and colleagues.[6,7]

The method has seven steps.

1. Identify the problem.
2. List all possible solutions.
3. Choose one.
4. Try it for 2 weeks.
5. If that doesn't work, try another.
6. If that doesn't work, find a resource.
7. If that doesn't work, accept that the problem may not be solvable now.

The first step, problem identification, may seem straightforward, but it may take some reflection on the part of the patient to identify the real problem. If patients have trouble coming up with potential solutions, the physician remembers to offer additional solutions after asking for permission. "I work with other patients who have your condition. Would you like to hear what some of them have tried?" This phrasing avoids having the physician resume the position of expert.

The long-term goal of chronic illness care focuses on building an individual patient's capacity, depth, and strength for his or her own disease self-management. This capacity will change, to some degree, over time and will also vary somewhat depending on the physical state of the illness itself. On the other hand, a patient's capacity for highly functional levels of disease self-management depends to some extent on the physician's and his or her medical team's application of some of the basic and advanced self-management support skills described in this text. As the physical illness itself evolves and the patient's life context changes as well (occupation, social role, family, emotional needs), the specific self-management support (SMS) needs of every patient will change as well. The competent physician needs to recognize and respond to these evolving SMS needs in a way that meets the patient's current need and continues to build capacity for the future. Working with patients with chronic illness over time and helping build their self-management skills remains one of the most gratifying parts of medical practice for many clinicians.

Often a clinic visit with someone with a chronic condition involves the caregiver as well. It is important to address the caregiver when the patient has given permission. The same techniques are used with the caregiver.

> **PHYSICIAN:** *John, is it okay if I ask your wife a few questions now?* (John nods assent.) *What has it been like caring for your husband?*
>
> **WIFE:** *Since the Alzheimer's diagnosis, I've had to learn a lot of new things. See, he used to do all the banking. I didn't know anything about where our money was. Now we do it together. Sometimes he loses his temper when he can't do something. That's not like him at all.*
>
> **PATIENT:** *Oh, I know all about our accounts. We have money at the downtown bank and the one by the mall. What's that one called?*
>
> **PHYSICIAN:** *Thank you, John.* (To wife) *I was wondering if you ever get a break from caregiving. Is anyone helping you?*
>
> **WIFE:** *Yes, my daughter comes over every Thursday afternoon so I can run errands.*

The physician has elicited the caregiver concerns and is paying attention to caregiver burden.

Caring for patients with chronic illness can be very rewarding when a partnership is formed between the professional and the patient. A slightly expanded framework for Function Three in collaborative management for chronic illness care includes the three broad areas of goal setting, action planning, and problem solving. Keeping all three areas in mind leads to improved outcomes.

## Summary

This chapter provides recommendations for longitudinal and evolving care and communication over time with patients who have chronic medical conditions using the framework of the three function model of the medical interview.

### References

1. Anderson G: *Chronic conditions: making the case for ongoing care*, Baltimore, MD, 2004, Johns Hopkins University.
2. Corbin J, Strauss A: *Unending work and care: managing chronic illness at home*, San Francisco, 1999, Jossey Bass.
3. Moos RH, Holahan CJ: Adaptive tasks and methods of coping with illness and disability. In Martz E, Livneh H, editors: *Coping with chronic illness and disablity*, Memphis, 2007, Springer.

4. Barlow J, et al: Self-management approaches for people with chronic conditions: a review. *Patient Educ Couns* 48(2):177–187, 2002.

5. Glasgow RE, et al: Implementing practical interventions to support chronic illness self-management. *Jt Comm J Qual Saf* 29(11):563–574, 2003.

6. Lorig K, et al: A comparison of lay-taught and professional-taught arthritis self-management courses. *J Rheumatol* 13(4):763–767, 1986.

7. Lorig K, et al: *Living a healthy life with chronic conditions (2nd Edition)*, Boulder CO, 2000, Bull Publishing.

## *Endnotes*

A. Medicare data and Harris polls of Medicare recipients
B. Partnerships for Solutions
C. For detailed discussion of 8 different strategies that patients use to cope with chronic physical illnesses, see Moos RH, Holahan CJ: Adaptive tasks and methods of coping with illness and disability, In Martz E, Livneh H (ed), *Coping with chronic illness and disability,* Springer, Memphis, 2007

# CHAPTER 20

# Health Literacy and Communicating Complex Information for Decision Making

Connie Davis ■ Khati Hendry

## OVERVIEW

If a physician wants to successfully communicate complex health information, health literacy must be taken into account. This chapter provides techniques to help patients understand basic and complex health information and to make choices.

## Why Health Literacy Matters

Health literacy has been defined as "The degree to which individuals have the capacity to obtain, process and understand basic health information and services needed to make appropriate health decisions."[1] Capacity refers to innate abilities as well as skills obtained throughout life; therefore educational level, culture, language, and the health care environment all play a role in determining a patient's health literacy. Health literacy includes spoken information, written information, and information from numbers (numeracy), including concepts of risk and benefit.

This definition has been criticized because it does not convey the demands placed on the patient from the health care system or the environment and does not consider the patient's emotional state during the interaction. Perhaps a better description of health literacy is when the patient's ability to understand, process, and use health information is equal to the demands placed on that person in an environment in which the patient feels respected and trusts the health care professional.

Surveys in the United States indicate that 93 million people have only basic literacy skills, but the majority of information (medication package inserts, pamphlets, consent forms) is written well above this level. Of those 93 million, 15% are functionally health illiterate.[2] Studies of numeracy among patients with diabetes indicate that 1 in 10 patients with diabetes have trouble understanding glucometer data.[3]

Low health literacy decreases the patient's ability to make treatment decisions, lowers adherence to treatment, increases the likelihood of poor disease control, lowers self-reported health status, lessens use of preventive services, and increases health care use.[4] Lower health literacy makes it harder for people to navigate health care environments and access needed services.

Health literacy problems contribute to safety and quality problems and are expensive. It is estimated that by not addressing health literacy, health care costs are increased by $106 to $238 billion dollars.[5]

# Health Literacy and the Three Function Model

Concepts and skills from the Three Function Model can help the physician address issues of health literacy.

## FUNCTION ONE: BUILD THE RELATIONSHIP

### Conveying Respect

Shame is common among patients with low health literacy and it is critical for the physician to acknowledge this issue and convey respect.

Example:

> PHYSICIAN: *I work with many patients who did not have a chance to attend much school and who are very successful in managing their health.*

## FUNCTION TWO: ASSESS AND UNDERSTAND THE PATIENT

Along with eliciting problems during the patient interview, the physician can follow universal precautions for health literacy. This concept, like universal precautions for infection control, implies that anyone may have difficulty understanding information in a health context. Physicians can be alert to cues that indicate low health literacy, such as reluctance to complete forms.

> PHYSICIAN: *I forgot my glasses so I'll take this form home".*

or

Patient nodding but not asking questions or speaking much during an interview.

Physician skills in checking or summarizing contribute to increased understanding and decrease barriers caused by low health literacy. Schillinger et al. have described this skill as "closing the loop" and found that it increases the number of patients with better control of their diabetes, as reflected in lower HbA1c levels.[6]

Example:

> PHYSICIAN: *Can you tell me how you will take this medication so I know that I made it clear?*
>
> PATIENT: (repeats his or her understanding)
>
> PHYSICIAN: *Yes, you will take it daily. Just make sure to take it in the morning 1 hour before you eat breakfast so the medicine can already be working by the time you eat.* (reinforcing what was understood and clarifying any misunderstood information)

It is very important that the onus of making the information clear rests with the physician.

## FUNCTION THREE: COLLABORATE TO MANAGE

elicit-Tell-Ask-Care-Counsel-Tell Back ((e)TACCT) provides an excellent method to provide information to the person with low health literacy. Avoiding jargon, limiting the amount of information provided to essential points, focusing on short, action-oriented phrases, using plain language, incorporating drawings into explanations, and relating information to prior knowledge will improve communication.

Terminology familiar to physicians may be foreign to patients. Studies indicate that in some populations, two out of three patients misunderstand common medical terms such as orally, terminal, and biopsy.[7] Stating that a test result was negative may not sound like a good thing to patients with low literacy. To avoid these sorts of problems, physicians must choose words carefully and then have the patient "tell back" what he or she understood.

# Communicating Complex Information for Decision Making

Communicating risk or options for treatment presents unique challenges. In this section, examples are given on how the Three Function Model can be used to communicate complex information for decision making, adapting it to accommodate a low health literacy level. The goal is to share decision making to the degree that patients desire to be involved, balancing the physician's power with the patient's choice.

## FUNCTION ONE: BUILD THE RELATIONSHIP

Health care decisions are often life altering. A close, respectful working relationship between patient and physician makes difficult conversations possible and has been shown to enhance decision making.[8]

## FUNCTION TWO: ASSESS AND UNDERSTAND THE PATIENT

Several of the skills in Function Two deserve special emphasis.

### Elicit Expectations

When information regarding risk or treatment decisions needs to be discussed, eliciting the patient's experience with the illness or treatment will help set the stage for a useful conversation and can help to assess his or her health literacy. Choose appropriate words and examples that the patient can easily understand.

Examples:

> **PHYSICIAN:** *Have you ever had this or something like this before?*
>
> or
>
> **PHYSICIAN:** *Has anyone you know ever had this before?*
>
> or
>
> **PHYSICIAN:** *What are you expecting will be the results of the treatment?*

After gaining an understanding of the patient's expectations and experience with the kind of risk or treatment being discussed, it can be useful to emphasize the partnership (Function One).

Example:

> **PHYSICIAN:** *Making this decision might make you feel uneasy. I will do my best to provide you with information so we can work on this decision together.*

Eliciting expectations also includes eliciting patient values. Here are some examples of discussions designed to elicit values, including a discussion about resuscitation:

Example in an office setting:

> **PHYSICIAN:** *Sometimes in health care we are faced with decisions that are difficult. This may be one of those times. I'd like to know a little more about what matters the most to you in your life.*
>
> or
>
> **PHYSICIAN:** *If your heart were to stop this very minute right here in my office, would you want me to do CPR?*
>
> or
>
> **PHYSICIAN:** *What, for you, makes life worth living?*

Example with a hospitalized patient:

**PHYSICIAN:** *Tell me what you understand about your medical condition.*

**PATIENT:** *Well, something is wrong with my pancreas. The doctor in emergency asked me lots of questions about my drinking, so I guess it's because of that. You know, times have been hard lately. I have been hitting the bottle more. But I'm not an alcoholic.*

**PHYSICIAN:** *So you understand that you have a problem with your pancreas. We call it pancreatitis. It is linked to your drinking. We expect you to recover from this illness. Have you ever thought about what you would like to have done for you if in the future you had an illness that was much worse? I want to be clear, I am not thinking about right now, but in the future with a more serious illness.*

**PATIENT:** *You mean like if I needed to be hooked up to machines to breathe or something like that?*

**PHYSICIAN:** *Yes, something like that.*

**PATIENT:** *Well, that happened to my dad and it was awful. He just laid there for days after his stroke and I thought we should just let him go. My sister, though, she was hoping for a miracle.*

**PHYSICIAN:** *Would you want us to do everything for you?*

**PATIENT:** *Not if I'm not going to get better! If I can't go out with the boys to a game or go back to my job, I think it's over.*

**PHYSICIAN:** *So it would be important to you that care be given if you could recover. You wouldn't want extra measures, like a breathing machine, if it wasn't going to help.*

**PATIENT:** *That's right.*

**PHYSICIAN:** *Thanks for sharing this information with me. Now let's focus again on what is happening now and helping you get better.*

Notice how the physician used simple questions to elicit the patient's views, used simple and reassuring words to convey information, summarized and checked back with the patient, and emphasized the partnership at the end of this example.

## FUNCTION THREE: COLLABORATE TO MANAGE

Before beginning any educational intervention, it is reasonable to elicit a patient's current level of understanding. For example:

**PHYSICIAN:** *Before I discuss things you might be able to do to help prevent a stroke or heart attack, I thought I would ask what ideas you have about things you can do to prevent a heart attack or stroke, so I don't go over things you may already know about.*

Several techniques may be helpful when providing complex information for treatment decisions or risk reduction.

A technique recommended by some experts is to provide basic information before determining how involved in decision making a patient would like to be.

Example:

**PHYSICIAN:** *There are three choices for treatment to decrease your risk of having a heart attack or stroke. The risk is there because of your blood pressure and cholesterol levels. One choice is to make changes in your daily life. The second choice is to take pills. The third choice is to combine life changes with pills. How would you like to make this decision?*

**PATIENT:** *I'd like to hear more about these treatments and think it over for a while.*

Another technique is to state that uncertainty exists when conveying complex information requiring choices.

Example:

> PHYSICIAN: *There has been a lot of research on this treatment, but it is not totally clear what to do next. Here is what we know now about the choices.*

Patients are sometimes surprised that a treatment that was formerly recommended is no longer practiced. To help explain this discrepancy, it helps to use the technique of acknowledging and briefly explaining the change.

Example:

> PHYSICIAN: *We used to always treat an ear infection with a medicine to kill the germs. Studies show that when the pain lasts less than 2 days, the medicines do not help and may cause problems.*

The physician can present his or her viewpoint during the conversation if the patient has indicated he or she prefers the professional to make decisions or collaborate on decisions—another useful technique.

Example:

> PHYSICIAN: *I think it is fine to hold off on medicine for now, but if the ear pain continues, we can start the medication.*

To convey the benefits and risks of a treatment, the physician can use the technique of presenting benefits and risks together.

Example:

> PHYSICIAN: *I would like to suggest this medicine to decrease your chance of having another blood clot. It could make you more likely to bleed, so we will need to follow it carefully by having regular blood tests and watching for signs of bleeding.*

Tips for improving communication of numerical data include using absolute risk instead of relative risk and providing information in different ways to avoid the bias for one choice over the other. In some studies, patients have been shown to prefer ratios over percentages, such as:

> *1 out of 10 people will have this problem.*
>
> *compared with*
>
> *10% will have this problem.*

Ratios can also be displayed with stick figures or faces to indicate the numbers affected, although it has been noted that people tend to identify with the healthier proportion.[7]

Examples:

> PHYSICIAN: *We have been checking your blood pressure over several visits now. For people like you with high blood pressure, if it stays high, 1 out of 10 of them will have a stroke or heart attack in the next 10 years.*
>
> or
>
> PHYSICIAN: *If we treat your high cholesterol, we can reduce your risk of having a heart attack in the next 10 years from 10 chances out of 100 down to 7 out of 100.*

Occasionally patients have heard risk reduction presented in the media as relative risk reduction, such as "treatment A reduces fractures by 30%." Using the technique of a familiar analogy, such as a sale discount, may help patients understand this statistic.

Example:

> PHYSICIAN: *Saying that the reduction in fractures is 30% only tells part of the story. Would you buy a car if it were 30% off?*

**PATIENT:** *That would depend on how much the car was in the first place.*

**PHYSICIAN:** *Exactly. If it were a $10,000 dollar car, 30% off would make the price $7000. If it were a $100,000 motor home, 30% off would make the price $70,000. That's a big difference. In your case, we have calculated your risk of having a fracture in the next 10 years as 12 chances out of 100. This medication could decrease that by 30%, which would make your risk of having a fracture 8 chances out of 100. The report you heard also didn't mention that the medication has some possible side effects, as all medications do. The chance of having a side effect with this medication is 15 out of 100.*

Providing complex information can be a challenging task, but the physician who has developed a caring relationship with the patient will find it well worth the effort.

## Special Considerations Using Written Materials

Written materials can be useful tools for providing education during the Tell-Act-Care-Counsel-Tell back process. Several groups have developed guidance for presentation materials.[9] Important tips include:

- Use a minimum of 12-point font (14-point if the document targets seniors).
- Use a sans serif font (e.g., Verdana, Helvetica, Arial, Tahoma).
- Avoid special effects for fonts (outlining, shadows).
- Use dark letters on a light background.
- Use left justification and ragged right text.
- Use bold text for emphasis instead of underlining or italics.
- Use upper and lower case normally.
- Increase the amount of white space on the page.
- Use simple line drawings.
- Use basic punctuation.
- Avoid abbreviations.
- Use the simplest words possible.
- Aim for sentences no longer than 20 words.
- Use few words with more than three syllables.
- Field-test your document on the population that will be using it, and make modifications based on feedback.
- Although word processing programs may feature estimates of reading levels of written materials, this does not ensure that a person will be able to understand and make use of the information. These assessments also do not consider numeracy. That said, these programs may be the only tool available to the busy clinician. There are also some interactive web-based tools available to determine reading effectiveness.[10]
- Written documents supplement spoken explanations, they do not replace them.

Because a physician is likely to work with patients of differing levels of health literacy, a useful strategy is to make sure that printed materials begin with simple, basic information on page 1 and progress to more detailed information on page 2 so that patients can choose the level of detail that suits their needs.[11] It is very important not to make low literacy level materials childish. For example, cartoons are not well accepted by many members of the public for conveying health information, but photo-novellas or comics are welcome by certain age and ethnic groups. Usability testing with the target audience will aid in determination of appropriate materials.

The skilled physician adjusts his or her delivery for each patient and is able to communicate the preferred amount of information in an understandable manner. This is done in an atmosphere of trust and respect. Physicians can use the concepts and skills of the Three Function Model to efficiently address common tasks and challenges of health literacy.

## References

1. Ratzan SC, Parker RM: Introduction. In Selden CR, et al, editors: *National Library of Medicine: Current bibliographies in medicine: health literacy.* NLM Pub. No. CBM 2000-2001. Bethesda, MD, 2000, National Institutes of Health, US Department of Health and Human Services.
2. Kutner M, et al: *The health literacy of America's adults: results from the 2003 National Assessment of Adult Literacy (NCES 2006-2483), US Department of Education*, Washington DC, 2006, National Center for Education Statistics.
3. Montori V, et al: Validation of a diabetes numeracy evaluation tool. *Diabetes* 53(suppl 1):A224–A225, 2004.
4. DeWalt DA, Berkman ND, Sheridan S, Lohr KN, Pignone MP: Literacy and health outcomes. *Journal of General Internal Medicine* 19(12):1228–1239, 2004.
5. Nielsen-Bohlman L, Panzer AM, Kindig DA, editors: *Health literacy: a prescription to end confusion.* Washington DC IOM, 2004, National Academies Press, pp 28–29.
6. Schillinger D, et al: Closing the loop: physician communication with diabetic patients who have low health literacy. *Arch Intern Med* 163:83–90, 2003.
7. Davis TC, Dolan N, Ferreira MR: The role of inadequate health literacy skills in colorectal cancer screening. *Cancer Investment* 19:193–200, 2001.
8. Epstein RM, Alper BS, Quill TE: Communicating evidence for participatory decision making. *JAMA* 291(19):2359–2366, 2004.
9. Plain English guide to design and layout. 2001: Plain English Campaign, www.plainenglish.co.uk.
10. Reading effectiveness tool: www.castendliteracy.on.ca/clearlanguageanddesign/readingeffectivenesstool.
11. Morrow DG, et al: Patients' health literacy and experience with instructions: individual preferences for heart failure medication instructions. *J Aging Health* 19(4):575–593, 2007.

# CHAPTER 21

# Sexual Issues in the Interview

Mary DeGenaro Cole ■ Steven Cole

## OVERVIEW

This chapter provides recommendations for addressing issues of sexuality in the medical interview.

Sexual behavior is part of the human experience and unique to every individual. Talking about sex openly and freely has not yet become a socially acceptable topic of conversation in all cultures. Despite the continual presence of sexually explicit images in magazines, on Internet sites, and on television, the issue of sexuality remains cloaked in secrecy, poor education, misunderstanding, and lack of knowledge. The reluctance to discuss sex extends to medical and nonmedical members of our community alike, creating the need for a separate chapter in this book to open discussion for physicians, medical students, and other health care professionals (i.e., clinicians).

Even though sex may be considered a private matter, sexual profiles are part of a patient's medical history, health status, treatment plan, and follow-up. Although clinicians tend to circumvent both subjects that risk embarrassment to themselves or patients and questions that trigger distress, shame, and humiliation, avoiding these issues leads to bad medical care. Good interviewing skills regarding sexuality require intellectual as well as emotional effort.

## Why Are Sexual Issues Important?

Clinicians deal with issues of sexuality because they commonly affect patients of all ages, from contraception to infertility, sexually transmitted diseases (STDs), erectile dysfunction (ED), and in some cases, rape and abuse. A patient's illness may be a consequence of sexual contact, as with human immunodeficiency virus (HIV), hepatitis B, and human papillomavirus. Knowledge of a patient's sexual orientation tells the clinician something about the person as an individual. Sexual behavior guides medical screening, diagnoses, and education.

It is no longer difficult to convince medical students in the world of HIV and acquired immunodeficiency syndrome (AIDS) that interviewing patients about sexuality is important to medical care. The prevalence and severity of these conditions create a mandate that all patients must be educated and evaluated about this epidemic. Therefore interviewing about sexuality remains a core component of clinician-patient communication.

Besides HIV and AIDS, numerous other STDs cause significant morbidity and mortality. Health care practitioners must understand these conditions and develop the ability to obtain appropriate information during the interview to assess risk.

The importance of interviewing about sexuality goes far beyond the ability to assess and manage STDs. Most important, sexuality is one of the core dimensions of a patient's quality of life. Primary sexual disorders are common (e.g., anorgasmia and impotence), and sexual dysfunction secondary to chronic physical illnesses (e.g., spinal cord injury, coronary artery disease, hypertension, depression) or its treatment is almost universal.

Few patients with chronic illness escape the sexual problems commonly associated with the condition or its treatment. Typical problems include decreased libido or decreased competence (e.g., impaired erection, impaired ejaculation, or impaired orgasmic function). These problems can result from illness or medication used to treat illness. Patients do not typically discuss these problems unless asked about them. Unfortunately, sexual dysfunction often leads to a significant impairment in quality of life and relationship problems with a spouse or significant other.

Sexual problems often become crucial to determining patients' overall adjustment to their illnesses. Evaluation of sexual dysfunction thus is one of the core competencies of good medical interviewing.

In general, interviewing regarding sexual issues is most effective when the basic skills of the Three Function Model are applied to the sexual dimension of health and illness.

## Function One: Build the Relationship

Because discussions surrounding sexuality can cause great embarrassment, it is usually helpful for the clinician to address potential emotional discomfort even before difficult subjects are raised. For example, at the start of this part of the interview, the clinician might say something such as the following:

> I need to ask you some questions about your sex life. These questions often make patients uncomfortable, but I want to assure you that they are a routine part of the medical evaluation. I ask them of all my patients, and they often provide information that is important to good medical care.

With this type of introduction, most patients are better able to discuss their sex life without great distress. If it becomes clear that the patient is uncomfortable, the physician can use the relationship skills discussed earlier in the text: reflection, legitimation, support, partnership, and respect. For example:

> PHYSICIAN: *I see these questions are making you uncomfortable.* (**reflection**)
>
> *This is understandable.* (**legitimation**)
>
> *Most people do find them difficult.* (**legitimation**)
>
> *I appreciate your efforts to be open.* (**respect**)
>
> *You should understand that I am only asking about what I consider to be important for your medical care.* (**support**)
>
> *Do you think you and I can proceed along this line a bit further to complete what is needed for a thorough medical assessment?* (**partnership**)

Building the relationship is important for successful interviewing about sexual issues. If the patient does not feel comfortable or agree to this line of questioning, it is generally useless for the student or physician to proceed; without a cooperative patient, the information obtained will be suspect—either incomplete or incorrect. Thus relationship building must continue until the physician has a willing partner.

Sensitivity to patients' cultural and religious values is essential. Patients of different cultures have radically different views regarding the propriety of discussing sexual activity with others. Religion also dictates what is considered acceptable behavior. The only way to be relatively confident that you are not offending a patient's cultural or religious sensitivity is to make sure you inform the patient about what you are about to ask before you proceed at each step, assuring him or her that these are routine questions you ask all your patients. If the patient objects to any line of questioning, you should honor his or her objections and omit the questions. Proceeding "over" objections will impair rapport and rarely lead to honest replies anyway.

It is important to determine and use the patient's own language and point of view at the beginning of the interview. Does he or she have a partner, husband, or wife? Be careful not to casually use opposite sex language that assumes heterosexuality, and be aware that age, education, and culture impact patients' understanding of certain terms, such as "safe sex" or "birth control." Another caveat is the place of sex within each patient's culture and religion.

## Function Two: Assess and Understand the Problem

Efficient and effective data gathering about sexuality requires use of the same skills discussed earlier in the text: open-ended questioning, facilitation, surveying, and checking. Because of the sensitive nature of these topics, the skilled interviewer usually relies more heavily on attentive silence (as a facilitative technique), surveying, and specific closed-ended questions. The content of data gathering about sexual issues generally falls into one of two domains: (1) basic evaluation of risk (for STDs, primary sexual problems, use of protection, and history of abuse); and (2) evaluation of the impact of chronic illness on the sexual quality of life.

### BASIC EVALUATION OF RISK

A basic evaluation of risk (for STDs, primary sexual problems, use of protection, and history of sexual abuse) is now considered a standard part of the routine medical examination. This separate chapter has been added to discuss the challenging dimensions of the interview process because these topics raise anxiety for both medical students and patients.

As discussed, the clinician should lessen patient apprehension before beginning this line of questioning by making it clear that he or she asks all patients these questions. Questions about sexuality should begin in an open-ended manner and proceed to closed-ended questioning for purposes of clarification. Attentive silence is a particularly useful facilitative technique to help patients overcome their reluctance to speak about potentially embarrassing issues. Surveying about potential sexual issues is also a useful technique. Finally, specific closed-ended questions may be useful to identify specific information.

Throughout the sexual interview, the clinician should monitor the patient's emotional responses closely. When questions seem to increase a patient's anxiety, the interview should address this concern directly. In general, complete medical interviews should include an evaluation of the patient's sexual orientation, sexual history, exposure to STDs, and use of protection during sexual intercourse, as well as a screening for sexual problems. In light of emerging data linking childhood sexual abuse with later unexplained physical complaints, patients should also be screened for a history of sexual abuse.

> PHYSICIAN: *As I mentioned earlier, I need to ask you some questions about your sex life that sometimes cause patients embarrassment. I need to assure you that I ask everyone these questions and the information I obtain may be important for your medical care.* (Function One)
>
> *Can we start with you telling me something about your sex life?* (Function Two)

In response to an open-ended question like this, patients frequently answer with a question, asking the clinician to be more specific. For example:

> PATIENT: *What would you like to know?*

Depending on the age, sex, or interview situation, the clinician can use one or more of the following suggestions. If the patient has a chronic illness or specific symptoms, a useful opening often focuses on the impact of the illness or symptoms on the patient's sex life.

PHYSICIAN: *Can you tell me how this illness has affected your sex life?*

or

PHYSICIAN: *Can you tell me a bit about your sex life? Tell me about your partner or partners?*

Surveying can be helpful in the domain of sexual interviewing:

PHYSICIAN: *Perhaps you can tell me if you have any issues, concerns, or problems regarding your sex life.*

Attentive and supportive silence is particularly valuable after a question like this because the patient typically needs a few moments to decide on disclosing potentially embarrassing information. In response to a combination of open-ended questioning, surveying, and attentive silence, most patients give the clinician some basic information that can guide follow-up questions.

Eventually, open questioning will need to be followed by closed questioning to obtain very specific answers to very explicit and sometimes distressing questions. For example:

PHYSICIAN: *This information you have given me is especially helpful. I do need to ask a few more detailed questions now.*

*How often have you had unprotected sexual intercourse in the last 2 years? How many different sexual partners have you had in the last 2 years? Have you experienced any difficulties in your sexual desire or activity in the last 2 years? Have you ever experienced any unwelcome sexual advances, perhaps long ago during your childhood?*

## IMPACT OF CHRONIC ILLNESS ON SEXUAL QUALITY OF LIFE

Most chronically ill patients suffer sexual dysfunction but feel reluctant to discuss the experience. Despite embarrassment caused by discussing sexual issues, it is an important part of medical evaluation. If possible, try to detoxify the issue by "normalizing" dysfunction during data gathering.
For example:

PHYSICIAN: *Most patients with your type of illness experience some sexual problems. What kind of difficulties have you been having?*

The judicious use of facilitation, such as attentive silence, head nodding, and the use of certain phrases ("uh-huh," "tell me more") can be enormously helpful at this point, leading to patient disclosure of important and sensitive information.

Because patients tend to provide sensitive information in small chunks, checking helps confirm accuracy and also serves as a facilitative technique for obtaining more information from the patient. For example:

PHYSICIAN: *Let me see if I understand you correctly. You have noticed that the chest pain seems to have gotten in the way of your sex life. You don't seem to have intercourse as often as you did before your illness began. Can you tell me more about … ?*

Clarification is essential in interviewing about sexuality because embarrassment often leads to vagueness. Physicians must become very concrete to help their patients be specific. For example:

PHYSICIAN: *I do understand your point about the decreasing frequency of intercourse. But it would help me understand you better if you could be more specific. How often were you and your partner having sexual intercourse before you got sick and how often are you having intercourse now?*

Many patients with chronic illnesses notice that sexual issues, among other problems, can impair relationships with their partners. This can lead to a crucial loss of social support, which in itself is a risk factor for further morbidity and mortality. It is important for physicians to assess these potential problem areas:

> **PHYSICIAN:** *You have told me a little about the sexual problems that have emerged as a result of this illness. How have these problems interfered with your relationship with your spouse?*

## Function Three: Collaborate for Management

Education and action planning for sexual problems rely on the same Function Three interviewing skills discussed earlier (see Chapter 5). Because of the concerns of sensitivity and embarrassment, extra attention must be paid to patient understanding and commitment. Clinicians should not say things such as, "Do you understand what I have been saying?" or "Remember to practice safe sex, okay?" It is far better to use checking, (e)TACCT. techniques of "tell-back" (see Chapter 5), and explicitly elicit statements of commitment from the patient:

> **PHYSICIAN:** *To make sure that I have communicated clearly, could you please review for me what we have been discussing about safe sex techniques?*
>
> or
>
> **PHYSICIAN:** *Just to make sure I understand what you would like to do about safe sex, could you review for me what it is that you are planning to do?*

## Managing Your Own Anxiety or Attitudinal Barriers

Talking about sexual issues causes most students and physicians significant anxiety, particularly as you first learn these skills. This discomfort is normal. Students are simply not accustomed to asking people intimate details about their sex lives.

The difficulty of sexual interviewing, of course, varies among individual clinicians and patient groups, depending on personal psychology and experience. There are some general patterns, however. Most individuals find asking older patients of the opposite sex questions about their sexual lives particularly difficult. Some interviewers may specifically feel this is like asking their own parents about their sex lives. Others find it difficult to conduct sexual interviews with a patient to whom they feel attracted.

These issues are common. Mastery requires an attitude of self-acceptance and understanding. The interviewer must assume that this is a standard part of clinical practice and yet, as a professional, must learn to develop appropriate emotional distance and at the same time a sense of absolute boundaries. Flirtatious, suggestive conduct is not acceptable; nor are any questions or any overt physical contact that are not clearly medically necessary ethically permissible.

Many students and physicians bring personal biases about sexual orientation or behavior to their work with patients. Such prejudice should not be part of medical care. In fairness to their patients, students or physicians who are burdened with negative attitudes should use self-examination and discussion with colleagues or supervisors to overcome these barriers to objective care. Role-play is a convenient and effective way to practice interviewing about sexuality. Using role-play to practice interviewing skills, with feedback from instructors and peers, offers an unequaled opportunity to gain proficiency and master anxiety or other barriers. All clinicians owe this to their patients: to bring to them an unbiased, objective ability to elicit, assess, and manage sexual issues in medical practice.

## Managing Specific Problems

Numerous sexual problems require intervention by the physician. A failure to practice safe sex (as discussed previously) is only one example. Others include the patient who is suffering from sexual problems related to illness (e.g., the stroke patient with physical obstacles to intercourse), the patient with decreased arousal secondary to the use of antidepressant medication, or the patient who is currently at risk for sexual abuse. Physicians must develop knowledge of initial management strategies (when, how, and where to make appropriate referrals) for these and other common sexual problems. A discussion of specific management approaches is beyond the scope of this text. However, the interviewing skills necessary to uncover the problems need to be acquired at an early stage of every medical career.

## Conclusion

Interviewing about sexuality and sexual problems remains a complex and difficult dimension of the medical interview. Understanding its importance and relying on the basic skills of the Three Function Model can help most beginning interviewers become adept in this domain. In particular, use of initial rapport-building techniques to establish partnership, along with the use of attentive silence, surveying, direct questioning, and checking, can help interviewers reach a high level of competence in sexually oriented interviewing.

# CHAPTER 22

# Interviewing Elderly Patients

Catherine Nicastri ■ Steven Cole

## OVERVIEW

Interviewing elderly patients presents particular challenges to the beginning student, as it also does for physicians in practice. In particular, common patient disabilities and problems such as hearing or vision loss, cognitive impairment, social isolation, personal loss, and physical impairment present obstacles that must be overcome to have a successful interview with the elderly patient.

Careful and sensitive application of the basic skills of the Three Function Model can meet most of the complex challenges associated with interviewing elderly patients. This chapter examines each of the three functions separately, with analysis of the ways the basic skills and communication techniques can be applied to maximize efficiency and effectiveness in the interview with elderly patients.

## Function One: Build the Relationship with the Elderly Patient

Because elderly patients often find the medical setting cumbersome, insensitive, and unresponsive to their needs, it is often helpful to anticipate this difficulty by screening for elderly patients' frustrations early in the interview and to take a few extra moments to build initial rapport. Even a few moments finding out patients' experiences and difficulties with the health care system can be particularly revealing and help cement the relationship for the future. An effort should be made to understand the patients' predicaments and empathize with their personal troubles. Elderly patients are often perceived as being homogeneous because of age, but in fact their life experiences have created a very heterogeneous patient population. It is important to recognize this when communicating with your patients so as to understand their individual needs. When people have lived to an old age, chances are they have experienced personal loss; for example, death of a loved one, loss of function and independence, and they may have feelings of worthlessness secondary to an inability to work and contribute to society as they did in the past.[1] They can be experiencing frustration, grieving, and insecurity, among other emotions.[1,6] The skills of reflection, legitimation, support, partnership, and respect should be used when listening and communicating with them to acknowledge that you are hearing about their frustrations, loss, and concerns. The value of the initial investment of a few extra minutes in this endeavor will be the efficiency it will bring to later visits.

A physician recently saw an elderly patient with Parkinson's disease and depression. The patient began the interview by noting that he had had numerous bad experiences with physicians and the health care system. The physician listened attentively and used rapport-building skills liberally in the initial 5 minutes. Although this patient had numerous criticisms of other physicians whom he had seen previously, the interviewer did not have to join in this criticism to build rapport. Straightforward empathic communication was sufficient.

*It certainly seems like you have had some troubling experiences with the medical system.* (**reflection**)

*I can understand how you felt insignificant and unimportant.* (**legitimation**)

*I want you to know that I care about your difficulties and I will do the very best I can to work with you to develop a plan to bring you some relief.* (**support and partnership**)

These relatively brief relationship-building interventions led to a meaningful, long-lasting relationship with this patient. The sense of caring communicated by this brief exchange facilitated the development of trust that was essential to ensure optimal clinical outcomes.

Often the elderly patient is accompanied to the medical visit by a family member or caregiver, creating a complex triadic relationship among the physician, patient, and third person. This third party may impact the interview and the physician-patient relationship in either a negative or positive way. This third party in the interview can positively facilitate the encounter by offering more information, voicing the patient's views, serving as a translator, or offering another opinion. On the other hand, the third party may hinder the relationship or encounter by suppressing the patient's ability to communicate freely or drawing the physician's attention away from the patient during the encounter when the physician addresses the third party. The third party may take on many roles during an encounter based on the length of the visit, content, and ability of the patient to communicate. Regardless of whether the third party's role is positive or negative, it changes the physician-patient interaction and relationship.[2,3]

Elderly people, when accompanied by another person, "raise fewer topics across all content areas (medical, personal habits, psychosocial and physician-patient relationship),"[2] are less responsive to topics raised, are less assertive, ask fewer questions, and are not forthcoming with personal information.[2] Therefore it is important to address all parties during the interview rather than directing questions and answers exclusively to the patient or the third person. Avoid only making eye contact with the third person even if he or she is answering most of the questions, for example, when a patient has cognitive impairment or other communication barriers. The physician may strategically position himself or herself between the patient and the third person to allow eye contact and direct communication with both.

To ensure that the encounter is not negatively affected by the third party, the physician should ask the third party to step out of the exam room for the physical exam. At this time the physician may encourage further questioning and conversation with the patient. There are also instances in which the physician may need to speak with the third party alone to discuss sensitive issues such as patient safety in the cognitively impaired individual, which may or may not warrant the permission of the elderly person. The relationship between the physician and family and/or caregiver is often necessary to gather information to help care for the elderly patient and help build rapport with the elderly person and the family. This relationship between physician and caregiver/family member is particularly useful when the patient has limitations in communicating such as cognitive impairment, low health literacy, psychological impairment, or language barriers. The physician must meet with and build a relationship with the caregivers and family. When conflict or difficulty arises, it is important to meet with the significant others and listen to their difficulties too. Again, the initial investment in relationship building will pay enormous dividends later.

For example:

**PHYSICIAN:** (to caregiver) *I would like to hear your thoughts on how your husband (father, grandfather ... ) is doing. How has it been for you?*

**FAMILY MEMBER:** *Well, it has been very difficult.*

PHYSICIAN: *I can certainly understand why this has been so hard. I think you've been doing a terrific job coping with these problems under the circumstances.* (**respect**)

Triad:

PHYSICIAN: (to elderly patient in private) *Now that your son (daughter, caregiver) has left the room, are there any concerns that you would like to address?*

PATIENT: *I do not feel I can talk freely in front of my son (daughter ... ) because he always has an opinion.*

PHYSICIAN: *I can understand why you would feel this way. I would like to reassure you that whenever you come in with another family member I will take the time to meet with you alone so you will be able to speak freely.*

## Function Two: Assess and Understand the Elderly Patient

The assessment of the elderly patient uses the same skills that are used in assessing younger patients. When multiple disabilities and dysfunction come into play, however, more thoughtful attention to use of the basic skills becomes increasingly important. Careful listening is essential. With the elderly patient, as with all patients, the physician must use open-ended questions, facilitation, surveying, and checking. It is important to note that open-ended questions do not work on patients with expressive aphasia. Rather the physician should ask yes-no questions to help elicit a history. Because the prevalence of cognitive impairment increases with age, all elderly patients must receive the cognitive screen as part of the mental status examination (see Chapter 14). Pointing out that questions about orientation and memory are routine for all patients can help diffuse patient anxiety and resistance.

As discussed in earlier chapters, when communicating with your patients there are certain rules one must follow. For many reasons, checking (or summarizing) is particularly important in interviews with elderly patients. Because of hearing, vision, cognitive, or communication difficulties, elderly patients may not succeed in transmitting information accurately to the physician the first time. Similarly, when cognitive deficits may be present, checking information received helps confirm the reliability of the information. Checking is important with the elderly because the narratives of their medical histories are generally complex. These complexities multiply the possibilities for errors, misunderstandings, and omissions. Given the potential problems of the interview, the interviewer of elderly people should take sufficient time to check his or her accurate understanding of the problem(s). This can save enormous time down the road. Checking is the most important data-gathering skill to use with elderly patients.

For example:

PHYSICIAN: *With so much going on in your life, let me repeat back to you what I have just heard to make sure I have understood your problems correctly.*

After relying on the skill of checking, the interviewer should pay special attention to the family and caregivers as sources of key information. An adequate assessment of the elderly patient must always include input from the family.

PHYSICIAN: (to family) *I have spent some time with your spouse (father, grandmother ... ). Please let me know how you think she's been doing.*

## Function Three: Collaborate for Management

Just as the first two functions require some particular attention and focus, so too does the third function when dealing with elderly patients. Education and self-management support require careful use of all the skills discussed earlier in this text. For elderly patients with significant disabilities, however, special attention to some of the basic skills becomes particularly pertinent. Perhaps the most important management skill for the elderly is *checking of understanding, or using the Teach-Back Technique.*

In addition to the physician checking that he or she understands the information the elderly patient is relaying, it is also important to check that the elderly patient understands what he or she needs to know about his or her own health. The Teach-Back Technique has been used to assess understanding of medical information at the office visit. By using the Teach-Back Technique we can ensure that we are communicating to elderly patients in a way that is understandable to them.[4] The physician is essentially asking the patient to relay back to him or her in the patient's own words the information that's just been given. If the patient is unable to reiterate the information, then the physician will need to change the teaching method until the patient understands. (Note: Teach-Back is the last step of (e)TACCT, the acronym for educational messages in Function Three; see Chapter 5).

Confirming that your patient understands necessary health information is especially important given the high prevalence of limited health literacy in the elderly population.[5] In 2003, the National Assessment of Adult Literacy (NAAL) reported that 39% of Americans have limited health literacy, whereas other studies have shown that more than two thirds of people older than the age of 60 have inadequate or marginal literacy skills.[6] Individuals with low literacy have less knowledge about their health problems, make more medication or treatment errors, are hospitalized more, and have poorer health status.[7] Given the high rate of limited health literacy, physicians need to communicate in clear and plain language to limit the complications that low health literacy may cause our patients (see Chapter 20).

Example of using the Teach-Back Technique:

> **PHYSICIAN:** (Do not use the phrase "Do you understand?" Instead, place the focus on how well you were able to explain the information to your patient.) *I have just given you a lot of information. In order to make sure I did not leave anything out, can you repeat back to me in your own words how you will take your pain medications?*

or

> **PHYSICIAN:** *Just to make sure I have made myself clear, could you repeat back to me what I have told you about your condition?*

If the elderly patient is unable to correctly reiterate the necessary information, then you need to reteach him or her using other techniques, which may include using visual cues, drawing diagrams, making medication charts, written instructions in plain language, or including another person such as a family member, friend, or caregiver.[7] It is also important to determine if a family member or caregiver to the patient has low health literacy and assess his or her understanding also. When it comes to management, the role of the family member and/or caregiver is just as essential as it is for the successful completion of Functions One and Two, relationship building and assessment. Adherence to a medical treatment plan increases whenever the family is involved; therefore it is important that they also understand.[9]

> **PHYSICIAN:** *We have just discussed the plan for controlling your mother's pain. I would like to take time answering your questions and hearing from you how you can assess your mother's pain and then give her the pain medication.*

## Conclusion

Efficient and effective interviewing of elderly patients involves particular focus on and attention to some of the same skills that are recommended for use with younger patients: early development of rapport, checking of information and understanding, and involvement of the family throughout.

Because of elderly patients' high levels of anxiety and frustration with the medical system, early and systematic empathic interventions are essential to building effective rapport. The frequency of multiple disabilities necessitates checking to corroborate details of data gathering. To enhance understanding and adherence, physicians should rely again on checking and Teach-Back Techniques to verify that the essential facts have been communicated and that patients are likely to follow the treatment plan.

In all stages of interviewing elderly patients, physicians may need to involve the family or caregivers for maximum efficiency and effectiveness. This is especially imperative when you are dealing with a cognitively impaired patient or one with mental illness. Effective relationship building, accurate assessment, and pragmatic management depend on family and caregiver involvement from the beginning of the care process.

Successful interviewing of the elderly also requires patience and overcoming the students' or physicians' own attitudinal barriers. Students and physicians with biases against the elderly should use self-examination and discussion with peers and teachers to overcome these attitudinal barriers to unbiased care. Approaching the elderly with respect and focused attention to the skills emphasized in this chapter can minimize the time (and sometimes frustration) associated with interviewing the elderly and maximize physician, patient, and family satisfaction as well as improve clinical outcomes.

## Addendum

Robinson et al. has provided a list of recommendations for communicating better with elderly patients. It is included here in this addendum because it parallels and supplements the messages in this chapter.

## 10 Tips from the Literature for Improving Communication with Older Patients

The physician should use communication techniques to aid in the transfer of information to increase understanding.

Adapted from *Improving Communication with Older Patients: Tips from the Literature.*[6]

1. **Sit face to face:** One should always sit face to face with the elderly person because many have hearing or visual impairment. Without raising your voice, speak clearly and slowly.[6] An easy low-tech way to help those with hearing impairment is to use the reverse stethoscope technique. Have your patient wear your stethoscope while you speak into the diaphragm.

2. **Avoid excluding your patient from a conversation.** When another person accompanies your patient, strategically position yourself in between the patient and third person to allow eye contact and direct communication with both.

3. **Listen.** Listen carefully and show the patient you understand.[6] Use the check back technique described in the preceding. Make sure that you address your patient's concerns and encourage questions at the end to ensure you covered what is important to them.

4. **Limit distractions and a noisy environment.** Avoid phone calls, pages, and interruptions involving other patients during the visit. Let your patient know that you are paying attention to them.[6]

5. **Provide enough time for the office visit.** Because of the complexity of elderly patients, which includes multiple medical and sociopsychological issues, an office visit often takes

longer than that for a younger patient. Schedule enough time for the visit so that you and your elderly patient do not feel rushed through the visit and important information is not left out.[6]

6. **Use plain language and avoid medical jargon.** Be careful to speak in clear, simple, and plain language as if you are having a conversation with your grandmother. Try not to use too much medical terminology and if you do, define medical terms in a language patients will understand.[7]

7. **Avoid giving too much information.** Studies have shown that only 40% to 80% of information presented by the physician is recalled after the visit and only half of what is recalled is correct. Too much information at a visit will often confuse a patient and be forgotten. Make sure you cover the most important information that is needed for your patient to carry out the treatment plan.[8]

8. **Write it down.** Back up the information you are relaying to your patient with written words in a checklist or task form.[6,7] Remember to write legibly in clear and simple language. Avoid medical jargon, acronyms, or symbols.

Example:

*For your pain: take 1 pill of Tylenol in the morning and one pill at night* rather than writing *Take Tylenol 1 tab po BID.*

9. **Use different learning techniques to aid in understanding.** Visual aids including pictures, audiovisual, computer programs, and diagrams can be used with written and verbal instructions to enhance understanding.[7]

10. **Use the Teach-Back Technique.** Always confirm that your patients understand what you are trying to communicate to them. Remember to leave time for questions and concerns your patients and/or family may have.

### References

1. Obrien S. How to have more effective communication with the elderly. www.about.com. http://seniorliving.about.com/od/lifetransitionsaging/a/communication.htm?p=1
2. Greene MG, et al. The effects of the presence of a third person on the physician- older patient medical interview. *J Am Geriatr Soc* 42:413–419, 1984.
3. Adelman RD, Greene MG, Charon R. The physician-elderly patient-companion triad in the medical encounter: the development of a conceptual framework and research agenda. *Gerontologist* 27(6):729–734, 1987.
4. Williams MV, et al. The role of health literacy in patient-physician communication. *Fam Med* 34(55):383–389, 2002.
5. Williams MV, et al. Inadequate functional health literacy among patients at two public hospitals. *JAMA* 274(21):1677–1682, 1995.
6. Robinson TE, White GL, Jr, Houchins JC. Improving communication with older patients: tips from the literature. *Fam Pract Manag* 73–78, 2006.
7. Weiss BD. *Health literacy and patient safety: help patients understand. Manual for clinicians,* ed 2, 2007, American Medical Association Foundation.
8. Kessels RPC. Patients' memory for medical information. *J R Soc Med* 96(5):219–222, 2003.
9. Adelman RD, Greene MG, Ory MG. Communication between older patients and their physicians. *Clin in Ger Med* 16(1), 2000.

# CHAPTER 23

# Culturally Competent Medical Interviewing

David J. Steele

## OVERVIEW

Global migration patterns over the past several decades are leading to increasing and unprecedented levels of diversity throughout the industrialized world. In the United States alone, the US Census Bureau projects that by the mid-twenty-first century, non-Hispanic, Euro-American whites will no longer be in the majority.[1] As Betancourt[2] notes:

> Sociocultural differences between patient and physician influence communications and clinical decision-making ... when sociocultural differences between patient and provider aren't appreciated, explored, understood, or communicated in the medical encounter, patient dissatisfaction, poor adherence, and poorer health outcomes result.

This chapter provides guidelines to help students and physicians maximize their effectiveness in caring for patients in a culturally appropriate manner. It describes specific strategies for interacting with patients who are members of cultures different from those of the physician; and it offers recommendations for working effectively with interpreters when interviewing patients who speak a language that the physician does not speak. The premise underlying this chapter is well stated by Johnson and his colleagues[3]:

> The overall goal of culturally sensitive care should be empathic understanding of the relationships among symptoms, distress, and the interpersonal life of the patient. One should show clear consideration of the culturally mediated personal meanings in the course of treatment of illness.

Meeting the objectives of the core functions of the medical interview—build the relationship, assess and understand the patient, and collaborate for management—requires the physician to be alert to the cultural beliefs and explanatory systems and models influencing the patient's behavior. Once the physician has elicited the patient's beliefs and sought to understand the behaviors associated with those beliefs, he or she is in a much better position to make effective use of the skills and strategies described in this book.

## The Culture Concept

Culture may be defined as the patterns of beliefs, values, understandings, and normative behaviors shared by an identifiable *group* of people. Culture is socially transmitted and acquired through learning over time. Culture provides a framework for viewing the world, for interpreting events, and for making value judgments about these events.[4] Because every individual belongs to many different identifiable and distinctive groups, every one of us is a member of many different cultures. Consider the following hypothetical person:

> Maria Sanchez Smith is a 37-year-old woman of Mexican descent who was born and raised in El Paso, Texas, in a middle-class family and neighborhood. She is bilingual in Spanish and English. A graduate of Baylor University College of Medicine, Maria is an associate professor of internal medicine at a major medical school on the east coast of the United States. Maria is married to a physician of Euro-American descent and she is the mother of two small children to whom she speaks Spanish at home in an effort to enable them to achieve proficiency in that language as well as English. Raised a Catholic, Maria converted to a Protestant faith while attending college and she is an active member of her congregation. Thus, Maria can be seen as being simultaneously a member of several groups (ethnic, linguistic, gender, class, occupation, religious, family), each having its own particular set of beliefs, values, norms, and behavioral expectations. Maria's perspective on life, her values, her attitudes, and her actions at any given time will represent a unique blend or amalgam of the various cultures to which she belongs.

Culture should not be seen mechanistically as a "thing" that simply determines how a patient will behave. To do so is to risk acting on stereotypical beliefs about patients based on assumptions about "the culture" to which they belong. An important task for the culturally competent interviewer is to identify for each and every patient he or she interviews what beliefs, values, expectations, and behaviors informs a particular patient's perceptions of health and illness, and how these perceptions influence the patient's responses to diagnostic information and treatment recommendations. Culturally competent care "is a system that … is sensitive to intragroup variations in beliefs and behaviors, and avoids labeling and stereotyping."[4]

In a real sense, every medical encounter should be viewed by the physician as a cross-cultural experience. As a result of physicians' training and enculturation into the "culture" of Western biomedicine, they speak their own language and see disease and illness in a particular way. What a patient may refer to as a "cold" is transformed into an "upper respiratory infection." A patient's "racing heart" becomes "tachycardia" in the lexicon of the physician. These common conditions may have very different meanings and implications for the patient and the physician beyond differences in vocabulary. Practitioners of medicine employ touch, sound, and sight in ways that are foreign to the patient not steeped in the traditions of Western biomedicine. Physicians rely on technologies that are unique to their professional cultures and may be unfathomable to those who are not members of that culture. By being alert to inherent differences in the perspectives of physician and patients, the interviewer is taking the first step in providing culturally competent and culturally appropriate care. The second step is to actively and systematically elicit the patient's perspective (his or her explanatory model) and interpersonal context. The third step is to explore with the patient the implications of his or her perspective and context for the treatment the physician wishes to provide.

## Importance of Understanding the Patient's Explanatory Model and Social Context

The physician-anthropologist Arthur Kleinman has been a pioneer in teaching the importance of eliciting and understanding the patient's explanatory models of illness.[5] An explanatory model consists of ideas about the nature and cause of the illness, notions about its seriousness and prognosis, expectations about how it should be evaluated and treated, and beliefs about how the individual and those around him or her should respond. It is on the basis of the explanatory model, often in conjunction with other individuals in the patient's network of relationships, that the patient makes decisions about whether to consult the physician in the first place and, having made this decision, about whether to accept the physician's explanations and advice. Because individuals construct their explanatory models out of their unique experiences and the influences of members of the various groups to which they belong, it should not be surprising to find that these models can be highly variable, even among individuals who are ostensibly members of the same culture or group. Explanatory models vary in content, coherency, and organization. Some are highly structured and elaborate. Others are largely implicit and changeable.

## Strategies for Eliciting Explanatory Models

In what has become a classic in medical anthropology, Kleinman[5] has proposed a menu of questions that can be useful for learning about the patient's explanatory model. These include the following:

- What do you call your problem? Does it have a name?
- What do you think is causing your problem?
- Why do you think it started when it did?
- How does this illness work? What is going on in your body?
- Is there anything in particular that you think needs to be done to figure out what is wrong?
- What kind of treatment do you think would be best for this illness?
- How has this illness affected your life and that of the people around you?
- What worries you most about this problem?

It is important to note that it is not necessary to ask each of these questions of every patient. For some patients a question or two may be all that is necessary to establish that the physician and patient are in substantial agreement about the problem, its meaning, and how it should be approached. In other situations, the physician may be surprised by the patient's responses and will need to spend more time and select more items from the menu to gain a fuller appreciation of the patient's beliefs and how they influence the patient's behavior.

Medical students and physicians sometimes assume that necessary information about the patient's explanatory model will emerge spontaneously during the visit. As Levinson and her colleagues[6] found in a comprehensive study of patient encounters, a majority of patients employed rather subtle cues to convey some of their worries and concerns. Physicians should make a point of conveying to their patients their interest in understanding the patient's perspective on the illness. But in addition, they should be particularly curious about the patient's experience and explanatory models when the patient appears to be skeptical of the physician's explanations, when the patient fails to adhere to a previously prescribed treatment plan, and when the patient seeks advice from different physicians or providers.

Eliciting the patient's explanatory model may be challenging. For a variety of reasons patients may be reluctant to give voice to their perspective. Some may be embarrassed and self-conscious about sharing their ideas with the "all-knowing" physician. Others may take it for granted that their views and that of the physician are congruent. Still others may think that the physician doesn't care about their point of view. Consequently, the application of many of the skills described elsewhere in this book designed to establish rapport and build a firm relationship with the patient coupled with the artful use of questioning and facilitation skills are necessary for acquiring useful information about the patient's explanatory model and context. In particular, the interviewer should approach the issue with genuine interest, humility, and nonjudgmental curiosity. The interviewer will also need to be flexible and persistent in asking questions. It is not uncommon for patients to deny that they have ideas about their illness when first asked. When this occurs, the interviewer should ask again using different phrasing or a different line of questioning. Consider the following example of a family physician interacting with a patient who is concerned about menstrual irregularities and her difficulties conceiving a child. After a discussion of her symptoms and past medical history, the following exchange took place:

PHYSICIAN: *What do you think might be going on?*

PATIENT: *I don't know. I'm confused.*

PHYSICIAN: *Confused? Well is there anything that you've wondered about or been worried about?*

PATIENT: (After a brief pause) *Tumors or something like that.*

PHYSICIAN: *Tumors. Is this something that your mother or sisters talked to you about?*

PATIENT: *No. My mother is back in Columbia. It's just something that I've heard about.*

This exchange took only seconds but provided important information. Had the physician not inquired about the patient's beliefs, he might not have discovered so early in their relationship that she was concerned about "tumors" as well as her difficulties conceiving. Had he simply accepted the patient's first response—"I don't know. I'm confused"—he might not have known how best to attempt to allay the patient's fears. In this case, persistence, flexibility, and genuine nonjudgmental interest in the patient's perspective paid dividends for patient and physician alike.*

Medical students and experienced clinicians often feel awkward about asking patients for their ideas about what might be wrong with them, or about their expectations about how the problem might be investigated or treated. This is understandable given the fact that it is not uncommon for the patient say something like—"that's why I came to the doctor"—in response to a query about their ideas. When this happens, one or more of the following responses from the physician might help with the exploration of the patient's culturally mediated beliefs or worries.

PHYSICIAN: *I find that many of my patients have their own ideas or things they've heard about and it's helpful for me to know what they have been considering.*

or

PHYSICIAN: *Is there something that you've worried about with these symptoms that you'd like for me to particularly address?*

or

PHYSICIAN: *Have you known anyone else with a problem like this? What did it turn out to be in their case?*

or

PHYSICIAN: *Is there something that your (mother, wife, husband …) thinks might be causing this problem and thinks we should check out?*

The patient's response to the last two options is likely to not only provide information about the explanatory model and illness belief system, but provide data about the social dynamics of the patient's context and how it influences patient behaviors as well.

## Continuum of Illness Beliefs

When considering patients' explanatory models it is useful to understand that these beliefs exist as a continuum.[7] On one end of this continuum are beliefs and explanatory models that are highly consistent with the Western, biomedical perspective of the culture of medicine. At the opposite end of the continuum are those explanatory models describing conditions that do not correspond with biomedical precepts. These are sometimes referred to as "folk illnesses" or "culture bound syndromes" associated with membership in a particular ethnic or national cultural group. These

---

*The author would like to thank Dr. Cynthia Haq, Department of Family Medicine, University of Wisconsin School of Medicine and Public Health for access to the teaching trigger tape from which this example interaction is extracted.

are the conditions that people often think of when considering issues of cultural sensitivity and awareness. Examples of folk illness include *empacho,* a gastrointestinal ailment recognized by some Latino ethnic groups, and the illness referred to as *gaz,* or gas, by some Haitians that can cause pain and discomfort in the head, shoulders, arms, or stomach. At the midpoint on our continuum are those illness episodes in which the patient and physician perspective shares elements but diverge in some ways. Examples of midpoint divergences include those situations in which the patient with a viral illness insists on being treated with antibiotics to cure the infection; or the patient diagnosed with hypertension who feels that the condition is a stress-induced disorder that only needs to be actively treated in the face of acute stressors. Regardless of where an explanatory model falls on the described continuum, it is important for the clinician to remind himself or herself that there is considerable variation in these belief systems, and even within identifiable cultural or ethnic groups not every member subscribes to exactly the same set of beliefs. There may be as much variation within a given group as there is between groups. Again, this provides the rationale for actively assessing the beliefs and understandings of the individual patient rather than presuming beliefs based on membership in any particular group.

The distinction between ideological and behavioral ethnicity may be useful in anticipating the salience of ethnic cultural factors as potential influences on patient beliefs and behaviors. Ideological ethnicity exists when a person acknowledges and identifies with a particular ethnic or national group heritage without that heritage being a dominant force in shaping ones beliefs, attitudes, or normative behaviors. Millions of Americans take great pride in being Irish, for example, but come no closer to actually being Irish than a plate of corned beef and cabbage on Saint Patrick's Day! Behavioral ethnicity is another matter. Here cultural roots are much deeper and are a major influence on individual beliefs, values, attitudes, daily behaviors, and social relationships. The potential mismatch between the culture of medicine and the patient's culture is much greater among behaviorally ethnic patients. Pachter[4] lists several factors associated with "adherence to ethnocultural beliefs and behaviors," including the following:

- Recent immigration to the host country
- Residence in ethnic enclaves or neighborhoods
- A preference for speaking a "native language"
- Formal education in the country of origin
- Frequent return visits to the country of origin
- Frequent contact with people from the native country

When the interview reveals that one or more of these traits are present, the physician needs to be particularly alert to the possibility that the patient may not share the beliefs, behaviors, or taken-for-granted assumptions held by the physician.

## Working with Interpreters in the Medical Encounter

Language differences add a whole new level of complexity to the medical interview. Trained interpreters should be employed whenever the physician and patient do not speak the same language.[8,9] The interpreter's job is much more than merely translating from one language to another. Rather, it is to "describe and explain terms, ideas, and processes that lie outside of the linguistic system" of both the physician and patient.[8] As Hardt[10] notes, "Regardless of how the provider phrases a question or provides an answer, an effective interpreter is able to express the content of the message on the appropriate level of the patient's language."

All too often the task of interpreting falls to anyone who happens to be available who is conversant in the language of physician and patient. Frequently, this is a family member, even a child, or a friend, or staff member—none of whom have been trained for this important role. Nonprofessional interpreters should be avoided if at all possible not only because they lack the requisite knowledge and skills of interpretation, but because it may be difficult for them to remain neutral. Family members may have their own concerns or agenda because of the impact of the patient's illness on the family. The patient may also be reluctant to divulge information that may be pertinent but which he or she does not want the family or members of the community to know about. A staff member or friend of the patient who is drafted into this role may take editorial license based on their interest in conveying a particular image of the patient or the group to which the patient belongs.[8] One study of the use of interpreters in a pediatric setting found that interpretation errors were common regardless of whether the interpreter was a professional or ad hoc.[9] However, ad hoc interpreters made many more errors than those trained for the task and their errors were significantly more likely to lead to potentially adverse clinical consequences.

Interpretation should be performed by a person who has been carefully selected and trained in all three major functions of the interview. Consider the simple example of conveying a concept like "allergy" or "allergic reaction" to a patient who speaks a language for which there is no linguistic equivalent for the word or phrase. A person who has not been trained to make such conversions would find it very difficult to do so.

## Enhancing the Patient-Interpreter-Physician Interaction

Hardt[10] describes a series of guidelines that have proved to be effective in facilitating effective interactions between patients, interpreters, and the clinician. Before the actual interview, the physician should spend a few minutes with the interpreter reviewing the goals of the forthcoming visit. This can save time in the long run as it can reduce the risk of misunderstandings. If using someone other than a trained interpreter is unavoidable, it is imperative that the physician try to learn about the nature of the relationship between the patient and the person who has been brought to the visit for that purpose. Doing so may enable the physician to anticipate potential biases that will need to be addressed. If the person providing the translation is a family member, the physician should attempt to find out that person's own agenda and concerns before the interview with the patient begins. The physician should make it clear that the full and accurate translation is the best and only way to adequately address the patient's illness.

The physician should make it clear that he or she and the interpreter are partners in meeting the patient's health care needs. It can be useful to invite the interpreter to share his or her sense of the interaction and the patient's story. Does the interpreter get the sense that the patient is anxious, angry, worried, or holding back? The interpreter should also be invited to share his or her insights about the patient's culture and community, which may help the physician better understand the patient's context, challenges, or resources.

If the physician's practice includes patients from a particular ethnic or linguistic group, it is advisable to make the effort to become familiar with health-related words or phrases in these patients' native language. Knowing the labels used for body parts, systems, and regions and native terms for common illnesses and folk remedies can help the physician track the interaction between the interpreter and the patient. This knowledge will also suggest avenues for further investigation and convey to the patient that the doctor is truly interested in his or her beliefs and traditions. Also, this knowledge can facilitate building rapport and promote the development of a good relationship that will enhance data gathering and collaborative management.

During the encounter the interviewer should arrange the seating in the examination room so the physician, patient, and interpreter all have face-to-face contact. The interviewing physician should direct all of his or her questions and comments to the patient throughout the visit. Once a question has been asked or a comment made, the physician should signal the interpreter to commence with the translation. This helps to regulate the pace of the interview and the flow of information. When the patient is speaking, the physician's gaze should be directed at him or her. The physician needs to observe the patient carefully during the interpreter-patient interaction, watching for nonverbal behaviors and cues. The physician should be on the alert for signs of emotional reactions (e.g., the patient appears sad, smiles or laughs, changes voice tone) and share these observations with the interpreter so he or she can assist the physician in assessing the significance of the patient's emotions based on the content of the interpretation.

If the physician suspects that something may have been omitted in the interpretation—for example, when the interpreter offers a brief translation following a lengthy exchange with the patient—he or she should ask the interpreter if more was said and remind him or her how important it is to get the full story. Problems of this sort are less likely to occur with well-trained professional interpreters. Clearly, sharing expectations of the interpreter before the visit can also be useful in reducing such occurrences.

The clinician should check his or her understanding with the interpreter and invite him or her to offer corrections or alternative understandings. If the interviewer does not understand the interpretation, he or she should ask for clarification.

## Guidelines for Language Use When Working with Interpreters

There are a number of things the physician should do when working with interpreters to make the interpreter's task more manageable. Questions should be brief and to the point. Similarly, when the physician is sharing information with the patient, he or she should use short sentences and pause frequently. Medical terminology should be avoided as much as possible because these terms may interfere with the interpreter's ability to translate accurately and efficiently. Idiomatic expressions or culture-bound metaphors should also be avoided. When translated literally, a statement like "Let's make sure we're in the same ball park" may produce little more than a puzzled stare from a patient who is unfamiliar with the expression.

Above all, when working with an interpreter, the physician needs to be patient. These encounters take more time, and the physician must try to avoid taking shortcuts out of a sense of time urgency.

## Collaborative Management and the Negotiation of Culturally Appropriate Treatment Plans

Through the effective use of the data-gathering skills described in Chapter 4, the culturally competent physician will have elicited information about the patient's explanatory model and context and will be in a better position to make more appropriate judgments about the implications of the patient's cultural context for subsequent treatment. When adherence to a particular model or system of beliefs poses risks for interfering with the patient's willingness or ability to accept a plan that is medically necessary, care must be taken to negotiate a course of action that will be mutually acceptable for the patient and the physician. This must be done with great sensitivity and tact so as to preserve and build upon the relationship and provide opportunities to develop a partnership with the patient. The following two case examples are illustrative.

CASE 1

Mrs. Jones is a 57-year-old woman of European-American descent who is being treated for hypertension. Her family history is significant for high blood pressure and premature death caused by heart disease. Mrs. Jones has a bachelor's degree in business administration and works full time managing the office of a small but busy legal practice. She enjoys a good relationship with her primary care physician and always keeps her appointments with her doctor. When nonpharmacologic methods proved ineffective in controlling Mrs. Jones' blood pressure she was placed on medications. In two subsequent follow-up visits in a 6-month period her blood pressure remained high and her physician suspected that she might not be taking her medications. He wisely decided to spend a little more time exploring her beliefs and understanding of her condition and how she was implementing the plan they had agreed to earlier in the year. This discussion led to the discovery that Mrs. Jones thinks of hypertension as a stress-related disorder ("hyper-tension"). She also believes that she can accurately tell when her blood pressure is elevated by the presence of tension headaches and when she feels "stressed out." At these times, Mrs. Jones acknowledged, she takes her blood pressure medications. But when she is feeling fine and not feeling stressed, she does not feel her blood pressure requires treatment. Armed with this information, Mrs. Jones' doctor was able to explain to her that hypertension is a biomedical condition that has multiple causes and that one's blood pressure can be persistently high even in the absence of perceptible stress. He was also able to explain to her that hypertension frequently does not produce symptoms, like headaches, that can be reliably linked to blood pressure elevations. He went on to propose that the two of them conduct an experiment in which Mrs. Jones would agree to faithfully take the medication for the next 6 weeks regardless of how she was feeling or whether she was experiencing headaches and that she would return following this trial to see how her blood pressure was doing. Mrs. Jones agreed to this, and on her return to clinic 6 weeks later her blood pressure had improved significantly.

---

**CASE 2**　　**(Based on a case described by Hardt and colleagues[10])**

Mrs. Gonzalez is young Puerto Rican woman who resides in a large urban center in the northeastern United States. She arrives at the clinic in obvious distress about her 3-year-old son who has been treated for the past 3 months for asthma. Mrs. Gonzalez speaks some English but feels more comfortable using Spanish, a language that the pediatrician does not speak. At this visit the pediatrician arranged for a Spanish language professional interpreter to be present who also is a native of Puerto Rico. During the course of the visit, Mrs. Gonzalez admitted to the interpreter that she did not believe the medications prescribed by the doctor at their last visit were helping her child. She also disclosed that her own parents felt that the child's illness was most likely the result of evil spirits and that he should be seen by an *Espiritista* for proper treatment.

Mrs. Gonzalez was at a loss. On the one hand she was worried about her child and wondered if her parents might not be right in their assessment of the situation. On the other hand, she liked the doctor and did not want to do anything that might offend him. On learning this information through the interpreter, the pediatrician reached an agreement with the patient that she would continue giving her son the medications he had prescribed, *as prescribed*, and that she would consult an *Espiritista* as suggested by her family. Following that consultation, Mrs. Gonzalez agreed to return to the clinic and tell the doctor what form of treatment the *Espiritista* had recommended so he could assess whether the folk remedies posed any kind of risks for the child. If they did not, he was happy to have Mrs. Gonzalez employ both Western and folk medical traditions in caring for her child. Mrs. Gonzalez left her encounter with her child's pediatrician reassured that she could trust him to be open and respectful of her beliefs, willing to continue the treatments he had prescribed, and relieved that she could also consult with a healer valued in her cultural community.

---

Although the cultural traditions of the patients described in these two cases differ considerably, the strategies employed by the physicians are similar. In each, the physician made an effort to elicit and understand the patient's beliefs in a respectful and nonjudgmental manner. Rather than dismissing the patients' explanatory models and trying to convince them to accept the physicians' biomedical perspectives, each entered into a partnership with the patient enabling them to collaborate in the development of a mutually acceptable plan. For Mrs. Jones, the physician was able to negotiate a trial period during which she would take her medications regardless of how she was feeling. He did not simply negate her belief that she could tell when her blood pressure was elevated by monitoring symptoms of headache and stress, but he provided her with an alternative understanding of her illness *and* a way for her to "test" this alternative.

In the case of Mrs. Gonzalez, the physician worked out a compromise that enabled her to visit a folk healer without abandoning the biomedical care he was providing. By having Mrs. Gonzalez return to the clinic and report the treatment proposed by the *Espiritista*, the physician was in a position to assess whether the treatment might be harmful to the child. If that turned out to be the case, he would then have to negotiate another compromise with the patient's mother. In this case the services of the Puerto Rican Spanish language interpreter would no doubt come in handy. Fortunately, most folk treatments have been found to be relatively safe. For those that pose a risk, if is often possible to work with the folk practitioner to find alternatives that do not produce harmful side effects. In this case the physician not only enters into collaboration with the patient, but with other members of the cultural community who are important to the patient.

## Conclusion

Providing culturally competent and appropriate care poses unique challenges and unique opportunities to learn from and serve our patients. This chapter closes by reviewing two acronyms that can help students and physicians elicit and work effectively with patients' explanatory models and culturally rooted beliefs and behaviors. The first of these is *LEARN*.[11]

**Listen** with sympathy and understanding to the patient's beliefs and concerns.

**Explain** your own perceptions, understandings, and beliefs.

**Acknowledge** and explore differences and similarities in beliefs.

**Recommend** treatment plans and options.

**Negotiate** agreement.

A second useful acronym to deliver culturally appropriate care is summarized by the *ETHNICS* framework.[12]

**Explanation:** Elicit the patient's explanation for the illness or problem.

**Treatment:** Ask the patient what he or she has tried or what needs to be done.

**Healers:** Ask, "Who else have you consulted or would you like to consult?"

**Negotiate:** Work to achieve a mutually accepted plan.

**Intervention:** Indicate what needs to be done now.

**Collaborate:** With patients, family members, other healers and the community.

**Spirituality:** Discover whether there is a religious or spiritual dimension to the illness.

Culturally competent interviewing requires awareness, sensitivity, and the mastery of the basic behavioral skills described throughout this text. Recognizing that all medical encounters, to varying degrees, involve differences in cultural beliefs and understandings is a necessary first step in the process. Physicians who act on this recognition by eliciting, clarifying, and exploring the patient's beliefs, experiences, and context will be in a position to achieve deeper levels of understanding of their patients and the many cultural influences that make each a unique individual. This understanding also contributes to improved medical outcomes by enabling the physician to present information in ways that will promote shared understanding and commitment to treatment recommendations. Most important, expressing a genuine interest in one's patients by exploring their beliefs, attitudes, values, and experiences will contribute to the development of the kinds of relationships that motivated the physician to become a healer in the first place.

## References

1. Swartz MH: *Caring for patients in a culturally diverse society, Chapter 3, Textbook of physical diagnosis: history and physical exam*, ed 5, 2006, Sanders Elsevier.
2. Betancourt JR: Cross-cultural medical education: conceptual approaches and frameworks for evaluation. *Acad Med* 78(6):560–569, 2003.
3. Johnson TM, Hardt EJ, Kleinman A: Cultural factors in the medical interview. In Lipkin M, Jr, Putnam SM, Lazare A, editors: *The medical interview: clinical care, education, and research*, New York, 1995, Springer-Verlag.
4. Pachter LM: Culture and clinical care: folk illness beliefs and behaviors and their implications for health care delivery. *JAMA* 271(9):690–694, 1994.
5. Kleinman A: *Patients and healers in the context of culture: an exploration of the borderland between anthropology, medicine, and psychiatry*, Berkeley, 1980, University of California Press.
6. Levinson W, Gorawar-Bhat R, Lamb J: A study of patient clues and physician response in primary care and surgical settings. *JAMA* 284(8):1021–1027, 2000.
7. Buchwald D, et al: Caring for patients in a multicultural society. *Patient Care* 28(11):105–123, 1994.
8. Putsch RW: Cross-cultural communication: the special case of interpreters in health care. *JAMA* 254(23):3344–3348, 1985.
9. Flores G, et al: Errors in medical interpretation and their potential consequences in pediatric encounters. *Pediatrics* 111:6–14, 2003.
10. Hardt EJ: *Discussion leader's guide: the bilingual medical interview I and II*, Boston, 1991, Boston Department of Health and Hospitals.
11. South-Paul JE: Negotiation with patients. In Mengle MB, Fields SA, editors: *Introduction to clinical skills: a patient-centered textbook*, New York, 1997, Plenum Medical Books.
12. Kobylarz FA, Heath JM, Like RC: The ETHNICS mnemonic: a clinical tool for ethnogeriatric education. *J AM Geriatr Soc* 50:1582–1589, 2002.

# CHAPTER 24

# Family Interviewing

Kathy Cole-Kelly ■ Thomas L. Campbell

## OVERVIEW

Interviewing patients' families is an important skill for all physicians. This chapter discusses how the Three Function Model can be applied to diverse medical situations to help clinicians improve outcomes for individuals by addressing the family environments in which they exist.

Families are the primary context within which most health problems and illnesses occur. Research results have demonstrated that the family has a powerful influence on health and illness.[1] Most health beliefs and behaviors (e.g., smoking, diet, exercise) are developed and maintained within the family.[2] Marital and family relationships have as powerful an impact on health outcomes as biologic factors.[3] Family interventions have been shown to improve health outcomes for a variety of health problems.[4]

Family members, not health professionals, are the primary health care providers for most patients. Outside the hospital, health care professionals give advice and suggestions for the acute and chronic illness, but the actual care is usually provided by the patient (self-care) and family members. With the aging of the population comes a significant increase in the prevalence of chronic illness and disability and a rise in family caregiving. For example, most patients with Alzheimer's disease are cared for at home by family members.

Unfortunately, families are often neglected in health care. Our culture focuses on the individual and emphasizes autonomy over connectedness. The effect of serious illness on other family members is often ignored. Recently, family-centered models that actively involve parents and siblings in the child's care have been developed for hospitals and outpatient clinics from within the specialty of pediatrics. Family practice has developed around the concept of caring for the entire family and treating the family as the patient. However, in most of the medical community, the family is rarely engaged as an active partner in health care. The ability to work effectively with families and use them as a resource in patient care is an essential skill for all physicians, regardless of specialty.

## Situations in Which Family Members Are Often Present

Although at times arranging or convening a family meeting to discuss health issues is important, the most frequent opportunities for interviewing family members are the times they accompany the patient to the hospital or physician's office. Family members are usually the ones who bring a patient to the hospital, and they can serve as valuable informants about the patient's health problem. Unfortunately, family members are usually excluded from the emergency room, where they could serve as informants. During outpatient visits it can be useful to inquire whether family members are in the waiting room and include them in the initial interview.

With more liberal visiting hours in hospitals, family members are often at the bedside of patients. Family members may be present during morning rounds or the initial hospital evaluation. Rather than routinely requesting that the family member leave during the evaluation, finding out about the family member and the role the patient would like the person to take is helpful. For example, most spouses would like to remain with the patient during medical interviews and examinations (except pelvic and rectal examinations). They often feel better informed about their spouse's condition and treatment and reassured by the care that the spouse is receiving. Studies have shown that even during distressing procedures such as cardiopulmonary resuscitation, family members would prefer to observe what is happening.[5]

In the outpatient setting, family members are often present in several situations. During pregnancy care the father of the baby frequently attends a prenatal visit and should be actively involved in the interview. Involving fathers in pregnancy and infant care can help increase the father's sense of connection and involvement with both the pregnancy and the infant. Thus involvement can have beneficial effects for the infant and the entire family. During well- and ill-child visits, one and sometimes both parents routinely accompany the child. After assessing the developmental level of the child, the clinician can decide how to balance the interview and talk with both the child and the parent. For infants and very young children the entire interview is with the parent(s). When a parent accompanies an adolescent to a medical visit, the physician must decide when to meet separately with the adolescent and how much to involve the parent.

An increasingly common situation occurs when an elderly patient is brought in by a family member who may serve as the primary family caregiver. This is usually an adult child, often a daughter, or the patient's spouse. Deciding how to involve the family caregiver in the interview is parallel to interviewing parents and children. The goal is to include the patient as much as possible, depending on the patient's cognitive abilities. For severely demented patients the interview is mostly with the family caregiver.

## The Three Functions of Family Interviewing

The principles of interviewing an individual patient also apply to interviewing families, but there are additional complexities. The physician must engage and talk with at least one additional person, and the opportunity exists for interaction between the patient and family members. In general, the physician must be more active and establish clear leadership in a family interview. This may be as simple as being certain that each participant's voice is heard ("Mrs. Jones, we haven't heard from you about your concerns about your husband's illness. Can you share those?") or acting as a "traffic cop" with a large and vocal family ("Jim, I know that you have some ideas about your mother's care, but I'd like to let your sister finish talking before we hear from you."). The next sections of the chapter contain a discussion of how the three functions of interviewing can be applied systematically to interviewing families.

## Function One: Build the Relationship

When working with families, establishing rapport and developing a relationship is known as "joining." An essential component of joining is making some positive contact with each person present so that each feels valued and connected enough to the physician to participate in the interview. Family members have often been excluded from health care discussions and decisions, even when they are present. They may not expect to be included in the interview or to be asked to participate in decision making. By making contact with each person, the physician is making it clear that everyone is encouraged to participate in the interview.

There are several other important reasons for joining with family members at the beginning of the interview. The clinician often has an established relationship with the patient but not with other family members. The family member may feel left out or that his or her role is merely that of an observer. One common example of this occurs during hospital rounds when there is a family member by the bedside. The usual approach is either to ask family members to leave during the interview or ignore them. This approach is not respectful of families and fails to use the family as a resource. This alternative approach is suggested:

1. After greeting the patient, greet and shake hands with the family member and introduce yourself.

   PHYSICIAN: *Good morning, Mrs. Janeway (the patient).* (Turn to family member and shake hands.) *Hello, I'm Frank Medcoci. I'm the medical student on the team taking care of Mrs. Janeway.*

   Usually family members will introduce themselves and state their relationship to the patient.

   FAMILY MEMBER: *Nice to meet you. I'm Mrs. Janeway's daughter, Mary.*

   It is helpful to learn what the family member's relationship is to the patient because the physician may deal differently with a son, daughter, or spouse than with a nephew or someone who is not a family member. If the family member does not provide this information, you can usually obtain it by asking, "And you are?" or, "And how are you related to Mrs. Janeway?"

2. Obtain the patient's permission to talk with the family member who is present. This can usually be done quickly and easily.

   PHYSICIAN: *Mrs. Janeway, before I ask you about how your night went, I'd like to talk with your relative (or husband, daughter, etc.) for a minute. Would that be okay with you?*

   Asking for the patient's permission, which is rarely denied or even questioned, is respectful to the patient and reassures him or her that the physician will be spending time talking with the patient as well.

3. Involve the family member in the interview from the beginning by asking a question such as the following:

   PHYSICIAN: *How do you feel your mother (or Mrs. Janeway) is doing?*

This question involves the daughter in the interview and communicates that the physician is interested in her viewpoint. It can also provide some important medical information. For example:

FAMILY MEMBER: *She looks okay now, but earlier this morning she threw up a bunch of blood.*

A similar situation involving a family member's presence often occurs when fathers attend prenatal visits. Fathers commonly feel marginalized during a pregnancy and may view themselves as merely observers, not as active participants and partners. They may sit in the corner of the examination room and remain silent and uninvolved if not invited to participate. It is important to greet the father of the baby at the beginning of the interview and recognize his role.

PHYSICIAN: *Hi, I'm Dr. Campbell (shaking hands). You are?*

FATHER: *Darrell.*

PHYSICIAN: *It's very nice to meet you, Darrell. I'm really glad that you came in with your partner (or wife or fiancée). I think it is really important for a dad to be involved in the pregnancy and delivery. You are welcome to any of these visits. Can you tell me a little about yourself?*

An important step in joining is communicating respect for the family member and his or her opinions. For many men, this can be done by inquiring about their job and showing interest in their work:

PHYSICIAN: *What kind of work do you do, Darrell?*

If the father is unemployed, the physician can discuss the challenges of looking for work. This step usually takes only a minute or two but strongly communicates an interest in that person's life. As with Mrs. Janeway's daughter, the physician could then ask Darrell:

> PHYSICIAN: *How do you think your girlfriend has been doing during the pregnancy?*

Later in the pregnancy, it would be important to inquire about how he would like to be involved in the labor and delivery.

Special issues are involved when children are present during the interview. Children are often expected to be seen and not heard in a clinical encounter involving their parent or another family member. However, they may have many questions or misconceptions about the family member's illness.

> Jim and Betsy Werner brought their 9-year-old daughter Rachel with them to Betsy's appointment with her oncologist. After discussing the next stage of treatment for Betsy's breast cancer, the oncologist asked Rachel if she had any questions. She asked, "Can I catch breast cancer from my mother?"

Children are more likely to participate in the interview and ask questions if the physician takes just a few moments to connect with them and make them feel important. With small children, a quick comment such as, "Gee, I like your sweatshirt," or, "I wish I had cool barrettes like those" can be enough to signal that the physician is interested in them. With older children and adolescents, a respectful "Hello," "Glad to meet you," and "If you have any questions, I hope you will feel free to ask them" can give them the message that the physician is pleased to have them there, while giving them enough space not to feel pressured.

## When There Is Conflict in the Family

Establishing a positive relationship with family members is particularly important and more challenging when there is conflict in the family. In these cases the family member will usually assume that the physician has taken the side of the patient in the conflict. In situations of conflict the physician must take extra steps to join with the family members and establish his or her neutrality. The goal is to develop an alliance with each family member and the patient without taking sides in the conflict. An exception to this goal is a situation in which family violence threatens one person's physical safety. Dealing with family conflict and violence is discussed in more detail later in the chapter.

In addition to establishing rapport and building a relationship through verbal communication, the physician can make use of nonverbal strategies to enhance the relationship with the patient and family members. Just as it is important to be sure that the physician and an individual patient are in a comfortable sitting position and at eye level with each other, so is it important that other family members are sitting or standing (if the room doesn't have enough chairs) near enough that they can hear what is being said and can be easily seen by the physician. This proximity to voice and face will help the physician make eye contact with each person in the room.

On entering the room and seeing that one family member is sitting far from the physician or is isolated from other family members, the physician can gently motion that person to come closer. This will enhance everyone's sense of being included in the patient visit and being an important part of the encounter. If one family member seems to be sitting or standing particularly far from the center of the clinical action, the physician might want to take the time to encourage the person to come closer to the action in the room. Otherwise, the family member taking a more distant position might be harder to build a relationship with during the encounter. Similarly, one family member might dominate both the verbal and nonverbal space in the encounter, making it difficult for the other family members to have as much involvement in the action with the patient or physician.

To encourage a relationship with the quieter members and discourage domination by louder members, the physician can use both verbal and nonverbal cues to ensure a connection with all the family members present. For example:

> FAMILY MEMBER: *I'm so concerned about my mother. She has been in the hospital far too often. I don't think the doctors are doing much here. I am really not at all …*

> PHYSICIAN: *Ms. Jones, I think I have a good understanding of what your concerns are and I want to respond to them, but I'd first like to hear from your brother, Mr. Norton. Mr. Norton, this is the first time I've met you and I'm wondering what your perspective is on your mother's condition. I'd like to hear your opinion. Maybe you could move your chair in a little closer so I can hear you better.*

## Function Two: Assess and Understand the Patient and Family

As stated initially, family members are an invaluable resource to the physician. A family-sensitive interviewer sees the presence of other family members as the opportunity for gathering important information about the patient and his or her health care context. The physician can gather information about the patient's and family's understanding of the illness, important health history information, current stressors affecting the patient, and potential resources to help the patient's care. In addition, the physician can gather information from the family about who is currently involved in the patient's care. This can be important for the physician to know when making treatment plans.

The initial step in gathering this information has been accomplished by the first function of interviewing: joining and relationship building. Without this step, family members will not appreciate their importance in the medical interview. Part of this initial joining and relationship building includes finding out exactly who is in the room and how each person is related to the patient. Once this has been accomplished and contact has been made with each person in the room, the physician can begin to gather information from the family.

The physician's goal is usually to gather information that helps with diagnosis or treatment planning. The family members may have their own agendas, which could be the reason they have come with the patient to the visit. Thus it is helpful to elicit the reason that each family member has come to the visit.

> PHYSICIAN: *Hi, I'm Dr. White. I don't believe I've met you before.* (**joining**)

> FAMILY MEMBER: *Oh, I'm Joey's father. I'm out of town a lot but was worried when I heard he was in the hospital, and my mother-in-law let me know he was here.*

> PHYSICIAN: *Great of you to come. Are there any questions I can answer for you? I'd like to hear your perspective on how Joey manages his diabetes.* (**gathering the information**)

> FAMILY MEMBER: *Well, yes, I'm sort of worried about Joey's care because his mother has been so preoccupied with our new baby. I'm wondering if something else can be done so he doesn't keep ending up in the hospital.*

By seeing the father as a resource, the physician gathers information in this brief interaction about the relationship to the child, a beginning hint of his involvement (out of town a lot), and his major concern (wife being overwhelmed and thus less attentive to Joey's diabetes).

The physician faces a more delicate challenge when gathering information about an adolescent patient. Issues of confidentiality are heightened during adolescence. Adolescents' attitudes span a continuum from determined to retain a strong sense of independence to comfortable with parents involved in both their health care and the interview. This has implications for the way the physician conducts the family interview. The physician first needs to inquire about the adolescent's comfort with questions being asked in the presence of his or her parents. Once this has been established, the physician can proceed by gathering information, either separately or with the family and adolescent together.

In addition to the verbal information the physician can gather from the family members present in the room, he or she can also gather important information through observations of where people sit and how they participate in the interview. Where family members sit in the examination room often tells the clinician something about relationships and roles in the family. For instance, how close a couple sits together is often a measure of their emotional closeness. A family member who sits across the examination room in the corner may reveal a sense of being an observer or a nonparticipant in the patient's care.

In addition to observing where family members place themselves relative to the patient in the room, noting where the family members sit or stand relative to the physician can be revealing. A family member taking the chair closest to the physician often indicates that the family member feels he or she is or should be in charge of the patient's care. This can give the physician information about differing levels of involvement in the patient's care. This observation could be useful information, triggering questions about relationships among members of the family and the patient.

Noting where patients and family members sit when the physician enters an examination or hospital room is important; however, this seating arrangement should not necessarily be accepted as the structure for conducting the interview. Just as the physician asks the patient to sit or lie on the examination table to facilitate the physical examination, so should the physician arrange chairs and family members to facilitate involvement of all family members in the interview. This might include asking a shy family member to pull up a chair next to the patient, or having the child sitting on the examination table move to the chair next to the physician, with the parent next to the child. By rearranging where the patient and family members are sitting, the physician is also making a statement about what roles he or she would like them to play, that is, "who the patient is" (sitting next to the physician) and how the accompanying family members should participate. This is analogous to asking the passive patient who sits on the examination table waiting to be examined to sit next to the physician and assume a more participatory role.

> Mary McCarthy is 11 years old and has come into the hospital because of an exacerbation of her asthma. In the room are her mother Susan, her father Bill, and her brother Toby. Mary and her dad are sitting on the bed (or examination table), and her mom is sitting as far away as possible from them both.
>
> PHYSICIAN: *Susan, why don't you come closer to us so I have you all in a single range of vision? That's great. Now, tell me what you noticed about Mary last night before you brought her into the hospital.*

Although there are significant advantages to having the family as a resource for gathering information about the patient and the context of care, the physician's fear of losing control of the interview can be a compelling disincentive. On walking into a roomful of family members, the physician may naturally feel overwhelmed and think it would be easier to interview the patient alone. However, several family-interviewing strategies can help the physician feel that he or she is able to gather information without relinquishing total control.

1. The physician can explain at the beginning that he or she is interested in each person's perspective and will be sure to hear each one.

2. If one person begins to dominate the interview, the physician should think of himself or herself as a benevolent traffic cop, putting up a hand to indicate time is up and interrupting the family member by saying something like the following:

PHYSICIAN: *Mr. Goodman, I'd like to hear more from you, but I want to be sure to hear your wife and daughter's perspective. Then, if there's time, I'll get back to you.*

3. In case a child begins to interrupt too much, the physician should make sure there are some toys in the office. The physician can also have the child sit near him or her, so that the physician may place a hand on the child's shoulder or leg and signal the child to "hush" if necessary.

4. The physician should avoid questions that might make family members feel blamed or create divisiveness between family members. In the course of gathering information about the patient's illness or treatment, discrepancies in family members' beliefs or approaches inevitably surface. It is important to avoid asking questions that could pit one family member against another.

Reframing information questions as queries that the physician would like clarified elicits the desired information while minimizing the potential for interpersonal explosions.

PHYSICIAN: *It seems that you and your mother had different approaches to the feeding of the baby. Can you help me understand how that worked?* (Special considerations for handling conflict or intense emotional responses during the family interview are discussed in the Special Circumstances section.)

## Function Three: Collaborate to Manage

All of the principles for education, negotiation, and motivation with an individual also apply to family members, with two important considerations. First, when delivering information to more than one person, it is important to recognize that each person is likely to have different knowledge, beliefs, and expectations about the medical problem and the prognosis and treatment. This must be taken into account when working with families. Second, family members can be an enormous resource in motivating patients to adhere to medical treatments or change unhealthy behaviors. This family resource should be used to benefit the patient.

## Delivering Information

One of the most common and important reasons for bringing families together and convening a family meeting is to deliver important medical information to the patient and his or her family. This often involves the delivery of bad news, such as the diagnosis of cancer or other life-threatening illness or a poor prognosis. For several reasons, patients should be encouraged to have family members with them when bad news will be given. First, the family members can be an important source of support for the patient during this stressful time. Second, patients often misunderstand information when the content is highly emotional. For example, a patient may interpret cancer as a death sentence even when the physician explains that the cancer is curable. The family members who are present can help correct these misconceptions. Third, family members often receive misinformation when it is relayed secondhand by the patient. In the preceding case, the patient might tell his family that he has terminal cancer. Physicians often receive phone calls from family members who did not receive the information directly. Delivering bad news with family members present allows the physician to see how the family reacts and will cope with the problem. The physician can learn how supportive or emotionally expressive the family will be.

Before providing information to family members, it is important to assess their current level of understanding, their beliefs, and their concerns, just as it is with individual patients. Knowing their baseline level of knowledge allows the physician to tailor the information that is provided and correct any misunderstandings. Understanding family members' fears can facilitate appropriate reassurances. If the physician initially takes the time to elicit the family's knowledge, beliefs, and concerns, the rest of the interview will be more efficient and effective.

Dr. C. is meeting with Mrs. Goldman and her family after she has been admitted with an exacerbation of her chronic obstructive lung disease.

**PHYSICIAN:** *I want to update you on your mother's medical condition, but before I do that, I'd like to know what your understanding of your mother's condition is.*

**SON:** (provides description)

**PHYSICIAN:** *That's a very accurate description of what is going on with your mother. I want to come back to that, but first I want to know what others understand about what has happened.*

One of Mrs. Goldman's daughters believes that her mother's breathing is made worse by the air conditioning in her apartment and that she needs to get more fresh air. Before correcting this misunderstanding, the physician elicits other beliefs and concerns about the patient's health. He then gives a brief summary of her condition, addressing each of the family member's concerns and beliefs.

In general, medical information should be provided to family members with the patient present and with his or her permission. Most patients want their family members to be informed about their medical conditions, but consent must be obtained.

**PHYSICIAN:** *I'd like to inform your family about your medical condition. Is there anything that you don't want me to share with them?*

The patient may not want to have some sensitive information discussed with certain family members. The patient should be present during these family conferences whenever possible. This prevents misinformation or secrets from developing. In the hospital or nursing home, this means meeting with the family at the bedside. The family members may desire not to "burden" the patient with issues concerning prognosis or treatment plans. At an extreme, family members may not want the patient to receive the diagnosis of a terminal condition, believing, "It will just upset him too much" or "If she finds out, she'll just give up." These efforts to protect the patient should be avoided because they lead to secrecy and a breakdown in communication.

The Matthews family wanted to meet separately with Dr. K., their father's physician, and with the hospital social worker to decide on nursing home placement after Mr. Matthews' stroke. They knew that their father would be upset if he knew what they were talking about.

Dr. K. insisted that they all meet together because they were talking about Mr. Matthews' future. The patient was upset at first when he learned about their proposal. However, as he heard family members express their love and concern for him and their fear that they could not care for him at home, he began to accept the idea of placement in a nursing home.

## Using the Family as a Resource in Motivating Patients to Change

Family members play an important role in developing and maintaining health behaviors. They can be a valuable resource in helping patients adhere to medical treatments and change unhealthy behaviors. Almost every important health behavior is a family activity or is strongly influenced by the family. These behaviors are risk factors and tend to cluster within families because family members tend to have similar diets, physical activities, and use of substances (e.g., tobacco, alcohol, illicit drugs).[2] Parents' health-related behaviors strongly influence whether a child or adolescent will adopt a healthy behavior. In a Gallup survey of health-related behaviors, most adults reported that their spouse or partner was more likely to influence their health habits than anyone else, including their family doctor.

Support from family members has been associated with successful smoking cessation, weight loss, participation in exercise programs, and compliance with medical treatments. Family interventions have been successful in the treatment of cardiac risk factors, obesity, and compliance with hypertension treatment.[4] In one large study, providing family support to help with compliance with blood pressure medication resulted in improved compliance, reduced blood pressure, and a 50% reduction in cardiac mortality.[6] Based on this and similar compliance research, the National Heart, Lung and Blood Institute recommends that physicians use the following as one of three basic strategies for increasing adherence with antihypertensive regimens:

> Enhance support from family members. Identifying and involving one influential person, preferably someone living with the patient, who can provide encouragement helps support the behavior change and, if necessary, reminds the patient about the specifics of the regimen.[7]

Whether in the hospital or outpatient setting, the family can be used as a resource in the treatment plan anytime a family member is present. The goal is to negotiate a treatment plan not just with the patient, but with the family as well. This is particularly important when the plan will have an effect on the family or must be carried out by family members. For example, it makes little sense to counsel most middle-aged men about low-fat diets without including their wives, who are usually responsible for the menu and cooking.

During an office visit the physician can help the patient negotiate with family members how they can be helpful to the patient in making behavioral changes. Consider the following dialogue:

**PHYSICIAN:** *So Jim, how do you think Karen (his wife) could help you remember to take your blood pressure medication?*

**PATIENT:** *Well, for one thing, it doesn't help when she nags me about it.*

**PHYSICIAN:** *Okay, scratch that off the list. What could she do to help you?*

**PATIENT:** *Maybe if she put my pills out on the breakfast table, it would help me to remember.*

**PHYSICIAN:** *All right, that sounds pretty simple. Karen, do you think you could do that?*

**WIFE:** *Sure.*

**PHYSICIAN:** *What else could she do?* (**additional negotiations**)

**PHYSICIAN:** *Jim, what should Karen do if she notices that you have forgotten to take your medication?*

**PATIENT:** *Just forget about it and don't nag me about taking them.*

**PHYSICIAN:** *Karen, are you okay with that?*

**WIFE:** *I guess so.*

The goal of these sessions is to help couples and families come up with specific helpful and supportive interventions that are acceptable to the patient and the family. Marital or family conflicts or dysfunction can sometimes interfere with this process. One family member may sabotage the patient's attempts at changing unhealthy behaviors. It may be necessary in such cases to refer the family to a family therapist who can help with underlying family issues.

# Special Circumstances When Interviewing Families

Interviewing families can present special challenges or circumstances that are not usually seen when interviewing individuals. This section discusses a few of the more common and important circumstances and issues that can occur when interviewing families.

## WHEN TO CONVENE THE FAMILY

Although family members often accompany the patient to the hospital and outpatient appointment, sometimes inviting family members to a meeting or session to discuss medical issues is helpful. Research results have demonstrated that patients and families desire family conferences or meetings and request them for serious medical and psychosocial problems.[8] Although the physician should convene the family whenever he or she feels it might be helpful for the patient or family, there are four situations in which a routine family conference should be considered:

1. **Hospitalization:** It is helpful to meet with the family shortly after admission to explain the patient's condition and treatment and before discharge to discuss the family's role in outpatient care.
2. **Prenatal and well-child care:** Both parents should be invited and included in all prenatal and well-child visits.
3. **Death and dying:** It is important to meet with the family at the time of a terminal diagnosis, during the dying phase, and after death.
4. **Diagnosis of a serious chronic illness:** Anytime a serious illness is diagnosed, involving the family can be helpful.

Family members usually attend a family conference when invited by the physician if the physician is positive and direct about the need to meet with the family, emphasizes the importance of the family in caring for the patient, and stresses the benefits of a family meeting to the patient and family.

## AVOIDING TAKING SIDES OR TRIANGULATION

A physician seeing multiple family members needs to learn to avoid becoming triangulated—being pulled into an alliance with one family member at the exclusion of another. The physician can be pulled unwittingly into unresolved conflicts between family members. In the case of an ill child, one parent may try to form an alliance with the physician that excludes the other parent. Or, a wife can try to get the physician on her side, hoping that the physician's alliance will bolster her position against her husband. To avoid being caught in the middle of a triangle, the physician needs to be facile at reassuring each member of the family that the physician is there to hear each person's story but not to take sides. Furthermore, the physician can assert that it will not be helpful to the family if the physician is pulled into an alliance with one member at the exclusion of another. The physician can emphasize the importance of everyone working together as the most beneficial way to enhance the health care of the patient.

## WHEN THE CUSTOMER IS NOT THE PATIENT

The customer is the person who desires a service and is not always the patient. Sometimes a family member may want some medical service or intervention for another family member. An obvious example is when a mother (customer) brings her young child (patient) in for treatment of a medical problem. A common but subtler case occurs when a middle-aged man is sent for a checkup by his wife because she is worried that he is not taking care of his health. Unless the physician inquires closely, the man may say that he is there for a checkup and that everything is fine.

When the patient is not the customer, it is helpful to talk directly with the customer to find out what the concerns or requests are. The wife of the middle-aged man might report that he has been having chest pains when they go for walks but that he is reluctant to do anything about it. In some cases it may be helpful or even necessary to have the customer and patient in the examination room together. Consider the following phone call:

> PATIENT: *Dr. C., you are seeing my husband this afternoon and I wish that you would talk to him about his drinking. Recently, he has been getting drunk once or twice a week.*

> PHYSICIAN: *Mrs. James, I hear your concern about your husband's health. I'd like you to come in with your husband later today so we can talk about your concerns. I think he needs to hear this directly from you.*

Recognizing when the customer is not the patient and communicating directly with the customer can help the physician from becoming triangulated or caught in family conflicts.

## DEALING WITH STRONG AFFECT DURING THE FAMILY INTERVIEW

The potential for family members to become very emotional is heightened when dealing with a critical life event such as a diagnosis of a serious illness (e.g., a newborn with cystic fibrosis or a middle-aged woman with breast cancer), a difficult decision (e.g., nursing home placement), and uncertainty (the course of the illness; for example, how long someone with chronic obstructive pulmonary disease has to live). When family members are offering their opinions about these difficult issues, one or many family members may have intense emotional feelings in response to the medical situation. Sadness and anger are the two most commonly expressed emotions when family members are confronting difficult medical situations.

The principles for dealing with strong affect in families are the same as those used when interviewing a single patient. In families, however, expressed feelings often trigger strong emotions in other family members and may intensify the affect.

When the physician is delivering bad news or discussing serious health problems, family members commonly express sorrow or grief. This can be beneficial for family members because it allows them to share their feelings and obtain support from one another. Often it can be helpful to shift the interview to an affective level and encourage family members to share their feelings with a question such as, "How are you all feeling about this?" In response to such a question, one family member may start sharing his or her emotional reactions, which may trigger another to start crying. The challenge for the physician is to refrain from intervening or interfering with this process. Many physicians treat tears like blood and try to stop any crying, usually because it makes the physician uncomfortable.

A few approaches by the physician can help during intense and sometimes stormy moments:

1. The physician should have tissues available to give the family members. Often it can be nice to hand the box to one member and ask him or her to give it to the emotional member.
2. The physician should be patient during this period and remember that it is better for the emotions to be expressed in the physician's presence. The physician and the other family members can be a witness to the feelings of the one member and can provide reassurance.

When anger is expressed by one member about a health outcome, it is important for the physician to listen, reflect that he or she has heard how angry the patient or family member is, and ask if others share that feeling. It can be valuable for the family members to experience their anger being heard. However, the physician should also feel confident about maintaining control of the situation during this time. When one family member is expressing frustration and anger for a few minutes, the physician and other family members should patiently listen; however, the physician may ask the family member to lower his or her voice while expressing the feeling. After hearing a few angry sentences, the physician can turn to the rest of the family members to ask if anyone would like to briefly add to the information being offered.

> **FAMILY MEMBER:** (in a loud angry tone) *I just don't understand why no one told us before about my wife's illness. I mean, I've been asking for someone to help us with her and I feel that everyone just keeps beating around the bush.*
>
> **PHYSICIAN:** *Mr. Platt, I understand your anger and frustration. These are difficult situations to predict, and I know it is hard to watch your spouse in this condition.*
>
> **FAMILY MEMBER:** *Yes, but you and your staff just seem to …*
>
> **PHYSICIAN:** *Mr. Platt, I'm going to interrupt you and give your son and daughter a chance to speak. Brenda (adult daughter) or Jon (adult son), do you share your father's frustration?*

Listening to one member express frustration may trigger another family member to echo the feeling. Often families have a family member who takes the role of peacemaker and quiets the intense emotion in the room without intervention from the physician. However, if the anger is starting to intensify, the physician needs to interrupt as the physician in the preceding example did and turn to another family member.

In addition to the expression of anger by various family members toward the health care system or the uncertainty of the situation, having multiple family members in one room increases the risk of conflict between family members. The intensity of the situation with a loved one can mobilize the family members' unresolved feelings of resentment or irritation toward one another. Sometimes the hospital is the first setting in which many of these members have gathered together in a long time. If sparks begin to fly between family members, it is important to provide them with a safe, controlled atmosphere. The physician needs to assert a sense of control by saying something like the following:

> **PHYSICIAN:** *I think this is not the time to resurrect unfinished issues. I hope you can resolve them in some forum, but at this time I need to be able to have you help me in getting this information or making these decisions.*

If angry emotions persist, a physician can ask a family member to leave until he or she can return in a calm manner. The physician can offer to meet with that person individually at another time if that seems helpful.

## VIOLENCE IN THE FAMILY

If a patient is concerned about his or her personal safety, interviewing the threatening family members in the room at the same time as the patient is inadvisable. The threat of violence is something to take seriously. The physician can provide the patient a safe environment to explore his or her options. This is true whether it involves a child fearing abuse from a parent or an adult fearing harm from a partner.

## MENTAL HEALTH REFERRAL

Just as a depressed or anxious patient may need a mental health referral, some families dealing with illness may need to be referred for family therapy. The physician may decide to refer the family to a family-oriented mental health professional when certain concerns emerge. If significant anger or conflict erupts between family members and the physician believes this may interfere with the patient's treatment, a family-oriented mental health referral can be useful. Similarly, if the family mentions that the patient's illness has resulted in significant strains or stresses, the physician can offer a family therapy referral to help members cope. Finally, if the family members seem organized around the illness in a way that appears to solidify battlegrounds that were already in place (e.g., a mother so tied to a child's diabetes and its daily routines that she excludes her alienated husband from all interactions with the child and herself), a family therapy referral can potentially help family members resolve conflicts and gain healthier alliances based less on an individual's illness.

## Family-Oriented Interview with the Individual Patient

Although many benefits accrue from having the family present in the medical interview, the individual patient is often the only one present in either the office or hospital visit. The absence of other family members does not have to lead to a solely individually oriented approach to the patient. If the physician enters the room and sees only an individual, he or she can maintain a family orientation by remembering that this patient is part of a larger context. Several techniques can reinforce this orientation during the interview. First, the physician can gather a family tree or genogram to understand the family health history, the current family members in the patient's context, the stage of the family's life cycle, relationship patterns and how members are involved in the patient's illness, and current family stresses.[9] In addition to gathering the genogram, the physician can ask a series of family-oriented questions that metaphorically bring the family into the office or hospital visit. The following are examples of questions the physician may ask:

PHYSICIAN: *What do other family members think about how you are doing?*

or

PHYSICIAN: *What does your mother (father, spouse, daughter) believe caused this problem?*

or

PHYSICIAN: *Has anyone else in the family had a problem like this? How was it treated?*

or

PHYSICIAN: *Who else in the family is concerned and involved in your problem?*

or

PHYSICIAN: *Are there other current or recent stresses in your family that are making it difficult to deal with your health care needs?*

or

PHYSICIAN: *Who in your family can you rely on for help with your current health care needs?*

The responses to these questions could alert the physician to the need for recommending that other family members come in for a medical family interview.

## Conclusion

Working with families in medical practice can be personally and professionally fulfilling. Gaining the skills to work with families contributes to a physician's clinical comfort and effectiveness. Understanding the three functions of a family interview enhances the physician's ability to work with family members in clinical settings. The first function of establishing rapport or joining with family members is fundamental to family interviewing. Gathering information from multiple family members encourages family involvement in the patient's care and provides important information about family beliefs about the illness. Negotiating a treatment plan with the family and educating family members about the illness can improve patient compliance and family confidence in the health care team. Although learning how to interview more than one person presents some challenges, the benefits of hearing the multiple perspectives on the cause and treatment of an illness can be invaluable. The family is always part of the treatment team, whether acknowledged by the physician or not. The active inclusion of family members in the treatment team can be a rewarding clinical experience for every physician, regardless of specialty.

## References

1. Campbell TL: Family's impact on health: a critical review. *Fam Syst Med* 4:135–228, 1986.
2. Doherty WA, Campbell TL: *Families and health*, Beverly Hills, Calif, 1998, Sage Press.
3. House JS, Landis KR, Umberson D: Social relationships and health. *Science* 241:540–545, 1988.
4. Campbell TL, Patterson JM: The effectiveness of family interventions in the treatment of physical illness. *J Marital Fam Ther* 21:545–584, 1995.
5. Dracup K, et al: The psychological consequences of cardiopulmonary resuscitation training for family members of patients at risk for sudden death. *Am J Public Health* 87:1434–1439, 1997.
6. Morisky DE, et al: Five-year blood pressure control and mortality following health education for hypertensive patients. *Am J Public Health* 73:153–162, 1983.
7. National Heart, Lung and Blood Institute: Management of patient compliance in the treatment of hypertension. *Hypertension* 4:415–423, 1982.
8. Kushner K, Meyer D, Hansen JP: Patients' attitudes toward physician involvement in family conferences. *J Fam Pract* 28:73–78, 1989.
9. McGoldrick M, Gerson S: *Genograms in family assessment*, New York, 1986, Norton Press.

# CHAPTER 25

# Troubling Personality Styles and Somatization

## OVERVIEW

This chapter discusses communication strategies to help manage patients with compulsive, dependent, histrionic, borderline, narcissistic, self-defeating, and somatizing personality patterns.

Because of their troubling personality styles or interpersonal behaviors, some patients are particularly stressful to interview and difficult to manage. Physicians, however, vary greatly in their responses to these behaviors. That is, some behaviors are particularly troubling for some physicians and not so troubling at all for others. Nevertheless, a few characteristically difficult behaviors seem universally problematic for most physicians. Studies have shown that about 15% of patients seen in primary care clinics are viewed as "difficult" by their physicians, and sources of this difficulty often lie in very specific "difficult" personality traits[1,2] and/or tendencies toward somatization (e.g., patients with medically unexplained symptoms [MUS]).[3]

Patients with these difficult interpersonal behaviors can arouse such intensely negative feelings in physicians that startling characterizations like "hateful" patients[4] may emerge, or pejorative labels such as "crock," "troll," "turkey," or "dirtball" can appear as pseudo diagnoses or seemingly creative or humorous (gallows) acronyms like NARTBA (no apparent reason to be admitted), gomer (get out of my emergency room), and TOBASH (take out back and shoot in the head) emerge to relieve anxiety and tension around interpersonal conflict. Such labeling, on one hand, can be viewed as a higher level mechanism of defense in that it serves to relieve distress through humor; but the humor comes at a price because the whole labeling process is not only dehumanizing, it also leads to bad care.[5]

The reasons that such patients elicit intense feelings among physicians are complex. In general, however, physicians label a patient when the patient's behavior provokes feelings of anxiety or anger. Demanding, demeaning, angry, or dependent behaviors are examples of patient behaviors that can provoke physician anger, interfere with care, and lead to labeling in retaliation. Patients also are labeled when physicians feel anxious about remaining in a state of uncertainty about diagnosis and management and therefore reach for negative labeling in a somewhat nihilistic attempt to come to diagnostic and/or management closure.

This chapter reviews some of the common causes of troubling interpersonal behavior and discusses some interviewing strategies that can help physicians manage such behavior more successfully. It is hoped that such strategies can help avoid recourse to pejorative labeling. The discussion of each problem is organized under four headings: (1) general characteristics; (2) inner conflicts and needs; (3) stresses of illness and illness behavior; and (4) interviewing strategies.

After the discussion of troubling personality types, suggestions are presented for working with the patient presenting with medically unexplained symptoms (i.e., the patient with somatization). Although troubling interpersonal behavior and somatization are distinct conceptual entities and problems, they are both addressed in this chapter because they commonly overlap in actual practice. Patients with troubling interpersonal behavior often come to their physicians with unexplained or exaggerated physical complaints. Similarly, patients who somatize typically suffer from one or more of the other troubling interpersonal behaviors described in this chapter.

Understanding the general characteristics of troublesome personality types and somatizing patients will help physicians recognize these problems. Through early recognition, physicians can develop appropriate management strategies before falling back on negative labeling, which itself represents a defeat for good care. An awareness of the inner needs and conflicts of these patients can help physicians empathize with them and feel more compassion for their underlying distress. The specific suggestions for interviewing strategies can help physicians manage these patients more successfully, facilitate better doctor-patient rapport, and encourage better patient coping, which also will lead to increased physician satisfaction in the management of difficult patients.

It is important to make the distinction between personality traits (or styles) and personality disorders. Many people possess some aspects of the personality styles described here. In psychiatric nomenclature, however, constellations of traits become formal "disorders" only when the traits lead to persistent maladaptive behavior that compromises functioning.[6] Furthermore, when such patients develop a bona fide acute or chronic general medical illness, the stresses of the general medical illness usually exacerbate their troubling interpersonal behaviors or tendencies to somatize.

# Compulsive Patients

## GENERAL CHARACTERISTICS

Compulsive individuals tend to be concerned about details and lead rigid, highly structured, and predictable lives. Such people emphasize rational processes and disdain emotionality. They often pride themselves on their ability to solve problems. They like to break problems into manageable segments and solve them methodically, one by one. In the words of Sergeant Friday, compulsive individuals may ask for "the facts, just the facts."

Compulsive individuals function best when they feel in control of themselves and their circumstances or the people around them. When in danger of losing control (e.g., illness), these individuals strive for as much certainty as possible. They avoid ambiguity at all costs.

## INNER CONFLICTS AND NEEDS

Compulsive people feel threatened or anxious when confronted by ambiguity, uncertainty, or emotionality. They often experience inner conflict around the recognition and expression of their own emotional lives. Feelings of anger, anxiety, or sadness are often denied, displaced, projected onto others, or experienced as physical sensations such as pain (somatization). These processes often occur unconsciously. The compulsive person may honestly insist that he or she feels no anger, when it is obvious to others that anger is present.

It is probably this fear of their own inner emotional lives that leads compulsive individuals to favor rationality and control. The compulsive individual desires control of self, others, and events. When adequate levels of control are ensured, the compulsive person feels more secure and enjoys an increased sense of well-being.

## STRESSES OF ILLNESS AND ILLNESS BEHAVIOR

Illness creates special anxiety for the compulsive individual. The uncertainty of illness strikes at the core of the individual's strategy for life adjustment. This person can no longer count on rationality to solve life's problems. No longer can he or she predict what will happen day by day. The emotions associated with illness—anxiety, sadness, and anger—are themselves anathema to the compulsive patient.

The anxiety a compulsive patient experiences during illness may lead to a doubly difficult situation. The physical symptoms of illness are frightening to anyone because they present uncertainty. However, the compulsive patient is independently frightened by the emergence of disquieting symptoms because they represent loss of control. The loss of control itself engenders high anxiety. Such a state of high arousal amplifies the illness symptoms and brings physical symptoms of its own, creating a cycle that may be difficult to break.

Under the stress of illness the compulsive patient develops an embattled stance to attain—or rather regain—control. In the battle for control the patient may see not only the disease but also the people involved in his or her care as potential enemies. This can lead to many conflicts with the physician, nurses, family, and friends, often over seemingly insignificant issues.

The compulsive patient needs and desires information. If the information provided does not resolve enough of the uncertainty, the demand for more information can become insatiable. Question asking can become repetitive and circular in a desperate attempt to gain control. Submitting to a hospital routine can be humiliating for compulsive patients, and they often fight for control of minor and seemingly irrelevant details, such as insisting that a sleeping pill be delivered at 9:30 instead of 10:00. In their struggle for order, compulsive patients can experience emotional tension and anxiety when deviations from schedules occur; they become angry, even enraged and unforgiving, at even the slightest deviations.

## INTERVIEWING STRATEGIES

Compulsive patients, even more than other patients, must be treated as equal partners in the alliance against illness. Detailed, accurate, and specific information is essential for good coping by compulsive individuals. This information should be provided in as straightforward a manner as possible. The physician must be scrupulously honest, but care should be taken not to overemphasize the uncertainties of treatments or responses.

The physician should allow the patient as much control as possible in the planning of every stage of treatment. The options and recommendations should be presented, and the patient should be allowed to make as many choices as possible. When compulsive patients are hospitalized, every reasonable effort should be made to minimize the enforced dependency that accompanies patient status.

Compulsive patients must not be prematurely reassured. Unrealistic reassurance that is not based on accurate factual investigations will create more anxiety and mistrust. In general, such patients will not react well to a "fatherly" arm around the shoulder, a pat on the head, or the global, "Do not worry, everything will turn out okay."

Compulsive personality traits can interfere with patient management because patients are so frightened by uncertainty that they continue to ask repetitive questions, do not seem to listen to the answers, and become angry when providers get frustrated and begin to cut their answers short. Sometimes this drives compulsive patients to accuse doctors of not listening, not caring, or not explaining. In reality the physician may have spent a great deal of time and effort attempting to discuss the illness with the patient. However, when the answers never seem sufficient, the physician may have become irritated and say such attacking things as, "I just told you the answer to that question. You're not listening."

This type of physician comment usually raises the patient's anxiety or anger and creates dissonance in the relationship. A far better type of physician response addresses the patient's underlying anxiety about the uncertainty of the illness situation. For example, faced with interminable questions, a physician might say something such as the following:

> PHYSICIAN: *No matter how much information I give you, I don't seem to be able to provide you with what you're really looking for. Is there some other question that you might want to ask but that you really haven't been able to put your finger on yet?*

> or

> PHYSICIAN: *I don't seem to be able to provide you with as much information as you need. I have a feeling that this whole situation is simply very troubling for you, especially the uncertainty. You appear to be a type of person who likes to be able to understand what is happening and to know where things are heading. Being sick, with all its uncertainties, is just very difficult. And I'm sorry that I just can't give you all the anwers you want.*

When the physician addresses the patient's underlying anxiety in this way, the patient may be able to begin talking about underlying fears and recognize that the uncertainty and lack of control may be particularly disabling. Simply recognizing the source of this distress can be a relief in many instances and can actually help the patient cope.

## Dependent Patients

### GENERAL CHARACTERISTICS

As implied by the label, the dependent person finds life difficult to negotiate without outside assistance. Other people, usually one or more "special" people, are sought out to provide a steady fount of emotional support, as well as to help manage day-to-day affairs and important decisions. When this help and support is not delivered, the dependent person may feel deserted, hurt, and angry and may demand more assistance.

### INNER CONFLICTS AND NEEDS

The dependent person has powerful needs to be nurtured and protected because of underlying fears of rejection and being alone. The active caring and help of others provide comfort and relief from insecurity, but only temporarily. Thus the dependent patient's search for support can be relentless. As these demands for support escalate, the dependent person can, in a self-defeating manner, evoke the very rejection that was most feared in the first place.

### STRESSES OF ILLNESS AND ILLNESS BEHAVIOR

Illness is especially frightening for dependent people because they not only suffer the normal worries that illness brings, but also imagine that sickness will lead to a loss of love. This added anxiety can lead to increased and exaggerated dependency on their usual caretakers and to increased physical symptoms (somatization).

Dependent individuals often turn to their physicians and other health care providers to fulfill their general dependency needs, as well as to relieve the specific anxieties evoked by illness. Providers often accept and welcome this dependency at first, especially if (as is often the case) the dependent person expresses a great deal of gratitude. Dependent patients often thank their physicians profusely and make comments like this one:

> PATIENT: *Thank you so much for listening. You're the only doctor I've ever had who really understands.*

Some physicians feel proud to evoke such praise from their patients, but experienced caregivers learn that such laudatory testimonials often lead to later disappointments. Once such patients have become emotionally dependent on their doctors, they tend to experience persistent physical symptoms because of their fear of losing access to the doctor's care and attention. This process is often unconscious (true somatization) or only partly conscious. The nature and severity of the symptoms will become increasingly difficult to explain in purely physical terms. Thus the brief honeymoon between the satisfied patient and the doctor will come to an end as the doctor becomes increasingly puzzled and then frustrated and exasperated. Sensing this, the patient will become yet more afraid of losing the nurturing relationship and will often become even more clinging and demanding, which only makes matters worse. In this way, such patients may change from a physician's dream to a physician's nightmare.

## INTERVIEWING STRATEGIES

The dependent patient certainly needs to be nurtured. Any attempt to treat the dependent patient as an independent partner in the doctor-patient relationship will usually fail and lead the patient to feel rejected and to try to find another doctor who will really "care." Thus a "parental" stance of reassurance can often be successful with dependent patients.

When dependent patients become demanding or clingy, physicians must make special efforts to limit their demands in a gentle and supportive way that minimizes the patients' inference of rejection. Physicians should state their concern and caring very explicitly at the time that limits also are set clearly. For example:

PHYSICIAN: *I want you to know that I am concerned about your health, and I want to do everything I can to get you better and also to help support you through this difficult period. But I also need to let you know that I won't be able to spend 45 minutes with you every time we get together. I understand that this time has been helpful to you, but I can't spend this amount of time with you and also get everything else done that I need to do. I would like to spend about 15 minutes with you each time you come for a checkup. How does that sound to you?*

Because dependent patients will almost always interpret any firm limits as a rejection, it may be helpful for the physician to warn the patient to anticipate this feeling. The physician might say something like this:

PHYSICIAN: *It occurs to me that trying to keep to 15 minutes might make you feel bad, perhaps a little rejected. I am sorry if you feel this way, because I am not rejecting you. I'm just trying to let you know the framework around which I think I can be of most help.*

Scheduling periodic visits that are independent of physical symptoms is another helpful strategy. This gives the patient the assurance of having at least some ongoing support without needing to be ill.

PHYSICIAN: *To give you more effective support, I would like to see you regularly, regardless of whether your symptoms are better or worse. I suggest once a month (or once a week) for a while and then we can reevaluate how you are doing in about 6 months. What do you think?*

The frequency of such visits may need to be less or more depending on the patient but sufficient to break the cycle of emergency symptoms related to anxiety and dependency. Once this circle is broken, the frequency of regularly scheduled visits can be progressively lowered.

Regardless of attempts by the physician to engage the patient in a healthy dialogue about the dependency, the extremely dependent patient will continue to test the limits of the physician's support. Even if the described intervention seems to be helpful in the beginning, some dependent patients feel insatiable neediness and will continue to ask for more than can be reasonably given.

The challenge for the physician is to continue to set appropriate limits without becoming so angry or rejecting that the patient is frightened or forced away.

# Histrionic Patients

## GENERAL CHARACTERISTICS

Histrionic patients, also called "hysterical" patients, live life at a high emotional pitch. Most experiences, including illness, are intense for them, and they can vacillate rapidly between emotional and giddy highs and very distressed lows. They are often attractive and seductive in the emotional, interpersonal, and sexual sense. They can be flashy in the way they behave, as well as the way they dress, walk, and talk. Their emotionality is usually labile and is often perceived by others as shallow.

## INNER CONFLICTS AND NEEDS

Histrionic individuals are driven by a need for admiration as a substitute for love. They tend to confuse admiration with love, which they may not be able to recognize in any other form. At a deeper, usually unconscious, level they crave love and fear that they are unlovable. Histrionic women in male company will often flaunt their sexuality in their efforts to receive admiration from men in lieu of more meaningful intimacy. Histrionic men, depending on the circumstances, may use flirtation or displays of bravado, humor, or aggressiveness in their efforts to seek admiration.

## STRESSES OF ILLNESS AND ILLNESS BEHAVIOR

Even mild illness is likely to be an intense experience for histrionic patients. In addition to the concerns that any sick person is likely to feel, histrionic patients may feel a special threat to their physical attractiveness, on which they depend for their attention. When histrionic individuals become sick, they therefore make special efforts to gain the attention, caring, and affection of caregivers. These efforts may include exaggerated and dramatic accounts of their illness, grandiose and inappropriate compliments to the physician, attempts to present themselves only in the best light, and, if the physician is of the opposite sex, seductive dress and behavior. Male histrionic patients may attempt to intimidate the physician, especially if the physician is also male. The description of their symptoms will often be dramatic and intense. This is partly because they experience the symptoms intensely, but also because of their need for maximum admiration and sympathy from the physician. This amplification of symptoms may be partly or even entirely unconscious (somatization).

## INTERVIEWING STRATEGIES

The physician can help histrionic patients cope by appropriately admiring them when they demonstrate this need. Care must be taken to avoid any behavior that might be interpreted by patients as seductive, challenging, or belittling. If patients make sexual overtures, these must be politely refused. For example:

> PHYSICIAN: *Thank you for your interest in me. I am flattered, but I need to keep our relationship a professional one. I think I can be of most help to you that way. I hope that is okay with you.*

If the patient makes threats or in other ways tries to be intimidating in pursuing his or her demands, the best policy is usually for the physician to show respect and seek further exploration before considering a definitive response. In this way the physician can often avoid either confronting or conceding to a threat. For example:

> PHYSICIAN: *I can see you feel very strongly about this, and I respect that. Tell me more about what makes this such an important issue for you. If I can fully understand your needs and wishes, I expect we can find a way to help.*

The excessive somatic complaints of the histrionic patient may be reduced if the physician shows specific respect for, and interest in, the ways in which the patient copes with the discomfort he or she experiences:

> PHYSICIAN: *I want you to know that I think you're doing a good job coping, given the pain you're experiencing.* (**respect**)
>
> *We'll do all we can to figure this out and get you better as soon as possible.* (**support**)
>
> *Tell me more about the ways in which you've managed to keep going in spite of all these troubles.*

## Self-Defeating Patients

### GENERAL CHARACTERISTICS

Self-defeating patients suffer in life and need to continue to experience this suffering. They perceive themselves as always giving to others and always suffering. This need to suffer, however, is not the same as a need to be physically hurt. Self-defeating patients may become "addicted" to a career of self-sacrifice and suffering, but they do not actually seek pain, physical abuse, or punishment.

### INNER CONFLICTS AND NEEDS

Self-defeating patients have a psychological need to maintain the role of sufferer. Perhaps because of unconscious guilt or identification with long-suffering parents,[7] self-defeating patients are not able to escape from their suffering. They have a strong need to see themselves as self-sacrificing and suffering because otherwise they would have to face intolerable emotions such as hatred of a loved one or guilt or failure. The prospect of recovery or relief from suffering presents a conflict to such patients. Recovery is tempting because the suffering is real, but it is frightening because it would bring painful emotions and drastic changes of lifestyle.

### STRESSES OF ILLNESS AND ILLNESS BEHAVIOR

Long-suffering individuals adapt well to illness but may be threatened by recovery. They can adapt well to the sick role behavior but not so well to recovery. Such patients readily adopt sick role behaviors even when they have only mild physical illnesses or none at all.

Self-defeating patients often frustrate physicians because the patients do not seem to desire to get well. Whatever the doctor attempts does not seem to work. Such patients have been called "manipulative help rejecters" because nothing a physician can do ever seems to help.[2]

### INTERVIEWING STRATEGIES

When working with self-defeating personalities in the medical setting, it is important for the physician to respect their suffering and be wary of promising a complete cure. The physician should remember that illness is a way of life and the threat of an illness-free life is unconsciously troubling for these patients. Such patients genuinely suffer and do not consciously thwart attempts at recovery. Their symptoms may be caused mostly by somatization but are nevertheless real. Patients in this condition really do feel terrible and are unaware of their need to remain ill.

In general, a useful intervention strategy includes a physician's explanation that medical science has not been able to find a complete answer to all problems for all patients. The emphasis for the future should probably be away from any notion of complete cure and toward the notion of coping. Medications or other therapies might help to some degree, but the cornerstone of effective treatment should become the scheduling of regular appointments to check on general conditions and to focus on the patient's ability to function despite the physical problems. As always, the physician must keep an open mind and watch for any new physical signs that warrant further investigation.

The physician should never promise cures or complete relief from suffering because such hopes will usually be dashed and lead to frustration for the patient and the physician. In addition, patients should not be told to, "come back again when you feel sick," because this invites the patient to again use illness behavior to get attention from the physician. The patient should be encouraged to return to regularly scheduled appointments, "whether or not you feel sick." This strategy has been shown to decrease overall medical costs and hospital use for many patients with multiple, chronic, unexplained somatic complaints.[8]

This conservative management approach will not always lead to an easy doctor-patient relationship. Many self-defeating patients continue to suffer and have physical crises again and again. However, a physician who can set appropriate limits in a supportive way and stay with the patient for the long haul will be able to limit iatrogenic injuries, decrease medical care abuse, and contribute to the overall adaptation of long-suffering patients.

# Borderline Patients

## GENERAL CHARACTERISTICS

The term "borderline" refers to a group of patients with a relatively persistent set of personality characteristics, the hallmarks of which are instability in personal relationships, unstable moods, and impulsive behavior. This is a seriously disabling personality disorder. Although the name historically described a syndrome of psychopathology at the border of severity between neurosis and psychosis, the concept is now used to describe a group of patients who simply demonstrate the described characteristics in a marked and persistent way.

The patient with borderline pathology commonly experiences wide fluctuations of feeling in intimate relationships—intense affection and love alternating with dislike or hatred. This seesaw quality in the borderline patient's close relationships carries itself to other situations and other relationships, including the relationship with the physician. The alternating feelings of love and hatred toward others mirror feelings the borderline patient has toward himself or herself.

In addition to the characteristic vacillation of feelings toward self and others, borderline patients suffer from extreme mood swings, an inability to tolerate being alone, difficulty in completing tasks, and impulsive behavior. Although many patients possess some of these features, borderline patients demonstrate these problems to such a degree and with such intensity that a separate label is appropriate to help understand them and develop appropriate intervention strategies.

## INNER CONFLICTS AND NEEDS

Borderline patients feel unloved and threatened by people and circumstances. These feelings may derive from early psychic trauma, including insufficient emotional support from parental figures,[9] or from a lack of resolution of very early or traumatic childhood conflicts (i.e., before the age of

18 months).[10] Borderline patients need emotional support and consistency in their relationships with others, but their internal psychic distress and fluctuating temperament lead to characteristic interpersonal failures. As with the dependent personality, the interpersonal demands of the borderline patient often lead to the very rejection so feared in the beginning. This rejection then proves to such patients that the world is unreliable and unloving. This tragic circle of neediness, rejection, and bitterness in close interpersonal relationships often repeats itself in the doctor-patient or staff-patient relationship when the borderline patient becomes sick.[11]

## STRESSES OF ILLNESS AND ILLNESS BEHAVIOR

Illness presents special adaptive challenges to the borderline patient. In a world that is perceived as unreliable and threatening, illness or hospitalization becomes a stress that threatens further loss of love and support. The ability to tolerate anxiety, frustration, pain, or uncertainty may be severely challenged in the borderline patient with limited resources to cope. The tendency to vacillate between good and bad extremes can become intensified. The fear of being alone becomes more severe, and the tendency toward impulsive behavior can grow excessively.

The borderline patient may describe the physician or other staff in glowing terms one day and hate them the next. These dramatic variations may occur in response to trivial incidents of which the staff and the physician are unaware. Equally dramatic changes may occur in the severity of the patient's symptomatic complaints because these are greatly affected by whether the patient feels loved or hated at the time. These changes in symptoms, at least partly caused by somatization of negative emotions, may be difficult to explain on purely physical grounds and therefore will puzzle the physician. Furthermore, the borderline patient usually has little insight into his or her own exquisite sensitivity; borderline patients characteristically hold others primarily responsible for their own emotional state and often for their symptoms as well.

## INTERVIEWING STRATEGIES

Depending on the severity of the borderline pathology, the ability to develop therapeutic doctor-patient relationships can vary greatly. Nevertheless, the following general guidelines can be helpful.

Perhaps the most useful principle is to remember that borderline patients are like frightened children. They have a fear of the unknown, of strangers, and of illness that is akin to a child's fearfulness but that may be masked by more adult presentations of anger, demandingness, and bitterness. Attempts to understand the "frightened child" behind the storm of emotionality will help the physician manage his or her own feelings and develop a strategy for helping patients. The best strategy, just as with children, is to combine consistent support with firm structure and limit setting.

The borderline patient feels a deep and continuing need for reassurance. Thus supportive attention and concern can be soothing, although the emotional "supplies" that the physician possesses may be insufficient for the patient's needs. When these needs and demands escalate, the physician should try to be as supportive as possible but to maintain a firm sense of the limits of his or her own tolerance, as well as the limits of the hospital environment. If the demands are presented with threats or aggressiveness, the best response is usually along the lines already described for histrionic patients. The patient's legitimate concerns and fears should be addressed, but when unreasonable demands are made, the physician should set limits in as clear and supportive a way as possible. At times there may be no way to completely satisfy a borderline patient (just as there may be no way to meet all the requests of a demanding child). However, sensitive attention to the patient's underlying fear and insecurity may communicate enough support to facilitate more adaptive behavior on the patient's part.

Some other strategies may be helpful in the management of the borderline patient, especially in the hospital environment. Because the borderline patient is often frightened of being alone, it can be helpful for his or her room to be positioned near the nursing station and for nurses or other staff to make frequent room checks. It has also proved useful for one staff member to be assigned the task of communicating medical information to the patient and for discussing problems. Because the borderline patient can "split" medical providers into ones they see as "good" and others who are "bad," limiting medical and problem discussion to one provider can minimize the tendency for distortion in communication to occur and can also minimize the danger of splitting intense emotional reactions between different caregivers or different providers.[11] Specially called staff meetings may be helpful to develop a unified care plan for particularly disruptive borderline patients.

# Narcissistic Patients

## GENERAL CHARACTERISTICS

Patients with narcissistic personality traits feel that they have special qualities and experiences and are entitled to special attention and special treatment.[9] This is their perspective about illness, just as it is about all other aspects of life. They seem genuinely perplexed when their sense of entitlement is challenged. It is as if their expectation for special treatment is their birthright and they expect others to recognize this right implicitly, in the same way that they recognize it for themselves. Some patients with narcissistic features are from the upper socioeconomic class or are leaders in business, politics, religion, or the military. Their expectations for special treatment may thus be based on realistic experiences. However, other narcissistic individuals develop and retain their sense of entitlement even when the world has not acknowledged their uniqueness.

Narcissistic individuals generally cannot understand others' points of view. They can be so wrapped up in their own world of uniqueness and expectation that every experience is filtered and colored by their own point of view. They have little tolerance or flexibility for the reality of the functioning of complex social systems. They expect rules, policies, or procedures to be waived for their personal desires or comforts, and they become enraged at the thought of being treated like everyone else.

## INNER CONFLICTS AND NEEDS

Narcissistic personality traits and, especially, narcissistic personality disorders generally are built on an edifice of insecurity and ego deficits. Narcissists' self-esteem is actually extremely fragile, and their apparent self-confidence depends on the adoration, respect, or uniqueness with which others treat them. The overarching need is to be respected and treated as special.

Inner conflicts revolve around this insecurity about self-worth. These conflicts may be well defended, and narcissists are often unaware of their fragile self-esteem. This shaky self-esteem may become apparent to patients only when they are threatened by the loss of special treatment by the social world. When respect and uniqueness is lost or denied, narcissists may react with rage or depression.

## STRESSES OF ILLNESS AND ILLNESS BEHAVIOR

Illness and hospitalization present great threats to narcissists because illness confronts these patients with their own vulnerability. Narcissistic patients who become sick participate in a living nightmare; they feel powerless and lost in a system that cannot be controlled and that often treats them in the manner they most fear, as one of many. This can arouse primitive, childlike fears of abandonment and, in general, a loss of love. Narcissists' usual sense of self-confidence and pride can be deeply shaken. These patients may be tempted to elaborate or exaggerate their symptoms to establish their unique status. This may happen unconsciously (somatization) or consciously (factitious illness).

As narcissistic defenses become challenged, patients may react with depression and with rage at a medical system that refuses to treat them as special. Narcissists may also feel this rage against particular providers or institutions if they feel that the uniqueness of their symptoms and entitlement has not been recognized. This rage can present in the form of impractical or impossible demands on the system or in the form of bitter criticism about alleged failures of diagnosis or treatment. Narcissists may also be depressed about the threatened loss of esteem, efficacy, and power in the world.

## INTERVIEWING STRATEGIES

The treatment of the narcissistic patient presents a great challenge to the physician and the health care system in general. When this patient is articulate, educated, and powerful, the rage and implied threat (sometimes of lawsuits) can frighten the caregiver. The physicians and other caregivers may change their general procedures in ways that may compromise good care. On the other hand, some caregivers may never "give anything" to the narcissistic patient, because some physicians may not want to be "manipulated" and do not want to cede one iota of control to the patient, especially to an unreasonably demanding one.

An intermediate strategy between the two extremes may be helpful. First, the physician should understand the underlying fear of the narcissistic patient. This fear is greater than that of the average patient. Not only is the narcissistic patient afraid of all the normal events that might occur in illness, but the narcissistic patient suffers additional fear because of the loss of uniqueness that illness implies. When a hospital environment treats a patient as "one among many," the narcissist suffers a special humiliation that must be understood before he or she can be helped.

The general strategy suggested in this text focuses on supporting the patient's claim to uniqueness, within the limits that the system and physician can tolerate. It is usually helpful to ask the angry, demanding patient what specific changes would make him or her happier. If the requests are general, such as, "I just want to be treated with more respect," an attempt should be made to get the patient to be quite specific in these requests. Once a series of requests has been received, the physician or staff can try to meet as many of these requests as possible. This often temporarily mollifies the narcissistic patient. Some but not all of the requests can usually be reasonably met. The patient can be told this directly. For example:

> **PHYSICIAN:** *We can change the time that the blood pressures are taken in the night so you can get a better night's sleep. I will write a specific, special order to make sure that this occurs. I can also make sure that the visiting hours for your son are changed so that he can come visit you when he gets out of work. I won't be able to change the meal times, however, because the dietary service is obligated to deliver to this ward according to a fixed schedule.*

Furthermore, if the physician can meet some of these requests, he or she can often negotiate for some relaxation of the patient's difficult behaviors. For example:

> **PHYSICIAN:** *I have discussed your requests with the nurses. As I mentioned, there are several requests that we can happily meet, but a few that just can't work out. In return for our efforts to meet your special needs, I wonder if you would be willing save your requests and problems for discussion with the head nurse, who will come to see you every day between 1 and 2 PM. If you discuss these requests with every staff member who comes in, the hospital routine can get confused and disrupted.*

# Somatization

## GENERAL CHARACTERISTICS

Somatization has been defined as "the expression of emotional discomfort and psychosocial distress in the language of bodily symptoms."[12] By this definition, emotional discomfort includes emotional distress, as well as bona fide mental syndromes or disorders such as major depression or panic disorder. In most cases of somatization, the sufferer is entirely unaware of the psychologic or neurobiologic connection between the emotional psychiatric dysfunction and the experience of physical illness.[13]

It is of utmost importance that physicians understand that the physical suffering of somatizing patients is just as real as suffering that has a demonstrable pathophysiologic etiology. Furthermore, from a differential diagnostic or management point of view, *the patient's response to placebo is of no use in determining whether pain complaints are psychogenic or physical in etiology.* Some physical pain responds to placebo, and some psychogenic pain does not. For example, 30% of postoperative surgical pain responds to placebo.[14] Thus physicians should not conceptualize the somatization process (or psychogenic pain) as "all in the head" or "not real." This trivializes serious problems and implies conscious deception in a situation in which the patient's experience of the pain is real.

The physician should distinguish between somatization (which is an *unconscious* process, of which the patient is unaware) and certain other related syndromes in which physical symptoms are *consciously* manufactured. "Malingering" refers to the process of consciously producing or exaggerating physical symptoms in the effort to achieve some understandable external gain—for example, disability benefits, insurance claims, or potent analgesics. The rare and often very dramatic and self-destructive Munchausen syndrome (also known as factitious disorder) involves the conscious production of symptoms in response to a compelling psychologic drive to be a patient.

## INNER CONFLICTS AND NEEDS

In contrast to many of the troubling interpersonal behaviors described previously, somatization represents a final common pathway for numerous different forms of psychic disturbance. Some mental disorders, such as depression or panic disorder, are associated with demonstrable neurobiologic substrates.[15] In such conditions, the mind-body connection may lead to direct physical manifestations of the psychiatric problem, such as insomnia and fatigue. Such symptoms usually respond well to appropriate psychotropic medication (or, sometimes, targeted psychotherapy). For other somatizing patients, complex psychologic mechanisms play a psychodynamic or behaviorally conditioned role in perpetuating physical symptoms and interpersonal dysfunction.

In all cases somatizing patients experience genuine and distressing physical symptoms, of which the cause is obscure. As a rule, somatizing patients are eager to find explanations for their suffering and consume considerable amounts of medical time and resources in seeking answers. Such patients often remain dissatisfied with their care. Because of the intractable and persistent nature of their physical symptoms and their demands for relief, physicians often find them troubling to manage.[1]

Somatizing patients are stuck in a painful trap; they need and want relief, but they characteristically find it difficult to accept explanations or treatments of their symptoms that are based on an appropriate psychobiologic understanding of mind-body relationships.

Successful management of the somatizing patient usually requires that the physician possess considerable knowledge and skill. Besides mastering the knowledge base for appropriate assessment, the physician who attempts treatment of the somatizing patient must develop a highly effective set of communication skills for rapport development and partnership for treatment.

## STRESSES OF ILLNESS AND ILLNESS BEHAVIOR

Patients who somatize may also develop concomitant physical illnesses. Management of the somatizing patient usually becomes more difficult in the face of clear-cut physical illness. The tendency to somatize may persist, resulting in the amplification of symptoms that have been caused by an underlying physical illness.[16] This creates circular problems and increasing confusion and frustration for both the patient and the doctor.

In the context of an emergent and definable pathologic condition, there is often increasing pressure for both the patient and the doctor to latch onto any positive physical finding, however obscure, in the hope that it will provide a complete explanation for the symptoms. By the same token, there is the related pressure to try any physical treatment that seems even marginally relevant in the hope that it will provide a cure. Because of these pressures, physicians often undertake risky investigations and treatments of marginal relevance. Such investigations and treatments often lead to iatrogenic damage, both psychologic and physical.

## INTERVIEWING STRATEGIES

Many doctors find it difficult to deal with somatization. Even when physicians believe that somatization may be the principal problem, many find themselves colluding with somatizing patients in an endless series of physical investigations and specialist opinions. This fruitless search for answers has the effect of reinforcing patients' determination to find purely physical explanations. By the time the physician decides to call a halt to this process, it is virtually impossible to do so without alienating the patient.

Despite having the "benefit" of frequent unsatisfactory clinical experiences, such as that described in the preceding paragraph, most physicians feel unable to develop management strategies that can lead to better outcomes. On the other hand, physicians who recognize the possibility or probability of somatization early in the assessment process can implement an appropriate management strategy before iatrogenic damage has been done and before the physician-patient relationship has deteriorated beyond repair.

An evidence-based communication and intervention strategy that incorporates the five steps described in the following can be readily learned and effectively used by nonpsychiatrists.[17-20]

1. **Diagnose and treat depression and anxiety** when they are present. Up to 50% of patients with severe somatization have comorbid depression or anxiety disorders. As described in Chapters 16 and 17, management of somatization becomes less complex when these psychiatric syndromes are effectively treated (with medications or psychotherapy).
2. **Develop rapport.** Understand and empathize with the patient and his or her dilemma.
3. **Change the agenda.** Emphasize coping, not curing.
4. **See the patient regularly,** whether or not he or she is experiencing the physical problems.
5. **"Don't just do something, stand there!"**

## DEVELOP RAPPORT

Develop rapport requires physicians to try their best to experience the world from the point of view of the somatizing—but suffering—patient. Physicians must acquire a vivid and accurate picture of the symptoms themselves but do so while moving quickly toward understanding (and empathizing with) the effect of these symptoms on the patient's overall quality of life.

When interviewing somatizing patients, it is always important to start with the symptoms themselves (e.g. "symptom-oriented" interviewing), but also to make it clear from an early stage that the physician is interested in the impact of these symptoms on the patient's life.

PHYSICIAN: *I would like to hear more detail about your symptoms, starting with the first thing that went wrong and what the circumstances were when it happened.*

After listening to the patient's story, it is essential to empathize with the patient's suffering. The physician can do this by recognizing the patient's distress and legitimizing his or her suffering. This is important to developing an effective partnership with the patient.

When developing an effective partnership, the physician should never say, or even imply, that "there is nothing wrong" or that "it's all in the mind." Somatizing patients know there is something wrong, and they derive little comfort from being told that there is nothing wrong. This discounts their suffering and serves as a marker for lack of physician understanding. Physicians can and should make comments such as the following:

PHYSICIAN: *It is clear to me that these are very uncomfortable symptoms.* (**reflection**) *I can well understand how distressed you have been about them.* (**legitimation**)

Somatizing patients are typically frustrated by the medical care system, which has not produced any relief from suffering. Empathizing with this frustration can serve as an important building block for the relationship. For example:

PHYSICIAN: *I can certainly understand why you are so frustrated with doctors. You've been suffering with the stomach trouble for 5 years, and yet you cannot find anyone who has been able to tell you what is wrong and what you can do for relief.* (**legitimation**)

Part of the empathic process involves understanding the somatizing patient's life situation and fears regarding causation. When beginning the assessment of psychosocial issues with a somatizing patient, it is always best to first ask about the *effects* of the symptoms on the patient's emotional state and day-to-day activities. Without this introduction, somatizing patients may feel that the physician is discounting the physical suffering if the focus is turned onto the psychosocial life situation. The following approach often proves useful:

PHYSICIAN: *These are tough symptoms. How have they affected your day-to-day life (e.g., work, home life, relationships, sleep, energy, sex life, or mood)?*

Similarly, accurate empathy requires understanding the nature of the patient's concerns about etiology.

PHYSICIAN: *It would help me if you could let me know about your own thoughts and fears about the possible causes of these symptoms.*

When physicians elicit a patient's underlying concerns, it is essential to empathize with these concerns and, when possible, to offer clear, realistic reassurance:

PHYSICIAN: *I can well understand why you might suspect that and how worrying that would be.* (**legitimation**)

*Based on the history, the physical examinations, and the other studies we have done, I can tell you emphatically (and our consultants agree) that your symptoms are not caused by underlying heart disease (or cancer).*

*Let me review, again, my specific reasons for saying this.* (**reassurance**)

## CHANGING THE AGENDA

Changing the agenda requires introducing a change in the mindset of both the patient and the physician to focus on coping, not curing. This requires accepting that the symptoms are of a chronic nature and are essentially not life threatening. Acute interventions have not worked in the past, so the management of symptoms through coping mechanisms is the best strategy.

## SEEING THE PATIENT REGULARLY

Physicians must schedule regular visits with patients to monitor symptoms, assess the effect of symptoms on the patients' quality of life, and develop the interpersonal relationships that will help patients cope better with their chronic symptoms. Because somatizing patients often develop their symptoms under circumstances of high stress and they tend to use physicians as a significant source of social support, an alteration in this maladaptive cycle can be extremely effective. The physician should not wait for patients to develop new symptoms. Patients with chronic, unexplained symptoms need to be seen regularly, usually about once a month, *whether or not they are experiencing their symptoms*. When physicians are able to maintain a relationship with these patients and see them regularly, the psychosocial aspects of the patients' conditions often become more apparent. The intensity and severity of their physical problems often diminish.

## "DON'T JUST DO SOMETHING, STAND THERE!"

It is important for the physician to minimize new investigations; however, somatizing patients often demand new tests. Sometimes it is appropriate to agree to more tests, but more often it is better to say something that both deflects the patient from further investigation, at least for the time being, and gently introduces the possibility of a different approach. This is perhaps the most delicate and complex intervention of the whole process. Although this intervention naturally has to be tailored to each patient, it might be something like the following interchange between the physician and the patient:

> PHYSICIAN: *I can well understand your wish for further tests because naturally you hope that they might provide a definite explanation for your symptoms and therefore some hope of relief. Sadly, I have to tell you that the chance of further tests showing even a partial explanation is virtually zero. I feel confident of this, and all the consultants you have seen agree.*
>
> PATIENT: *So what do you suggest? I know something is the matter.*
>
> PHYSICIAN: *What I suggest is that we agree to have a temporary halt to the tests while we review the situation, watch you very closely, and consider a different approach that I think can offer at least a partial solution. At the moment, I feel that all the information we have from our tests and our consultants make it clear that we are not dealing with a dangerous medical condition that we are missing. Because I understand how much you are suffering and how these problems are affecting your daily life, I would like to see you regularly to help work out a way to manage these symptoms better. I will offer suggestions for treatment strategies that might be helpful, but I think we both have to understand that the goal right now is not one of complete cure. Rather, we are shooting for some slight improvements and for ways to help you cope better with the problem. The most important part is that I would like to see you regularly to monitor your progress and work with you to help with management strategies that help you feel better.*

This type of conservative management of chronic, unexplained physical complaints, using the doctor-patient relationship as the key ingredient for "treatment," has been shown in the randomized, prospective clinical trials to be effective in achieving improved clinical outcome and decreased medical expenditures.[19,20]

## Conclusion

Numerous clinical situations that involving troubling interpersonal behavior or chronic somatization have the potential to cause great distress for physicians and poor clinical results for patients. Interviewing strategies based on understanding the determinants of these troubling behaviors and somatization can lead to improved relationships with patients and better outcomes.

## References

1. Hahn S, et al: The difficult patient: prevalence, psychopathology, and functional impairment. *J Gen Intern Med* 11(1):18, 1996.
2. Hinchey S, Jackson JL: A cohort study assessing difficult patient encounters in a walk in primary care clinic, predictors and outcomes. *J Gen Intern Med* 26(6):588–594, 2011.
3. Kroenke K, Rosmalen J: Symptoms, syndromes, and the value of psychiatric diagnostics in patients who have functional somatic disorders. *Med Clin North Am* 603–626, 2006.
4. Groves JE: Taking care of the hateful patient. *N Engl J Med* 298(16):883–887, 1978.
5. Cohen-Cole SA, Friedman CP: The language problem: integration of psychosocial variables into routine medical care. *Psychosomatics* 24:54, 1983.
6. American Psychiatric Association: *Diagnostic and statistical manual of mental disorders*, ed 5, Washington, DC, 2013.
7. Levy ST, Lyle C, Cohen-Cole SA: Masochistic character pathology in medical settings. In Ross JM, Myers WA, editors: *Psychoanalytic psychotherapy*, Washington, DC, 1988, American Psychiatric Association.
8. Smith GR, Monson RA, Ray DC: Psychiatric consultation in somatization disorder: a randomized controlled study. *N Engl J Med* 314:1407–1413, 1986.
9. Adler G: *Borderline psychopathology and its treatment*, New York, 1985, Jason Aronson.
10. Kernberg O: *Object relations theory and clinical psychoanalysis*, New York, 1976, Jason Aronson.
11. Groves JE: Management of the borderline patient on a medical-surgical ward: the psychiatric consultant's role. *Int J Psychiatry Med* 6:337–348, 1975.
12. Katon W, Ries RK, Kleinman A: The prevalence of somatization in primary care. *Comp Psychiatry* 25:208–215, 1984.
13. Walker EA, Unetzer J, Katon WJ: Understanding and caring for the distressed patient with multiple unexplained symptoms. *J Am Board Fam Pract* 11(5):347–356, 1998.
14. Ford CV: *The somatizing disorders: illness as a way of life*, New York, 1983, Elsevier Science Publishing.
15. Belmaker R, Agam G: Major depressive disorder. *N Engl J Med* 358:55–68, 2008.
16. Barsky AJ: Amplification, somatization, and the somatoform disorders. *Psychosomatics* 33(1):28–34, 1992.
17. Gask L, et al: The treatment of somatization: the evaluation of a training package with general practices trainees. *J Psychosom Res* 33:697–703, 1989.
18. Smith GR, Monson RA, Ray DC: Psychiatric consultation in somatization disorder: a randomized controlled study. *N Engl J Med* 314:1407–1413, 1986.
19. Smith RC, et al: Primary care clinicians treat patients with medically unexplained symptoms: a randomized controlled trial. *J Gen Intern Med* 21:671–677, 2006.
20. Drossman DA: The problem patient: evaluation and care of medical patients with psychosocial disturbances. *Ann Intern Med* 88(3):366–372, 1978.

# CHAPTER 26

# Communicating with the Psychotic Patient

Guy Undrill

## OVERVIEW

Psychotic patients present some of the biggest challenges for the physician. Features of psychotic illness make forming a relationship, assessing and understanding the problem, and collaboratively managing the problem more difficult than in nonpsychotic patients. Of all the challenges, none is more difficult for both patient and doctor than the fear and stigma surrounding mental illness, which can lead doctors to treat these patients differently from their other patients. This chapter discusses strategies to help physicians communicate with psychotic patients.

## Psychotic Patients

### GENERAL CHARACTERISTICS

Psychosis is defined by an impairment of reality testing, typically in the form of hallucinations (perceptions in the absence of stimulus, such as hearing voices or seeing things) or delusions (culturally alienating beliefs, which may be bizarre). Although these symptoms are the most dramatic part of psychosis, they are often not the most handicapping: so-called "negative symptoms" of reduced motivation, social withdrawal, and blunted affect can (with their psychosocial consequences) have a major impact on quality of life. Underpinning both of these sets of deficits are a variety of cognitive defects,[1] including problems with attention shifting, working memory, and executive function. These last groups of impairments call for particular adaptations to the interview.

### INNER CONFLICTS AND NEEDS

Psychosis is a complex phenomenon that cannot be simply reduced to a single set of inner conflicts and needs. Psychosis often starts in the teens or twenties and may be overlaid on a variety of developmental stages. A 15-year-old patient presenting with first episode psychosis will have quite different needs from a patient with a 20-year history of hospitalizations. However, there are some recurrent themes. The patient may be terrified of perplexing inner experiences and have a need to be understood. Communication may be difficult because of cognitive impairments, and the physician may need to provide additional support and structure beyond his or her usual practice. In addition, it is often necessary to consider the setting carefully. Particularly if a patient is acutely psychotic, a busy, over-stimulating environment (such as an emergency room) is full of ambiguous stimuli that can be prone to misinterpretation. A quiet, uncluttered, and well-lit room is generally preferred.

## STRESSES OF THE ILLNESS AND ILLNESS NEEDS

Psychotic illnesses can be intensely traumatic. Patients may be fearful of losing their own sanity or may manage psychotic experiences by self-medicating with drugs or alcohol, or down-regulating social interaction in an effort to cope better. Social isolation can be exacerbated by others' fear of mental illness.

# Strategies

## SELF MANAGEMENT

Psychotic patients are at increased risk of suicide and of violence. The latter risk should not be overemphasized: The principal risk factors for violence are the same in both nonpsychotic and psychotic patients, and the relative risk of violence contributed by psychosis is far less than (for example) recent use of drugs or alcohol. Most psychiatry primers have information on risk and personal safety in the interview.[2]

It is important for the physician to learn to manage his or her own anxiety about dealing with psychosis. The interview may lead to long silences, odd behavior, or frankly bizarre content. Uncontrolled fears can lead to physicians abandoning their usual routine and missing comorbid illnesses, or letting opportunities for therapeutic interventions pass them by in their enthusiasm to move on from this difficult patient to someone who is easier to engage. Much of the large excess of mortality suffered by people with schizophrenia (who die on average 15 to 25 years earlier than the general population) is attributable to the same causes as the general population, although this group are less likely to receive secondary care interventions and more likely to receive less intensive treatment than nonpsychotic controls.[3]

The general approach to the psychotic patient should be calm, respectful, nonjudgmental, and empathic. This includes recognizing that for some psychotic patients, interpersonal detachment is a coping mechanism and a medical interview can be very stressful. Be flexible: Sometimes several short interviews may be preferable to one long interview.

Be honest and genuine. Paranoid patients are particularly sensitive to any hint of deceit or manipulation. Do not hedge awkward issues that you find difficult to address such as the need for compulsory admission or restraint: Explain what you are doing and why.

## COGNITIVE SUPPORT

In interviewing the psychotic patient, a not uncommon experience is to feel the sense of what the patient is saying slipping away. Even as each individual statement the patient makes seems understandable at the time, 5 minutes after the interview has finished it is difficult to recall what the patient said. This is a soft sign of mild formal thought disorder. When thought disorder is encountered, it is helpful to provide cognitive support. It is often helpful to start the interview with an outline of what you will be covering and why, then checking in with the patient to make sure he or she is in agreement. Continue to structure and signpost the interview more than you normally would. This includes using checking and summary liberally, but also other structuring interventions such as explaining the rationale for your approach and announcing that you are transitioning to a different segment of the interview (e.g., an accentuated transition).

> PHYSICIAN: *Thank you for telling me about the last time you were in the hospital and how that worked out for you. Now I'd like to move on to asking you some questions about your past medical history if that's okay.*

Cognitive deficits can include theory of mind deficits, which can make normal social cues difficult to read for the patient. Patients may misread social cues; for example, coming in to your office and sitting in your chair. More subtle social deficits sometimes can be experienced at the edge of conscious awareness. Sometimes it is possible to catch oneself unconsciously adapting to the patient and departing from one's normal style in a way that (if noticed) can provide one with important diagnostic information. It may be necessary to politely bring the interview to a close in a more unambiguous way than you might with a nonpsychotic patient who would read cues such as closing the patient's chart or shifting the interview to "closing small talk."

Cognitive support may also be helpful with patients who are overwhelmed by intrusive hallucinations and may find it difficult simply to attend to what you are saying.

Cognitive deficits often affect the patient's ability to plan and anticipate consequences of actions, which means that collaborative management must be done in simple steps, for example, chunking information into smaller pieces and repeating it more often. Chronically psychotic patients may lack flexibility in thinking and have difficulty conceiving of alternative futures or negotiating priorities, which may require time and tact to address. This can feel time consuming but is usually more effective in the long run than abandoning collaborative management for a paternal or controlling approach. Value small changes and play the long game. It is usually worth prioritizing tomorrow's therapeutic relationship over any particular piece of therapeutic work that your patient is refusing today. Despite this, one cannot be dogmatic about a collaborative approach. This group of patients can become very ill and lose the capacity to work with you in any meaningful way. Occasionally there may be dangerous levels of self-neglect or violence to others. In this situation, it may be necessary to use more forceful approaches to restrict freedom or give medication against the patient's will.

Open questions often create anxiety and elicit more thought disorder. If you have elicited thought disorder, switch to closed questions, but continue to support autonomy by offering menus of choices when possible.

## AFFECT MANAGEMENT

With nonpsychotic patients, building reflections around affect, meaning, or values often deepens the relationship productively. Psychotic patients can sometimes experience these kinds of reflections as invasive, or, in extreme cases, as mind reading—particularly if they have other delusions of thought alienation or interference. Try to keep proportionately more of your reflections at a simple, factual level, without neglecting the patient's affective experience. Use reflections more as structuring devices to build understanding and draw the patient back to the key issues of the interview. When possible, anchor the reflections more in reality than the patient's initial utterance, especially when thought disorder is present.

For paranoid patients, make each intervention smoothly flow from one to the other so the relationship between your successive interventions is clear to the patient. This can help to avoid inflaming a sense of persecution that can arise when the patient is unable to follow your line of thought and fills in the blanks with a paranoid interpretation.

> **PHYSICIAN:** *Other patients of mine who have been troubled by voices have sometimes felt that their thoughts weren't their own. Is this something that you have ever experienced?*

It is particularly important to try to avoid argument, confrontation, or criticism. Critical comments are often directed at negative symptoms by families or less skilled practitioners, who are frustrated by the patient's apparent laziness or inability to help himself or herself. Remember that symptoms of lack of motivation and apathy are part of the illness and that hostility and critical comments are predictive of relapse of positive symptoms.

## REALITY ORIENTATION

Traditional teaching in psychiatry was that it was either futile or positively harmful to talk about a patient's abnormal experiences with them. This is no longer considered correct by most experts.[4] It is perfectly safe to talk about psychotic experiences (although you shouldn't collude with them). Patients will often want to talk about their beliefs and their own explanatory models of what is happening to them and can become quite frustrated if their experiences are treated as of diagnostic significance only. The craziest-seeming ideas often have a kernel of truth in them, which sometimes only becomes apparent when you have spent considerable time with your patient and begin to know him or her well. This should inform your initial approach to the patient, which should be one of respectful interest and collaborative empiricism as you explore beliefs and later test out evidence for the ideas and the utility of beliefs together.

Build the patient's (and your own) capacity to acknowledge that there are radically different ways of seeing the world that may have validity. The real skill in interviewing psychotic patients comes in balancing reality orientation with avoiding argumentation.

> **PHYSICIAN:** *What you're describing is very real to you, and it's frustrating that I don't see things the same way. Let's take a look at what has led you to your conclusions.*

One way of avoiding argumentation is to try to develop a shared vocabulary of distress with the patient that avoids jargon. For example, a patient may not wish to describe his or her experiences in terms of psychosis but may be able to talk about the "difficult time" he or she is having.

## Conclusion

Patients with psychosis are among the most challenging to interview and test the communication skills of the most experienced clinicians. However, in an age of technological medicine, being able to apply purely clinical skills that make a real difference to your patients without leaving the consulting room makes these patients deeply satisfying to treat.

### References

1. Bentall RP: *Madness explained: psychosis and human nature*, 2003, Penguin.
2. Stern TA, et al: *Massachusetts General Hospital handbook of general hospital psychiatry*, ed 6, 2010, Saunders.
3. Wildgust H, Hodgson R, Beary M: The paradox of premature mortality in schizophrenia: new research questions. *J Psychopharmacol* 24:9, 2010.
4. Henry L, et al: *Cognitively oriented psychotherapy for first episode psychosis (COPE): a practitioner's manual*, Melbourne, 2002, EPPIC.

# CHAPTER 27

# Breaking Bad News

Geoffrey H. Gordon

## OVERVIEW

Breaking bad news is often challenging, partly because the three functions (build the relationship, assess and understand the patient, and collaborate for management) overlap and occur simultaneously. This chapter helps clinicians address the complexities of breaking bad news by applying the concepts and skills of the Three Function Model.

The main task is to give new and potentially upsetting information as part of collaborative management.

> *Mr. Jones, the test showed that the lump on your x-ray is a lung cancer. We have time to think about what to do next. I'd like to ask Dr. Smith to advise us on the best treatment, but I'll still be your main doctor.*

At the same time, the need to assess and understand the patient

> *What do you already know about lung cancer? What kinds of information would you like to have now? Is there anyone else you'd like to include in these discussions?*

and to build the relationship,

> *I can see this news is really hard for you. I'm wondering what you're most concerned about right now.*

are all equally important. Breaking bad news without attention to all three functions can severely impair patients' and families' coping.

Why a chapter on breaking bad news? Students are often surprised to learn that US physicians avoided the practice, study, and teaching of breaking bad news for decades. For example, the percentage of physicians who tell patients they have cancer rose from 10% in the 1960s to greater than 90% in the 1980s. Some of this change reflected increasing public awareness of cancer diagnosis and treatment, greater patient autonomy and self-determination, and greater scrutiny of physician practices. More recently, breaking bad news is often included as a part of competency-based training and assessment for medical students, residents, and oncologists.[1-5]

Breaking bad news is challenging for both physician and patient. For physicians, breaking bad news can mean acknowledging feelings of helplessness, sadness, or fear of death. Careful plans for breaking bad news can be derailed by other crises or simply lack of adequate time. For patients, bad news can signal loss of health, income, plans for the future, or even life itself. In addition, neither party knows quite what to expect from the other, creating more tension and uncertainty. These challenges inhibit the teaching and learning, as well as the practice, of breaking bad news.

Most of the published research on breaking bad news focuses on patients with cancer and their families. This chapter draws on this and other work including notifying parents of a child's developmental disability, giving the news of a positive HIV test, informing patients that all available and appropriate treatments have failed to control their disease, and notifying survivors of a loved one's death.

In the chapter that follows this one, Chapter 27A, Joseph Weiner presents an alternative, highly structured, nine-step model, which is a bit more simplified than the approach presented here, that reconceptualizes the process of breaking bad news as a process between physician and patient that is both transactional (information and emotional content flows back and forth) and transformational (these exchanges ideally lead to fundamental growth). Dr. Weiner's model is fully aligned with the other concepts presented in this chapter.

## Preparing to Break Bad News

Preparing the patient for bad news can begin early in the workup if the data suggest a potentially serious disorder.

> PHYSICIAN: *Mr. Virchow, your low blood count and blood in the stool really worry me. A lot of things can cause blood in the stool. Sometimes it's hemorrhoids, which are blood vessels in the rectum. Sometimes it's polyps, or little growths on the wall of your intestine. These can bleed, and if they've been there a long time, they can even turn into cancer. I think we should do some more tests to find out exactly what it is.*

> PATIENT: *Really? You know, I think my mother might have had that.*

> PHYSICIAN: *I'm not sure that's what it is. Like I said, we need some more tests. The most important test is to look and see if there is anything abnormal. If we see something, we can take a biopsy and then tell you what it is. How does that sound to you?*

> PATIENT: *Well, if that's what you have to do, I guess it's okay.*

This is a good opportunity to ask patients how they would like to receive results:

> PHYSICIAN: *Whatever we find, we're going to have to talk about what to do next. Is there someone you'd like to come with you to that visit?*

> PATIENT: *Yeah, my wife. She always wants to know what the doctor says.*

Another useful way to lay the groundwork for potential bad news is to elicit the patient's explanatory model (Function Two: Assess and Understand the Patient). Briefly, this is the patient's attributions (what might be wrong and why) and expectations (what should be done and what results to expect). These are based on the patient's prior experiences with self, family, friends, the media, and other sources. They often develop before the medical visit and influence the decision to seek care.

> PHYSICIAN: *Mr. Virchow, I wonder what you've been thinking about this blood in the stool and your low blood count. What do you think is wrong?*

> PATIENT: *I don't know, Doc. That's why I came to see you.*

> PHYSICIAN: *I understand that, and I'll tell you what I think, but it helps me to know what you've already learned about this, or what concerns you the most about it.*

> PATIENT: *Well, I did see a piece in the paper a while back about blood in the stool. It was all about colon cancer. They said sometimes it's too late to do anything about it. They said you should eat broccoli.*

> PHYSICIAN: *What would colon cancer mean to you?*

> PATIENT: *Well, my mother had some kind of cancer. They opened her up and saw it everywhere and just closed her up again. She died in agony 2 weeks later.*

> PHYSICIAN: *Okay. Let's make sure I understand. You've wondered if this might be colon cancer. And your experience tells you that cancer is painful and fatal. That must be really frightening for you. You did the right thing by coming in and getting checked out. You need to*

*know, though, that if we can find colon cancer early, there's a lot we can do to treat it and any symptoms it causes.*

Many patients worry that they have a serious illness but are too nervous to ask the doctor about it. Eliciting the explanatory model can help the physician anticipate what kinds of information and emotional support might be needed.

## Breaking the News

Delivery of bad news lends itself to the (e)TACCT (elicit, Tell, Ask, Care, Counsel, Tell Back) model for giving patients information and instructions (Function Three). Because bad news is usually emotionally charged, the (e)TACCT steps may not follow an orderly progression, and Care (Function One: Build the Relationship) often takes a prominent role. The process of eliciting the patient's explanatory model was described in the preceding. That can be followed by the other steps of TACCT.

## TELL

The first step in Tell is assessing what the patient is ready to hear. This can be done by reviewing the clinical data and asking the patient to update you on what he or she has already learned about the condition.

>   **PHYSICIAN:** *Mr. Virchow, you know that we saw a lump in your intestine and took a biopsy of it. What have you already learned about the results?*

Consider these possible responses:

>   **PATIENT:** *Well, is it cancer?*

>   **PATIENT:** *Could you wait till my wife gets here? She gets off work at 6 o'clock.*

>   **PATIENT:** (silent, stares at the doctor's face)

Patients who immediately ask if the diagnosis is cancer are ready to hear the news. Others may indicate, verbally or nonverbally, that they are uncomfortable proceeding. For these patients, techniques to slow down the message may be appropriate. Buckman[6] describes the "warning shot" (e.g., "I'm afraid I have some bad news") and then assessing the patient's readiness to go on.

Most patients in the United States prefer a clear, simple, and empathic statement of the news, followed by a pause to let the message sink in. The pause gives the patient time to assimilate the news and the physician to gauge the patient's response. This is not the time to give a mini-lecture because most patients remember little of what is said after receiving bad news.

Some patients want more information than others. One way to assess this it to simply ask:

>   *Are you the kind of person who likes lots of information and detail about your condition, or a sort of person who likes a brief summary and recommendations?*

Some patients, particularly those from family-centered versus individual-centered cultures, may prefer that you give information to their family members rather than to them:

>   *Do you prefer that I talk with you about your condition, or would you rather I talk with a family member?*

Basic information-giving techniques include using simple, clear words instead of medical jargon, giving small amounts of information at a time with pauses in between, and summarizing periodically. Drawings or simple metaphors can also be useful. Some oncologists make audio tapes of the bad news visit so that patients and families can listen more than once to the information they have been given.

## ASK

Even with the most careful explanations, many patients have trouble recalling or understanding information from a bad news encounter once they have left the physician's office. Check patients' understanding by acknowledging that sometimes doctors' explanations can be unclear and by asking them what they have understood so far. Preprinted materials should be personalized by highlighting information relevant to the patient's situation. Patients should also be encouraged to write down questions that come up between visits and bring them in at scheduled appointments. They may also want to hear from other patients who have "been through it" and have volunteered to share their experiences with other patients.

## CARE

The most common patient response to receiving bad news is an emotional one and requires empathy (Function One: Build the Relationship).

> PHYSICIAN: (sitting down and making eye contact) *The biopsy showed cancer of the colon.*

> PATIENT: *Oh, my God, doctor. Not cancer.* (weeps, wrings hands) *Oh, my God. What am I going to do now?*

> PHYSICIAN: (touching the patient's hand) *I know this comes as a shock. This wasn't what you were expecting at all. But I want you to know that we'll take it one step at a time and work on it together. What worries you the most right now?*

Some patients report feeling stunned or shocked by the bad news and don't have much of a reaction. These patients are challenging because their ideas and feelings are temporarily inaccessible. The stunned state should be acknowledged and the likelihood of future emotions and questions legitimized.

> PHYSICIAN: *I can see that you're feeling overwhelmed right now. I imagine you're quite stunned by this news and that it is hard to even think about. Have I got it right?*

> PATIENT: *Yes. I can't believe this is happening. I'm going to wake up in a minute and this will all be a bad dream.*

> PHYSICIAN: *I wish it were so. Is there anyone that I can call for you? Anyone at home that you can be with?*

> PATIENT: *Yes, my wife should be home by now.*

> PHYSICIAN: *You two will probably have some questions or concerns that you'd like to talk about with me. If you'd like, I can call her for you now. Then I'd like the two of you to come see me soon to talk about what to do next.*

Some patients become angry when receiving bad news and direct this anger toward the physician. Physicians can experience this as a personal attack and become defensive or angry in return. A more effective approach is to understand that anger is a normal reaction to bad news and that acknowledging and respecting angry feelings helps defuse them.

> PATIENT: *What do you mean, the cancer is back? I did everything you told me. I took all the treatments and followed all your advice. There's got to be some mistake!*

> PHYSICIAN: *I've double checked the tests, and I'm sure it's back. This was a surprise to me, too. This isn't what either of us expected. You did all the right things, and now this happens. I can see how you'd be angry.*

> PATIENT: (agitated) *Why didn't you find it sooner? I could have been cured!*

PHYSICIAN: *I know it just doesn't make sense. We did all the right things and it still happened. Being angry, even with me, is okay. But I'd still like to be your doctor and help you with this. Can we talk about that now, or would you like some time to think about it?*

Many patients are frightened and tearful about the news and need a physician with good relationship skills.

PATIENT: (trembling and weeping) *Don't let this happen to me, please! I've got two kids in grade school! You don't understand. I just can't have cancer now!*

PHYSICIAN: *I can see this is a terrible blow for you, and you're doing everything you can to cope. And I can see that your biggest concern is looking out for your family. I want you to know that I'll still be your doctor and stick with you on this.*

PATIENT: *Yes, please don't give up on me! My husband—he doesn't know what the kids need—he won't even be able to handle this himself. What can I tell him?*

PHYSICIAN: (touching her shoulder) *Why don't you ask him to come in with you? I know someone who can help the two of you deal with this together and also decide what to tell the kids. We can schedule it for later this week.*

Patients who receive bad news usually remember the physician's attitude and manner more vividly than the technical details of the news. Physicians must be able to convey an attitude of honesty and caring even in the face of strong and varied emotions. The greatest challenge for physicians is to remain with patients, accept strong emotional reactions as normal and understandable responses to bad news, and express support and partnership. Listening carefully to patients and not interrupting them with more questions, premature reassurance, or explanations is a powerful skill. Dame Cicely Saunders, originator of the hospice movement in the United Kingdom, said, "The real secret is not what you tell your patients, but what you let your patients tell you."

For patients whose response is mostly inquisitive rather than emotional, the physician can forecast that the patient may have some feelings come up after the visit.

PHYSICIAN: *We've talked about a lot of information today. I'm also wondering how you're feeling about all this. After all, that's an important part of you and your medical care.*

If the patient has been more emotional than inquisitive, the opposite applies.

PHYSICIAN: *I know this has been upsetting for you. I also anticipate you'll have some questions for me later on. Please write them down so you don't forget them.*

## COUNSEL

After breaking bad news and responding to the patient's emotions, the most important part of the bad news interview is to explore the meaning of the news to the patient, give information and advice, and then reach a shared understanding of the condition.

PHYSICIAN: *You told me about your mother's experience with cancer. So tell me, what do you think the biopsy result means for you?*

PATIENT: *I know what's coming. Her death was a nightmare. I can't face that.*

PHYSICIAN: *What bothered you most about her dying?*

PATIENT: *She was in horrible pain right up to the last. I don't know if I can take that.*

PHYSICIAN: *Given that experience I can see why you'd be scared. But in your case we don't know if the cancer has spread, and we certainly have more treatments to choose from, for both cancer and for pain. Your condition doesn't have to be like hers.*

PATIENT: *So I'm not going to die from this?*

**PHYSICIAN:** *I don't have any evidence for that right now. But we need some more information and then I can review the treatment options with you.*

Planning specific next steps for the immediate future is reassuring to patients who receive bad news. It demonstrates that something can be done for them and they won't be abandoned. The plan can include deciding who else needs to know the news and if the patient wants help sharing it. It can also outline immediate next steps such as diagnostic tests and consultations.

## TELL-BACK

This step is often omitted or relegated to a quick "Did you understand what I said?" and an embarrassed nod from the patient. However, it is a critical step in giving bad news. The proof comes when physicians ask the more appropriate question, "I want to make sure I was clear. Can you tell me the most important points we covered?" Physicians are often surprised at the answers, which can stray far from the intended message. A useful and less threatening question for patients is, "When you get home, and someone asks what the doctor said, what will you tell them?" Patients usually have no more than three or four take-home messages, and these can be quickly clarified in the last few minutes of the visit.

## Importance of Physician Self-Awareness

Breaking bad news affects physicians as well as patients. Physicians bring personal experiences, values, attitudes, and beliefs to their interactions with patients. When the bad news is life threatening, it challenges physicians' belief in the power of aggressive biotechnology to overcome disease and makes them vulnerable to feelings of inadequacy or guilt. For some physicians a patient's death means a failure of knowledge, responsibility, or dedication. Awareness of one's own hot buttons and blind spots is an important part of giving bad news.

Medical education has traditionally encouraged physicians to suppress their emotions for the sake of objectivity. This suppression is reinforced through intense work schedules and little time to reflect on personal reactions to patient care. Physicians who fear displaying their emotions can appear cold and uncaring to patients when giving bad news. For example, several studies show that parents receiving bad news about a child felt supported when the informant appeared appropriately sad and offended when the informant was detached and "professional." The refusal to acknowledge emotions in self and others, combined with poor training in communication and interpersonal skills, leads physicians to withdraw in response to patients' emotional responses to bad news. This withdrawal can lead to burnout and feelings of personal isolation and disconnection from the work of patient care. Many training programs now include activities that encourage reflection and self-awareness with the goal of improving clinical care and job satisfaction.

## Special Challenges in Breaking Bad News

### BREAKING BAD NEWS FROM A DISTANCE

Patients prefer to receive bad news in person, preferably from a physician they know.[6] Breaking bad news by telephone, voicemail, or e-mail can be upsetting to patients, but is sometimes unavoidable. The most common bad news to break from a distance is notifying someone of a loved one's death. Ideally this can still be done in person:

**PHYSICIAN:** *Mrs. Jones? This is Dr. Welby at Mercy General. I'm the doctor on call this evening, and I need to talk with you about your husband's condition. Are you able to come to the hospital?*

MRS. JONES: *Is this about Harold? Is he okay?*

PHYSICIAN: *Yes it is. I'm afraid his condition has worsened and we'd really like you to come. Do you have a way to get here?*

MRS. JONES: *I'll come right away.*

Death notification by telephone is sometimes necessary when families ask directly if death has occurred or they are unable to come to the hospital.[7]

MRS. JONES: *I'll come right away. He isn't dead, is he?*

PHYSICIAN: *Yes. I am terribly sorry to have to tell you this over the phone, but I am afraid he has just died. He died peacefully around 8 o'clock tonight. Is anyone there with you now?*

MRS. JONES: *No, but I can call my sister. She said to call if I need anything. I'm sure she would bring me to the hospital. I hate to lose him, but he was suffering so …* (sobbing)

PHYSICIAN: *I'd like to see you when you arrive. Please come right up to the seventh floor and ask for Dr. Welby. We can talk some more then.*

Survivors often want to see the deceased's body. This is an important part of the grieving process and should not be denied. Survivors are often concerned about whether their loved one was alone at the time of death, if he or she suffered, and if there was anything they could or should have done differently during the events leading up to the death. Most medical centers now have specially trained personnel who can screen for organ donation eligibility and talk with families about consent for donation. Families may find comfort in making an anatomical gift; however, certain conditions such as malignancy or infection may preclude the possibility of organ donation.

## DON'T BREAK THE NEWS

Some patients specifically request not to be told bad news. Ask what the bad news would mean to them, and what they fear might happen if they receive it (see Attributions and Expectations and Giving Information sections).

PATIENT: *Doctor, if the news is bad, I'd just rather not hear it. Do what you have to do, but don't tell me about it.*

PHYSICIAN: *If I understand correctly, you're saying that you don't want lots of information and explanations about what we've found and what we're doing. Many people feel that way, and I certainly won't force information on you. We know, though, that your job here is to create the best environment for our treatments to work. We think your ideas and feelings would help us plan the best treatment. So the more you know about it, the more we can tailor care to fit you individually.*

Sometimes family members will ask that a patient not be given bad news. Families should be reassured that information won't be forced on the patient but also advised that the patient's knowledge of and participation in care will increase its effectiveness. Families may have had unfortunate experiences with bad news in the past, or may have strong cultural beliefs about how bad news should be given and received. In some cultures, for example, bad news is routinely withheld from patients so that they don't lose hope or give up. In other cultures, giving bad news is traditionally a family event and everyone must be present when the patient gets the news. It may help to share your dilemma with the patient (e.g., "Your family has told me that you would prefer not to know some important facts about your condition. What are your thoughts about this?"). Cultural consultants in the form of translators or patient advocates can sometimes mediate cultural or ethnic differences around giving bad news, informed consent, and active participation in care.

## DENIAL OF BAD NEWS

Disbelief or denial is a normal psychological response that protects people from being overwhelmed by bad news. Most patients in denial are ambivalent, or of two minds about the news. Most doctors have experienced careful breaking of bad news to a patient, only to hear the patient tell others the next day, "They don't know what's wrong yet" or "I think I'm just run down." At this point, arguing, persuading, or proving the bad news can be counterproductive. It can be useful to ask the patient to consider what decisions might have to be faced if the condition worsens.

> **PHYSICIAN:** *What kinds of decisions and plans should we make now, in case you're too ill to make them in the future?*

Another useful approach to denial is to hope for the best and prepare for the worst. This allows the physician to acknowledge the patient's viewpoint while at the same time acknowledging the need to be prepared in case the facts prove otherwise.[8]

> **PATIENT:** *I know you think this is cancer, but it feels just like it did when I had pneumonia. They told my father he had cancer, and they were wrong, that was 10 years ago. Just treat me for pneumonia and I'll be fine.*

> **PHYSICIAN:** *I wish that this wasn't cancer. But it's always good to have a Plan B just in case it doesn't turn out the way we want.*

Note the strategic use of "wish" rather than "hope." "Hope" implies that an outcome is possible under unusual circumstances, whereas "wish" indicates that is unachievable.

# Honest Disclosure and Realistic Hope

One of the hardest conversations in medicine is telling patients that their life-limiting disease is progressing despite all available and appropriate treatment.[9-12] Physicians fear that the patient will lose hope and give up. In fact, up to 30% of physicians intentionally give patients a more optimistic prognosis than their actual estimates for fear of taking away hope.

Patients usually change what they hope for as illness progresses. Initially hope may be focused on a cure, then later on a response to treatment, then later on completing a specific goal or project, and finally to die in comfort surrounded by loved ones. Physicians can be of great service to patients by helping them clarify their goals, values, and concerns, and collaborating with them to find ways to pursue them despite a progressive illness. For example, a physician dreaded telling an elderly woman that her trouble walking resulted from progression of her previously treated metastatic cancer, now with spinal cord compression. In breaking this news to the patient he asked her what it would mean to her if she could not walk or travel. The woman replied that her greatest hope now was to attend her granddaughter's imminent graduation at a distant college. Together, they decided to create a video in which she could give a special message to her granddaughter and to have it delivered in time for the graduation.

Patients may ask tough questions, such as, "Am I going to die?" and "How long do I have?" These questions deserve direct and honest answers. In all cases, however, patients should be given hope for support and partnership.

> **PHYSICIAN:** *I think what you're asking is whether you will die because of this cancer. There are statistics on how long people with this kind of cancer live, with and without treatment, but they are just averages. Some patients live much longer and some shorter than the average. I can tell you the averages for your condition, but I can't predict how long you have. I want to tell you again that I am here to help and support you through this.*

## Teaching How to Give Bad News

Most physicians first give bad news as students and residents, when they have the least experience or training, and are haunted by their experiences. With the advent of competency-based learning and certification, a growing literature describes courses, web-based instruction, and objective structured clinical examinations (OSCE) on giving bad news for students, clinical evaluation exercises (CEX) for residents, and intensive experiential workshops for fellows and practitioners. Teaching methods include readings, skills practice with role-plays (using scripts, trigger videos, or simulated and volunteer patients), and reflection on the feelings this aspect of care generates. Program evaluations demonstrate improvements in self-rated knowledge, skills, and attitudes, but few studies demonstrate changes in practice or improvements in patient outcomes.[13-19] For example, Fallowfield described a 3-day intensive course on giving bad news for oncologists that includes specific time for didactics, skills practice, and personal reflection. Improvement in skills in the clinical setting persisted after a year with no further intervention.[5]

## Conclusion

Breaking bad news is receiving the attention it deserves, as research demonstrates the importance of communication skills on health outcomes and the developed world's population lives long enough to develop chronic and treatable diseases. Giving bad news requires that all three functions of the medical interview be used simultaneously: give information, assess and respond empathically to its emotional impact, and gather data to guide the giving of more information and collaboratively plan for next steps. Particular challenges include patients and families who ask that bad news not be given; physicians who lack the attitudes, skills, and self-awareness to give bad news effectively; and both parties when bad news is given without a plan for the future and a sense of hope.

### References

1. Krahn GL, Hallum A, Kime C: Are there good ways to give bad news? *Pediatrics* 91:578–582, 1993.
2. Iserson KV: The gravest words: sudden-death notifications and emergency care. *Ann Emerg Med* 36:75–77, 2000.
3. Schofield PE, et al: Psychological responses of patients receiving a diagnosis of cancer. *Ann Oncology* 14:48, 2003.
4. Baile WF, et al: Oncologists' attitudes toward and practices in giving bad news: An exploratory study. *J Clin Oncol* 20:2189–2196, 2002.
5. Fallowfield L, Jenkins V: Communicating sad, bad, and difficult news in medicine. *Lancet* 363:312, 2004.
6. Ambuel B, Weissman DE Fast Fact and Concept #6: Delivering Bad News: Part 1. July, 2005 and Part 2. September 2005. 2nd Edition End-of-Life Palliative Education Resource Center www.eperc.mcw.edu.
7. Osias, RR, Pomerantz DH, Brensilver JH: Fast Facts and Concepts #76: Telephone Notification of Death Part 1, 2nd Edition. October 2006, #76 Telephone Notification of Death Part 2, 2nd Edition, July 2006, End-of-Life Physician Education Resource Center www.eperc.mcw.edu.
8. Back AL, Arnold RM, Quill TE: Hope for the best, and prepare for the worst. *Ann Intern Med* 138:439–443, 2003.
9. Quill TE, Arnold RM, Platt F: "I wish things were different": expressing wishes in response to loss, futility, and unrealistic hopes. *Ann Intern Med* 135:551–555, 2001.
10. Evans WG, et al: Communication at times of transitions: how to help patients cope with loss and re-define hope. *Cancer J* 12:417–424, 2006.
11. Casarrett DJ, Quill TE: "I'm not ready for hospice:" strategies for timely and effective hospital discussions. *Ann Intern Med* 146:443–449, 2007.
12. Warm E, Weissman DE: Prognostication. Fast Fact and Concept #30; 2nd Edition, July 2005. End-of-Life Palliative Education Resource Center www.eperc.mcw.edu.

13. Ury WA, et al: Assessing medical students' training in end-of-life communication: a survey of interns at one urban teaching hospital. *Acad Med* 78:530–537, 2003.
14. Han PK, et al: The palliative care clinical evaluation exercise (CEX): an experience-based intervention for teaching end-of-life communication skills. *Acad Med* 80(7):669, 2005.
15. Rider EA, Volkan K, Hafler JP: Pediatric residents' perceptions of communication competencies: implications for teaching. *Med Teach* 30:e208–e217, 2008.
16. Farber NJ, et al: Using patients with cancer to educate residents about giving bad news. *J Palliat Care* 19:54–57, 2003.
17. Ameil GE, et al: Ability of primary care physicians to break bad news: a performance based assessment of an educational intervention. *Pat Educ Couns* 60:10, 2006.
18. Back AL, et al: Efficacy of communication skills training for giving bad news and discussion transitions to palliative care. *Arch Intern Med* 167:453–460, 2007.
19. Lenzi R, et al: Design, conduct, and evaluation of a communication course for oncology fellows. *J Cancer Educ* 20:143–149, 2005.

### Books

1. Buckman R: *How to break bad news: a guide for health care professionals*, Baltimore, 1992, Johns Hopkins University Press.

### Websites

1. Emanuel LL, von Gunten CF, Ferris FD: Module 2: communicating bad news. In *The education for physicians on end-of-life care project (EPEC) curriculum*, 1999, The Robert Wood Johnson Foundation. http://www.epec.net/
2. The End of Life Physician Education Resource Center (EPERC) is a peer reviewed clearinghouse for educational materials for physicians on all aspects of end of life care, including giving bad news. At http://www.eperc.mcw.edu.
3. URMC (University of Rochester Medical Center) ACGME Competency Project. Communicating bad news. One of 6 teaching modules from the University of Rochester; includes learning objectives, pretest questions, written text, slides with embedded videos, role-plays, readings, and evaluation forms. At: http://www.urmc.edu/smd/education/gme/acgme_competency_modules.
4. Doc.com is a web-based teaching resource for health care communication, published by the American Academy on Communication in Healthcare (AACH). Modules on giving bad news and related topics, and guides for using the modules, are available via www.aachonline.org.
5. Oncotalk is a program of intensive conference retreats designed to improve communication skills of medical oncology and palliative medicine fellows. Modules on giving bad news and related topics, as well as a toolbox for medical educators, are available at Oncotalk@u.washington.edu.
6. https://www.aamc.org/services/currmit/

# Sharing Difficult or Bad News: A Nine-Step Process of Transformation

Joseph S. Weiner

## OVERVIEW

This chapter presents a nine-step structured transformational process to sharing difficult or bad news.

The process of sharing difficult or bad news is a privilege for the clinician, because it is an opportunity to shepherd a patient and family through some of the most critical and vulnerable moments of their lives. When performed poorly, the experience can leave scars for the patient, the family, and even the physician. However when the physician implements some basic skills in a systematic and genuine way, even with the worst of news, the patient and family have an opportunity to successfully process difficult information, potentially moving forward with genuine strength and hope. In such situations, patients (if they survive) and families remember the good care they received for years to come with appreciation.

There are quite a few complexities involved in sharing difficult or bad news well, and Dr. Gordon discusses these in considerable depth in Chapter 27 within the broad context of the (e) TACCT approach (Function Three) of the Three Function Model for education. In contrast, this chapter presents an alternative, nine-step, highly structured, stepwise and systematic template that supplements (e)TACCT: Clinicians can readily use it to guide their efforts in this area that is fully consistent with Dr. Gordon's recommendations around (e)TACCT. Furthermore, the template in this chapter can be most effectively applied after the student has already mastered the concepts presented in Chapter 27.

First, this guide begins with the suggestion that clinicians change the language they use to describe the encounter itself—"breaking bad news"—because language influences the way we think and behave. To be specific, the word "breaking" suggests a physician-directed and -controlled experience. The words "bad news" imply that the information to be given is only "negative" or about something "wrong." Neither, however, represents the actual, ideal, or complete clinical reality of the recommended interaction around sharing difficult or bad news.

This chapter encourages a shift to a more transactional model in which information and reactions are shared reciprocally. The outcome of a transactional model is not just to ensure that information is clearly communicated and received, but that there is the potential for patient exploration and emotional growth, and from this, realistic hope may emerge as part of the process of not just hearing the news, but also understanding, processing, and dealing with the news.

A more clinically useful and patient-centered way to conceptualize this process would be to think of it as sharing difficult or bad news. The ideal process between physician and patient is both transactional (information and emotional content flows back and forth) *and* transformational (there is an opportunity for exploration and growth). The encounter involves numerous interpersonal events, most of which involve sharing:

- The physician shares a diagnosis or information, which may happen to be challenging or upsetting or even emotionally devastating.
- The patient shares an emotional reaction.
- The physician explores the reaction.
- The patient shares the reasons for the reaction.
- The physician and patient can begin to construct realistic emotional and medical hope while discussing treatment suggestions.

Much has been written about how to share difficult news, although there aren't large, rigorous, randomized, controlled studies of patient outcomes using manualized communication approaches.[1-4] Therefore the following represents a pragmatic, synthetic clinical approach based on the Three Function Model and current research to date and, in many respects, similar  Dr. Gordon's approach in Chapter 27. Like any other method, you will learn to depart from it to tailor your approach to your own individual style and the specific needs of the patient.

This method can be broken down into the following nine steps:

1. Prepare yourself for the discussion.
2. Make an introductory statement to prepare the patient for the news. (Functions One and Three)
3. Present the news in a concise, understandable manner. (Function Three)
4. Wait for the patient to have an emotional response. (Function One)
5. Reflect the response you see back to the patient. (Function One)
6. Legitimize the response. (Function One)
7. Explore the response. (Functions One and Two)
8. Provide realistic hope. (Functions One and Three)
9. Discuss next steps if the patient is ready. (Function Three)

This nine-step method is detailed more in the following; but first it is important to understand the recipient's experience of difficult or bad news and a common pitfall that physicians fall into when delivering this news.

## The Recipient's Experience of Receiving Difficult or Bad News

Patients and family members usually wait for test results with much anticipation, and even if they expect prognostically bad news, no matter how well they prepare, such news can still produce a significant emotional reaction, such as fear, anger, shock, confusion, or sadness.

It is extremely important for the physician to allow the patient and family to first process their emotional reactions to receiving difficult news before further education and treatment planning can be done. If the patient and family don't have this opportunity, the immediate physiologic stress response overrides their cognitive abilities. In neurophysiologic terms, the amygdala and locus coeruleus take over and prevent the cerebral cortex from properly analyzing the situation. For the physician to reengage the patient's cognitive coping mechanisms, the same empathic communication skills discussed in Chapter 3 can be applied here:

Empathic Communication to Deepen Understanding (ECDU) facilitates Function Three

Reflection + Legitimation + Exploration

# The Biggest Trap into Which Clinicians Fall

Physicians who share difficult or bad news are commonly anxious about causing the patient emotional discomfort from the news.[5,6] As a result, they prematurely try to ameliorate the patient's emotional reactions by moving the discussion too quickly to Function Three. This is such a common trap that, in my experience, most clinicians fall into it.

## AN INEFFECTIVE SHARING OF DIFFICULT NEWS

PHYSICIAN: *We got the biopsy results back and we have some things to talk about.*

PATIENT: *Uh oh, that sounds serious.*

PHYSICIAN: *Well, the biopsy shows that you have lung cancer.*

PATIENT: *Oh no! I can't believe this.*

PHYSICIAN: *It's okay. We have a lot we can offer you. I'm going to have you speak to a great oncologist. We will talk about options for surgery and chemotherapy. There is so much we can do for you. I don't want you to feel down or scared. The most important thing is that we have a lot to offer you …*

Why was this not effective? The patient heard very little of what the physician said after the words "lung cancer." The physician thinks he or she is offering emotional support by telling the patient all that he or she can offer, but in reality the patient is suffering through the emotional reaction to the news without processing it further. In addition, the physician is losing a valuable opportunity to understand specifically *why* the patient is upset. By knowing specifically why the patient is upset, the physician will be in a better position to more broadly attend to the patient's suffering.

Therefore one of the developmental skills for the learner to master when sharing difficult news is:

> **Emotionally Support the Patient with Reflection, Legitimation, and Exploration (Empathic Communication to Deepen Understanding, Chapter Three) Until the Patient Is Ready to Hear About Treatment Planning.**

## A MORE EFFECTIVE WAY TO SHARE DIFFICULT NEWS

PHYSICIAN: *We got the biopsy results back and we have some things to talk about.*

PATIENT: *Uh oh, that sounds serious.*

PHYSICIAN: *Well, the biopsy shows that you have lung cancer.*

PATIENT: *Oh no! I can't believe this.* (he cries)

PHYSICIAN: (After giving the patient a moment to express tearfulness) *This is really upsetting news.* (**reflection**)

PATIENT: *Of course, you just told me I have lung cancer!*

PHYSICIAN: *Yes, most of my patients get really upset when they hear this kind of news.* (**legitimation**)

PATIENT: *I'm sorry. I didn't mean to snap at you. Oh my, this is terrible news.*

PHYSICIAN: *I hear how upset you are. Now, people get upset for all different reasons when they receive a diagnosis of cancer. What upsets you the most?* (**exploration**)

PATIENT: *I'm the breadwinner for the family. How will we pay our bills if I'm out sick?*

or

PATIENT: *Will I lose my hair from the chemo? My friend did. I can't deal with that.*

or

PATIENT: *Will I die?*

or

PATIENT: *Will I be in pain?*

or

PATIENT: *How can I tell my children? They'll be so upset.*

At this point in the discussion, the patient is able to share what concerns him or her the most about the diagnosis. This will allow the physician to understand how to best help the patient. It will also put the physician in the position to express even deeper empathy (understanding) for the patient's suffering and provide realistic hope.

For example:

PATIENT: *Will I die?*

PHYSICIAN: *There is no cure for lung cancer that has spread like yours, but we do have treatments that can control the cancer and keep you alive for as long as possible. During that time, we may come up with better treatments.*

or

PATIENT: *How can I tell my children? They'll be so upset.*

PHYSICIAN: *I'd be happy to meet with you and your children so I can share the news with them.*

## Thoughts for Medical Students

From the medical student's perspective, very few of you will be called upon to tell a patient that he or she has advanced cancer, but you may be called upon to interact with patients who have important questions about their diabetes or high blood pressure or even recent myocardial infarctions. It is too early in your professional development to give answers to such patients' concerns. However, you can summarize your understanding of their concerns and make a list of their concerns to present to your preceptors. For example:

STUDENT: *I hear your question about whether your diabetes will cause your kidneys to shut down. I want to still further understand what causes you to have that concern. People ask that question for different reasons.*

PATIENT: *Well my sister had diabetes and she died from kidney failure. Will that happen to me?*

or

PATIENT: *My daughter's getting married next May and I promised to walk her down the aisle.*

At this point, the student is in the position to summarize the patient's concerns.

STUDENT: *So I'm hearing that one of your big concerns is whether you'll be able to walk your daughter down the aisle. I'm glad you can share that specific concern with me, because when I speak with Dr. Jones, I'll tell her about it so she can address it. As a medical student, I don't have the knowledge yet to answer your question, but the great thing is that I have the time to gather all your concerns so I can share them with Dr. Jones. What other concerns do you have?* (Explore the patient's concerns to completion.)

There is a common student reaction to all this. It may be a frustrating experience for you as a student to not be in the position to offer answers to the patient's questions and concerns, especially when you think you may know some of the answers. That's totally understandable. However, it's important to keep in mind that you will be serving an extraordinarily important role in gathering and further understanding the patient's specific concerns. This is for two reasons.

First, this level of understanding usually doesn't get done in enough detail by the practicing physician because of time constraints or other factors. Second, the process of guiding the patient through the articulation of his or her concerns will give him or her hope that someone understands the patient's most important priorities and his or her suffering can be addressed.

It can't be emphasized enough how helpful and important this level of empathic communication and understanding becomes for patients. It is all too common for a patient to receive generic treatments for generic diseases without addressing his or her specific needs and the needs of the family. By gathering the specific concerns of the patient, you will be helping improve the personalized health care your patient will receive. This will have a lasting impact on his or her life.

A detailed explanation of the nine-step approach to sharing difficult or bad news is outlined below.

## Nine Steps to Sharing Difficult or Bad News

### 1. PREPARE FOR THE DISCUSSION.

1. This can include:
    a. Reading about the situation (a rare disease or a complex clinical situation)
    b. Deciding what time you're going to speak to the patient (early in the morning or late in the afternoon when things are not backed up)
    c. Thinking about the conversation (what you might say, or role-playing it with a friend or colleague)
    d. Asking the patient ahead of the results if he or she wants someone with him or her when hearing the outcome of a test or procedure

### 2. MAKE AN INTRODUCTORY STATEMENT THAT IMPLIES YOU WILL DISCUSS SOMETHING IMPORTANT.

1. Make a brief, calm statement that you will be having a serious discussion.
    a. "We received the biopsy results back and we do have some things we need to talk about."
    b. "We got your blood test results back and we have some things to discuss."
    c. "We got the results of the CT scan. I want to talk to you about what it shows."
2. Wait a second or two until you have the patient's full attention. Often the patient will say, "So what did it (the biopsy, etc.) show?"

### 3. STATE THE NEWS WITH CLEAR, CONCISE LANGUAGE.

1. "The biopsy shows that you have cancer in your lung."
2. Avoid medical terminology such as "lesion" or "mass," which can be confusing.
3. Try to be as definitive as possible.
    a. If a biopsy reading definitely concludes that the patient has cancer, avoid phrases like, "The biopsy shows that you may have cancer" or "The biopsy shows that you probably have cancer."
4. If you can't be definite, be clear and honest.

a. "We're concerned about your blood tests and CT scan." (pause) "We need to do further tests."

b. When the patient asks, "What do you think it is?" you can say something like, "It may be an infection or it may be cancer. We can't know until we take a sample. That's called a biopsy."

## 4. WAIT FOR THE PATIENT'S REACTION.

1. While waiting, actively observe what the reaction is so you can be prepared to be empathetic (see the following).
2. If the patient moves quickly to "So what can we do now?" take a moment to explore first.
   a. "Before we talk about what our next steps are, what are your reactions to this news?"
   b. If the patient says, "Doc, I'm not an emotional person. I deal with things by taking action," then it's fine to move to treatment planning (Function Three), while continuing to observe for any emotional reactions that may later develop.

## 5. REFLECT THE RESPONSE OF THE PATIENT BACK.

1. Reflection has three steps:
   a. Observe the reaction.
   b. Name the patient's reaction in your head.
   c. Express the reaction back to the patient in a manner that would be acceptable for him or her to hear.
2. Examples of reflective statements:
   a. "You seem sad."
   b. "This news is very upsetting."
   c. "You look like you have a lot on your mind."
3. If you are not sure what the patient's reaction is, you can say, "What's on your mind now?" or "What does this news mean to you?"

## 6. LEGITIMIZE THE PATIENT'S REACTION, AS NEEDED.

1. Legitimation allows the patient to feel that his or her reaction is a normal or common one.
2. By legitimizing the patient's reactions, he or she will feel a little less alone when dealing with the situation.
3. Examples of legitimizing statements:
   a. "Many of my patients react exactly as you are doing."
   b. "It's understandable to be angry about your illness."
   c. "Of course you're upset. I would be too."

## 7. EXPLORE THE CAUSE OF THE PATIENT'S REACTION.

1. This will enable you to understand what the causes of the patient's suffering are, apart from the actual diagnosis.
2. For example, "Most people get upset about a cancer diagnosis, but everyone gets upset for different reasons. What upsets you the most about the news you have cancer?"
3. Take your time to gather a list of the biggest concerns the patient will have. This will help in collaborative management. (Medical students will need this list to present to their preceptor.)

4. (Medical students must not answer medical questions. Let patients know you will personally present them to the doctor and get the answers so "we can best address them as a team.")

## 8. PROVIDE REALISTIC HOPE (FOR MEDICAL STUDENTS, STATE THAT YOU WILL PRESENT THE PATIENT'S CONCERNS TO YOUR PRECEPTOR).

## 9. IF THE PATIENT'S IMMEDIATE STRESS RESPONSE HAS SUBSIDED ENOUGH, BEGIN COLLABORATIVE MANAGEMENT: NEXT STEPS IN DIAGNOSTIC AND TREATMENT PLANNING.

1. At this point, the physician can say, "May I address your concerns now and the next steps to treat the cancer, or do you need more time to take this news in?"

If you understand these principles and follow this protocol, often something surprising and deeply gratifying happens: After delivering bad news, providing empathic support, and discussing difficult treatment choices, in acknowledgment of what you've given to the patient, you'll hear the following two heartfelt words: "Thank you."

*The author wishes to thank Steven Cole for his important conceptual suggestions and editorial advice.*

### References

1. Baile WF, et al: SPIKES-a six-step protocol for delivering bad news: application to the patient with cancer. *Oncologist* 5:302–311, 2000.
2. Emanuel LL, von Gunten CF, Ferris FD, editors: *Education for physicians on end-of-life care (EPEC) curriculum*, Chicago, 1999, The Robert Wood Johnson Foundation.
3. Paul CL, et al: Are we there yet? The state of the evidence base for guidelines on breaking bad news to cancer patients. *Eur J Cancer* 45(17):2960–2966, 2009.
4. Weiner JS, et al: Manualized communication interventions to enhance palliative care research and training: rigorous, testable approaches. *J Palliat Med* 9(2):371–381, 2006.
5. Weiner JS, Cole SA: ACare—a communication training program for shared decision making along a life-limiting illness. *Palliat Support Care* 2(3):231–241, 2004.
6. Weiner JS, Cole SA: Three principles to improve physician training for end-of-life care: overcoming emotional, cognitive, and skills barriers to communication with seriously ill patients. *J Palliat Med* 7(6):817–829, 2004.

# CHAPTER 28

# Disclosure of Medical Errors and Apology

Steven Locke ▪ Toni Walzer ▪ Roxane Gardner

## OVERVIEW

This chapter provides physicians with recommendations to help them communicate with patients and families about medical errors. It describes in detail how to prepare for, conduct, and follow up an interview with a patient and family who have experienced a medical error.

In 2000, the Institute of Medicine (IOM) wrote in its authoritative report, *To Err Is Human*, that injury resulting from medical errors is a major cause of preventable deaths in the United States.[1] The IOM recommended that health care organizations and practitioners make the reduction of medical errors a priority and called for steps to promote safety through system redesign. This influential report fostered what is now called the Patient Safety Movement, with the goal that improvements in health care systems will lead to reductions in preventable error and improvements in patient safety.

Medical errors are an unfortunate but inevitable part of the health care process. Acquiring the ability to disclose a medical error and apologize appropriately to a patient who has suffered because of a medical error is an important communication skill often overlooked in medical training. Recent trends in medical education and the Patient Safety Movement reflect a sea change in recognizing the importance of training clinicians to manage medical errors and communicate with patients and family members in an effective and compassionate manner. This chapter describes how to prepare for, conduct, and follow-up an interview with a patient and family who have experienced a medical error.

Appropriate and prompt disclosure of medical errors and adverse events to patients and their families is now considered the standard of care, comprising an essential element of a successful program to improve patient safety.[2,3] Some state and federal laws require disclosure of medical errors. Patients consistently state that they desire full disclosure when errors occur, and physicians express support for disclosure. Nevertheless, it often does not occur.[4] Failure to disclose errors honestly is thought to be associated with a greater risk of malpractice litigation,[5-7] providing additional support for the benefit to physicians of learning how to develop necessary communication skills for this important patient encounter. A patient may interpret the lack of an explanation and apology as insensitive or defensive and feel that the physician who remains silent after a serious adverse event is trying to conceal what really happened. Consequently, the failure to disclose the error and apologize can be a powerful stimulus to complaint or litigation.[7] Some patient safety experts advocate that apology may be the most important thing a clinician does after a serious adverse event, both to help the patient begin to heal and to heal the provider.[8]

There is little direct research about the process of disclosure of medical errors, but what evidence exists suggests that the issues are complicated. Factors have been identified that have either facilitated or impeded physicians' error disclosure. Among the most important of 35 factors found to facilitate disclosure were honesty, accountability, and restitution. Forty-one factors were identified that impeded disclosure, such as concern about legal liability and blame.[9]

The importance of communication skills in the physician-patient relationship is reflected in research on medical malpractice. Interestingly, plaintiffs who have filed malpractice claims rate dysfunctional delivery of information and poor listening behavior of the provider among the main reasons for suing their physicians.[10,11] Patients are often seriously affected by medical errors. These can impact their work, social life, and family relationships, leading to intensely emotional reactions. As physicians, we often view problems and how to fix them in clinical rather than emotional terms, adding further injury to the patient. In a study of 227 patients and their families who were taking legal action, only 15% considered the communication after the original incident satisfactory, desiring a greater appreciation of the severity of the trauma they had suffered.[7]

There is evidence that significant gaps exist between how physicians disclose errors and what patients wish to hear during such disclosure. This indicates a need for the development of educational programs to teach physicians how to communicate more effectively with patients about errors.[12-14] Research is now exploring how surgeons approach error disclosure and apology, and how such training could be beneficial in situations involving wrong-site surgery, retained foreign objects, and other adverse surgical outcomes.[15]

Effective communication in the face of a medical error or adverse outcome is becoming a factor in health care system reform. Partly this is a reflection of a more patient-centric orientation in our changing care delivery environment. National leaders in health care reform have recognized the importance of medical error disclosure and apology to any successful medical liability reform in the United States.[16] Policies concerning apology and disclosure of medical errors and adverse events are rapidly changing. As of 2007, more than 34 states have "apology laws" that exclude expressions of sympathy as proof of liability, but only four states have the stronger protections that exclude admission of fault.[17] Our hope is that such legislation will foster a climate that encourages transparency, reduces malpractice claims, and decreases physicians' discomfort in participating in these difficult conversations. However, the impact of this legislation is still unclear.[18]

The Three Function Model and its associated skills offer a useful framework within which these recommendations reside: building and maintaining the relationship with the patient and family (Function One) (Chapter Three) serves as the foundation for successful resolution of communication about a medical error. Assessing and understanding (Function Two) (Chapter Four) the specific manner in which your patient and family is experiencing the error is key to your management approach. Finally, collaborative management (Function Three) (Chapter Five) holds the key to successful resolution of the problem.

## Learning Context

For the purposes of this chapter, assume that you are in the position of primary responsibility for the patient and a participant in the health care team.

## Preparing for the Initial Conversation

The aftermath of dealing with an adverse event or medical error is stressful for everyone involved—for you and the members of the clinical team as well as the patient and his or her family. Remember that patient care takes priority and it is essential that the patient not feel abandoned after a medical error or adverse event occurs. Once the patient is stabilized, time can be set aside to plan for this difficult conversation.

It is important to take time to plan what to say to the patient. As physicians, our highest ethical obligation is to admit error, take responsibility for it, apologize, and bear the consequences. However, immediately after an adverse event or medical error has occurred you will likely not know all the details about how or why it happened. A detailed investigation will be needed to sort through the issues leading up to the event and determine the steps necessary to prevent it from happening again. There may be tension between the ethical ideal and clinical practice in which questions of liability and legal protection arise. Consult with your institution's risk manager should such questions arise. Discussions you have about adverse events and medical errors with the risk manager at your institution have legal protection. In general, discussions you have with your clinical supervisor or other members of your team are not protected from legal discovery unless specifically sanctioned as such by your risk manager. Rules on legal protections vary from state to state, so in your clinical practice it is important to be familiar with the legal protections in your state and know how to access your institution's risk manager.

Reflect on your own feelings about the incident. When speaking with the patient you will want to convey sincerity, humility, empathy, and regret. These are the foundations for effective communication in this challenging situation. The impression you leave with the patient from this initial conversation may color the patient's recollection and affect the physician-patient relationship and the patient's perception of the quality of care. With the risk manager's guidance as needed, the health care team should meet and review, share, and reflect on what happened. During this meeting it is important to focus on the facts, avoiding speculation or arriving at premature conclusions. This is an opportunity to share understanding of events and their impact. We recommend two clinicians share the initial conversation with the patient and family; a risk manager or hospital administrator should not be included at this time. One clinician should be designated to lead the conversation and the other to provide support and corroboration. In our experience it is best to have no more than two members of the team share this initial conversation, as the patient can be overwhelmed and intimidated by having the entire team present. Be transparent and honest about the incident when disclosing to the patient that an error or adverse event has occurred. Explain what you know without speculating on what you don't know or about which you are unsure.

In planning this initial conversation, consider the patient's ability to understand what you will say, taking into account factors such as pain, sedation, language, culture, disability, and health literacy. Anticipate that patients may have a variety of responses to receiving bad news. The seminal work of Elisabeth Kübler-Ross taught us that patients have many similarities in how they respond to catastrophic news.[19] These include denial, anger, negotiation, depression, and acceptance. Awareness of the universality of these reactions can help prepare you to listen and respond with compassion and understanding. Anticipating the patient's responses and preparing for your conversation will decrease your own anxiety, leading to more effective communication.

### Examples of denial:

PHYSICIAN: *I would like to talk to you both about a problem with the surgery. When we encounter bleeding in surgery, we use special gauze pads called sponges, and we left one inside.* (education—simple, direct)

PATIENT: *What do you mean? You left something in to control the bleeding and it dissolves?*

PHYSICIAN: *No, unfortunately, it does not dissolve.* (simple, straightforward)

PATIENT: *So why do you leave it in?*

PHYSICIAN: *We didn't mean to leave it in. We just found out that it was seen on the x-ray.*

PATIENT: *Oh, that couldn't be me. They just did a chest x-ray, they weren't looking at my belly.*

HUSBAND: *And the x-ray lady was so cheery. They would have told us if they thought something was wrong.*

PHYSICIAN: *No, it is you. They were able to see it on the x-ray that you had taken.*

*Examples of* anger:

PATIENT: *I can't believe this happened! What's the matter with you people? Don't you keep track of your equipment? How can you be so careless?*

PHYSICIAN: *I can see you're angry* (reflection) *and I can understand why you would be upset.* (legitimation, empathic communication) *We do have safeguards to prevent this from happening, but they didn't work in this case. I'm really sorry that we let you down.* (simple apology)

HUSBAND: *We're really angry about this! Who's responsible for this mess?*

*Examples of* bargaining:

PHYSICIAN: *I am. I'm responsible for her care, and I take responsibility for fixing this situation.* (support) (simple apology and assumption of responsibility)

HUSBAND: *What do you mean, "fixing it?"*

PHYSICIAN: *We are going to need to go back to the operating room and take out the sponge.*

HUSBAND: *Can't we wait until she's recovered? She's so weak and exhausted now. Besides, I don't know if I would trust you to operate on her again. I might want to transfer her to another hospital.*

PHYSICIAN: *We could certainly have you speak with one of the other surgeons here for a second opinion. But Mrs. Jackson, I would like to continue to take care of you and see you through this.* (personal support) *I am sorry that we left a sponge in, and there is no excuse for it.*

*Examples of* depression:

HUSBAND: *I just can't understand how this happened to us. We're nice people. My wife has worked so hard raising our children and she was just starting to get back into a job that she loves. Now I don't know if they will keep it open for her for weeks. It's not the money. I just wanted her to be able to do something that she wants to do for herself. This is my fault—I told her we should come here.*

*Examples of* acceptance:

PATIENT: *Well, Doctor, so what happens now? What do you think is best for me to do? You need to make sure this never happens to anyone else.*

As we mentioned earlier, these conversations are stressful for clinicians, the patient, and their families. In making your plans, consider including other patient supports in addition to the family such as clergy, interpreters, and so on.

Planning the environment is essential to conveying to the patient that this is an important conversation. Choose a private location, turn off pagers and cell phones, and make arrangements to avoid interruptions.

# The Conversation

Sit down within touching distance of the patient (Building Rapport, Function One). This conveys a number of important messages. It conveys compassion and concern and reduces emotional distancing. It shows you have adequate time to address their concerns. Positioning yourself at eye level minimizes the power imbalance in the physician-patient relationship that can intimidate a patient who is already under duress. (See Chapter 30 on Nonverbal Communication.) It is important to begin the conversation in a way that focuses the patient and eases him or her into the coping process, for example:

> PHYSICIAN: *Mrs. Jackson, I have something important to discuss with you about your surgery.*

Often physicians will begin the conversation with idle chat, assuming that it puts the patient at ease. It works to the contrary, putting them off guard, and will make hearing about the adverse event even more overwhelming. Speak slowly and listen actively, allowing time for the patient and family members to process the information. Silence is very powerful. It not only gives patients a chance to absorb the impact of the disclosure, but also allows them time to think of questions of how this affects them. (See Chapter Four on the use of "attentive silence" to facilitate understanding.) Openly disclose the known facts of the adverse event, for example:

> PHYSICIAN: *Unfortunately, one of the surgical sponges that are used to wipe blood out of the way was left inside.*

Don't speculate about what happened because gaining the complete understanding of an adverse event takes time. Avoid long explanations, as in the following example:

> PHYSICIAN: *We have an elaborate system to track our surgical sponges. The nurses count the sponges before the incision is made and again when the peritoneum is closed. Do you know what the peritoneum is? That's the lining of the abdomen. The sponges are counted again when the incision is closed. I think there was a problem and they lost count when one group of nurses left at the end of their shift and a new group joined us in the OR at the beginning of the next shift.*

The patient is not likely to process all this detail so early, and it often gives the impression of the physician being defensive or blaming other members of team.

Instead, consider the following:

> PHYSICIAN: *We have a system in which the sponges are counted before and after the operation, but there was a breakdown in this safeguard.*

At this early stage in the process you are unlikely to know all the mitigating details of what led to this event. Do not guess. Sharing your conjecture with the patient may further damage your relationship and make the defense of a future case more difficult if the investigation reveals this to be incorrect.

Once you have disclosed the error and addressed the patient's questions and concerns, it is time to offer an apology. An effective apology should include the following four elements: (1) taking personal responsibility, (2) behaving in a sympathetic and empathic manner, (3) showing genuine remorse, and (4) trying to make amends.[20] Moreover, some evidence suggests that patients may be less likely to sue physicians when an honest disclosure and apology is accompanied by modest payment.[21]

It is important to apologize and say "I'm sorry" without assigning blame. Be clear and straightforward, such as:

> PHYSICIAN: *I am so sorry that we let you down.*

> or

> PHYSICIAN: *This never should have happened. I'm sorry we failed you.*

> or

> PHYSICIAN: *I'm sorry this happened. It's terrible.*

Blaming someone else is a poor practice and interferes with the important effort to rebuild trust. Avoid comments such as:

> **PHYSICIAN:** *The nurses count the sponges before we close the wound. They told us the sponges were all accounted for, but they must have counted wrong and so we didn't look for any left behind.*

Be sincere, showing respect and empathy for what the patient is experiencing. Validating the patient's feelings and eliciting his or her perspective will help you align with the patient and address his or her concerns. Saying "I know how you feel" should be avoided, as the patient is likely to become more upset and respond with: "You have no idea how I feel." Even if you have experienced a medical error yourself, you can't presume that you know how someone else is feeling. Basic relationship skills can be effective; for example, comments such as: "I can see how upset you are (reflection) and I feel terrible about it" are likely to be better received by the patient. (See Chapter Three.)

Take responsibility for the patient as his or her caregiver, again using basic relationship skills.

> **PHYSICIAN:** *As your physician, I am responsible for your care. I would like to continue to take care of you and see you through this, if you will allow me to.* (**personal support**)

This does not mean that you are assuming blame for the event. Assure the patient you will continue to provide care unless the patient chooses otherwise. Be aware that the patient and family may have lost trust in you and your team and listen for signs of that in the conversation.

> **PHYSICIAN:** *I can understand given what has happened that you might have concerns about my continuing as your doctor, but think it over and let's talk about it and see if we can work things out.* (**legitimation, partnership**)

If the patient or family expresses reservations about your judgment, skill, or experience, then offer to obtain a second opinion. This may return some control to the patient at a time when he or she is vulnerable. When offering a second opinion, it is important that you not imply abandonment.

> **PHYSICIAN:** *If you are so concerned about my judgment or skill that only seeing a different doctor will make you feel safe, I can arrange for another doctor to see you.* (**support**)

If the patient wants to transfer his or her care to a different hospital, avoid being defensive. Support the right to change, but also help the patient and family to understand your concerns if changing hospitals could lead to additional risks. For example, possible delay of corrective actions could lead to additional adverse consequences.

Once issues related to continuity of care have been addressed, assure the patient that an investigation will occur and that you will follow-up with the patient. Such investigation is usually performed together with the hospital risk management department and is called a "root cause analysis."

Let the patient know that action will be taken so that, where possible, this won't happen again. Patients need to understand what went wrong in their care and want to be sure that others won't suffer a similar fate, as in this example statement:

> **PHYSICIAN:** *I will be keeping you informed about what we find out and how we will use this information to improve our care so that other patients don't experience the same problem.* (**support**)

Focus the patient on the immediate clinical plan and decisions that need to be made.

> **PHYSICIAN:** *I think it is important to remove the sponge soon so you don't get an infection. Also, I think it makes sense for us to take you back to the operating room here, but I will help transfer your care if that's what you decide.* (**support**)

Confirm the patient's understanding of the information provided. (See Chapter Five, Educational Skills, "Tell-Back.")

> **PHYSICIAN:** *Mrs. Jackson, I know this news might be overwhelming to anyone, especially when you've just been through surgery. I would like to be sure that I explained it adequately. Can you tell me what your understanding of the situation is?* (legitimation, tell-back)

Acknowledge the patient's concerns if questions about his or her medical expenses or financial compensation are raised. Clinicians can assure the patient he or she will advocate on the patient's behalf even though the clinician is not usually in a position to make such financial decisions. Certain serious reportable events require the hospital to waive payment if the error was within the control of the hospital, was reasonably preventable, and caused patient injury.[22] Nevertheless, it is preferable to assure the patient that the issue of payment will be reviewed promptly and someone will get back to him or her with an answer.

> **PHYSICIAN:** *Mr. Jackson, I think these are important questions that I don't know the answers to. I would be glad to talk with the hospital administrators and have someone come and speak with you.* (**support**) *I think we need to focus on taking care of your wife right now.*

Patients may have concerns about the impact of the adverse event on their condition or recovery, especially after they've had some time to reflect on the information you've provided.

> **PHYSICIAN:** *I know that hearing that you need to be taken back to surgery gives you a lot to think about. Perhaps you would like some time to talk privately with your husband about what you would like to do next. Is there anyone else you would like to call? I'll come back in a few minutes and then we can talk more.* (**empathy, support**)

A patient recovering from an adverse event may require additional services, such as rehabilitation or home care, and be worried about their availability. Offer additional patient support services as indicated, including social services, patient advocates, and clergy.

## The Aftermath

After the disclosure conversation has concluded and an apology offered, carefully document the known facts in the patient's record. Avoid speculation or editorial commentary about what could have caused this event to happen. Naturally, you should follow-up with the patient clinically, providing care according to his or her current health circumstances and medical history. Respect the patient's need for quiet time to reflect on what has been discussed but don't avoid interacting with your patient and the family.

Error disclosures and their aftermath are stressful so be sure to take care of yourself and get the help you need for clinical coverage, emotional support, and legal advice. Remember to get guidance from your risk manager about which conversations about this matter are legally protected and which are not. In general, conversations that are legally protected are those you have with your hospital risk manager, your clergy or spouse, your personal physician or therapist, and, of course, your attorney.

When an adverse event or an error occurs and a patient is harmed, hospital risk managers may advise greater disclosure and transparency than physicians may find comfortable. However, in the event that advice from a hospital risk manager about what to disclose creates an ethical dilemma or other controversy, you should discuss your distress within the context of legally protected conversations. Remember, protected conversations are those you have with your hospital risk manager or the risk management supervisor or hospital legal counsel, your personal attorney, clergy, spouse, personal physician, or therapist. Other alternatives you may consider include consulting with your hospital employee assistance program or anonymously reporting your concern to the hospital's compliance hotline. Such hotlines were originally launched for employees to report suspected cases of financial fraud, but they have now come to be used for a variety of concerns.

If you are concerned about the details of the case and feel you must discuss the clinical scenario and its aftermath, do so within the context of the legally protected conversations listed in the preceding paragraph, or within the context of peer review proceedings. It is not possible to guarantee such conversations will have 100% legal protection, and you should consult with your state laws because there is variability in laws governing legal protection across the nation.

Most important, if you are upset and distressed by the situation, then it is better not to keep these feelings suppressed but to talk about how you feel with someone from your hospital employee assistance program or your designated hospital support person or program or your risk manager, personal counsel, therapist, clergy, or spouse.

Here is an example of how the mishandling of a medical error disclosure can create a second victim—the physician:

> *A second-year resident examined a female patient in the emergency room with abdominal pain and fever. The primary impression was that the patient had acute appendicitis. A white blood cell count was obtained. After seeing a normal white blood cell count, the resident discharged the patient with instructions to call her physician later in the day if the pain or fever worsened. The resident did not realize then that the lab result actually belonged to different patient with a similar name. The patient returned to the emergency room later that day in severe pain and underwent an emergency laparotomy for a ruptured appendix and septic shock. The patient survived and was eventually discharged home in good condition. The case was reviewed by the emergency room Chief as part of the hospital's Quality Improvement program. After reviewing the case, the Chief spoke with the resident to learn why the patient had been discharged to home in light of the lower abdominal pain, fever, and an elevated WBC count without further evaluation or observation. The resident realized the lab error and was remorseful and apologetic, feeling awful and worried about what would happen next. The Chief reassured the resident, who was known for being an excellent doctor, saying "I am not going to tell anyone about this incident and I suggest that you don't either." The resident reluctantly followed this advice but for years was troubled by guilt and shame at having hidden the mistake from the patient. As an older adult, professional counseling allowed the physician to confront and resolve residual guilt and shame over having kept quiet about the error.*

In contrast to the preceding case in which the failure to disclose a medical error led to years of distress by the participant physician, there is another story that is an inspiration to many. This story is about how the trauma of suppressing disclosure of an adverse outcome and the creation of a "wall of silence" (in an effort to protect the physician) can actually cause the clinician to suffer. Instead of accepting an aftermath of guilt and isolation, this clinician took actions that fostered an alliance between himself and his patient.

> *Anesthesiologist Rick Van Pelt has written and lectured about the emotional impact of having been involved in a life-threatening adverse anesthesia event during a routine orthopedic surgery. This event resulted in an outcome not only traumatic for the patient but also for him as her doctor. Following the adverse event, he was counseled by hospital administration and his medical colleagues not to communicate with the patient or her family. He considered this approach to be ethically unacceptable and wrote the patient a personal letter of apology. Months later the patient contacted him. He describes a successful resolution that permitted healing and led them both to found MITSS, Medically Induced Trauma Support Services (www.mitss.org), a nonprofit organization founded in 2002 whose mission is "to support healing and restore hope to patients, families, and clinicians who have been affected by an adverse medical event."*

# The Follow-up

Information as to the chain of events leading up to or triggering the error will become clearer as time passes and the investigation unfolds. Patients value information that will help them understand how and why the error happened to them. They also value knowing that changes will be made and that what they experienced will not happen again. Therefore keep the patient informed of the progress of the investigation. After the investigation has been completed, be sure to inform the patient what will be implemented to prevent this from happening again, especially if the root cause analysis confirms an error or a systems failure. This would be the time for the full apology: taking responsibility, showing remorse, and making amends.

# Conclusion

It is yet unclear whether apology laws that allow more openness about medical errors will result in system changes and ultimately improve patient safety.[23] Surveys have shown that patients want to be listened to, taken seriously, and respected as partners in their care. They want to be told the truth and supported emotionally as well as physically. Full disclosure and genuine apology where indicated can help strengthen the physician-patient relationship and facilitate the healing process between the individuals involved in such events.[24] James Reason wrote in 2000 that humans make errors, thus we know that physicians are not infallible.[25] The pressure to be perfect remains entrenched in the culture of medicine, and such self-directed pressure can facilitate efforts to conceal, cover-up, or deny that errors were made. Concealing, covering-up, or denying errors that occur in medical practice can further compound the harm experienced by patients and their family members and escalate the physician's risk of legal jeopardy. Taking time to learn and practice the elements of effective disclosure and apology during medical school will help improve the culture of medicine over time. Effective medical error disclosure and apology are among the essential skills and abilities that physicians of all specialties need to deliver high-quality, safe medical care throughout the lifespan of their patients.

## References

1. Kohn LT, Corrigan JM, Donaldson MS, editors: *To err is human: building a safer health care in America*, Washington D.C., 2000, Institute of Medicine, National Academy Press.
2. *When things go wrong responding to adverse events: a consensus statement of the Harvard hospitals*, Boston, 2006, Massachusetts Coalition for the Prevention of Medical Errors, http://www.macoalition.org/documents/respondingToAdverseEvents.pdf [Accessed: May 10, 2006].
3. Weinstein L: A multifaceted approach to improve patient safety, prevent medical errors and resolve the professional liability crisis. *Am J Obstet Gynecol* 194(4):1160–1165, 2006.
4. Mazor KM, Simon SR, Gurwitz JH: Communicating with patients about medical errors: a review of the literature. *Arch Intern Med* 164:1690–1697, 2004.
5. Liebman CB, Hyman CS: A meditation skills model to manage disclosure of errors and adverse events to patients. *Health Affairs* 23:22–32, 2004.
6. Vincent C: Understanding and responding to adverse events. *N Engl J Med* 348:1051–1056, 2003.
7. Vincent C, Young M, Phillips A: Why do people sue doctors? A study of patients and relatives taking legal action. *Lancet* 343:1609–1613, 1994.
8. Leape L: Understanding the power of apology. www.npsf.org. 8(4):1–3, 2005.
9. Kaldjian LC, Jones EW, Rosenthal GE: Facilitating and impeding factors for physicians' error disclosure: a structured literature review. *Jt Comm J Qual Patient Saf* 32(f):188–198, 2006.
10. Beckman HB, et al: The doctor-patient relationship and malpractice. Lessons from plaintiff depositions. *Arch Intern Med* 154:1365–1370, 1994.
11. Hickson GB, et al: Factors that prompted families to file medical malpractice claims following perinatal injuries. *JAMA* 267:1359–1363, 1992.

12. Bell SK, Moorman DW, Delbanco T: Improving the patient, family, and clinician experience after harmful events: the "when things go wrong" curriculum. *Acad Med* 85:1010–1017, 2010.

13. Chan DK, et al: How surgeons disclose medical errors to patients: a study using standardized patients. *Surgery* 138(5):851–858, 2005.

14. Carr S: Disclosure and apology: what's missing? A report based on an invitational forum held on March 13, 2009. Medically Induced Trauma Support Services (MITSS) http://www.mitss.org/MITSS_WhatsMissing.pdf. [Accessed February 26, 2012].

15. Gallagher TH, Studdeert D, Levinson W: Disclosing harmful medical errors to patients. *N Engl J Med* 356(26):2713–2719, 2007.

16. Clinton HR, Obama B: Making patient safety the centerpiece of medical liability reform. *N Engl J Med* 354:2206, 2006.

17. McDonnell WM, Guenther E: Narrative review: do state laws make it easier to say "I'm sorry"? *Ann Intern Med* 149:811–815, 2008.

18. Mastroianni AC, et al: The flaws in state "apology" and "disclosure" laws dilute their intended impact on malpractice suits. *Health Aff (Millwood)* 29(9):1611–1619, 2010.

19. Kubler-Ross E: *On death and dying*, 1969, Macmillan Publishing Company.

20. Leape L: *citing Lazare A. On apology*, Oxford, 2004, Oxford University Press.

21. Kraman SS, Hamm G: Risk management: extreme honesty may be the best policy. *Ann Intern Med* 131:963–967, 1999.

22. Serious reportable events in health care 2006 update, national Quality Forum, Item Number NQFCR-18-07, March 2007.

23. Dresser R: The limits of apology laws. *Hastings Cent Rep* 38(3):6–7, 2008.

24. Lazare A: Apology in medical practice: an emerging clinical skill. *JAMA* 296:1401–1404, 2006.

25. Reason J: *Human error*, Cambridge, 1990, Cambridge University Press.

# CHAPTER 29

# Risky Drinking and Interviewing About Alcohol Use

William Clark

## OVERVIEW

This chapter presents strategies for communicating with risky drinkers and patients who abuse alcohol.

Alcohol use disorders afflict at least 20% of adults. Death certificates, medical records, news outlets, and almost everyone's personal experience attest to the resulting litany of tragic family and social problems, preventable injuries, and death. Extensive research documents that people with this common disorder are widespread in office and hospital practices, physicians commonly fail to recognize alcohol use disorders, and physicians who do recognize them commonly fail to use strategies of proven effectiveness for assisting these patients.

This chapter defines *risky drinking* and other *alcohol use disorders*, and suggests tactics for maintaining relationships and giving therapeutic advice that respects patients' perspectives and preferences. Dialogue is difficult. Helping patients to reflect on their drinking behavior feels difficult not only because heavy alcohol (or drug) use produces toxic brain effects and thinking problems, but also because the stigma associated with alcohol problems encourages defensiveness, minimization, and lying. Patients frequently cannot see the problems you perceive, or they are unable to imagine or undertake action steps toward resolving problems, or both.

More than 50% of US adults abstain or drink less than 12 drinks in a year. More than 30% drink more than "moderately." Within this heavy-drinking group, roughly 10% will manifest alcohol abuse and 10% alcohol dependence at any given point in time (see the following).

Experience and research with the complexities of motivation, readiness, initiation of behavior change, and maintaining changes inform the ideas and tactics we suggest. When applying the skills we describe, students and seasoned clinicians in primary care or specialist practices can move from common feelings of dismay or irritation when working with patients with alcohol disorders and begin to celebrate the successes they will appreciate and foster.

## DEFINITIONS

### A drink

A 12 oz. beer, 5 oz. wine, 2 to 3 oz. of cordial or aperitif, or 1.5 oz. (bar shot) of hard liquor or brandy; each of these standard drinks contains approximately 0.6 oz. of ethanol. Alcohol is absorbed quickly from an empty stomach, and alcohol taken with food is completely absorbed, albeit more slowly.

243

## Normal or healthy or moderate drinking

Expert consensus holds that "moderate drinking" is defined by a low quantity of intake (less than 14 drinks weekly for men and less than seven drinks weekly for women), a social setting for drinking, and little intoxication (not more than four drinks per occasion for men and three for women).

## Risky or hazardous drinking

Drinking above moderate limits, whether more than the specified number per occasion or more frequently (or both) is variously called "at risk" or "hazardous" and is likely to cause harm, according to long-term studies.[1]

## Alcohol abuse

Alcohol abuse is a "maladaptive pattern of use leading to impairment or distress, manifested in a 12-month period by one or more of the following: failure to fulfill role obligations; recurrent use in hazardous situations; legal problems; continued use despite alcohol-related social or interpersonal problems."

## Alcohol dependence

Individuals with alcohol dependence suffer diverse medical and psychosocial consequences (such as health problems, legal problems, family dysfunction, and performance problems at school or work) from poorly controlled drinking. They are preoccupied with drinking, spend less and less time on other life activities, and continue to drink despite consequences, although they may attempt to cut down. A striking 5% to 10% of American adults develop this syndrome. What distinguishes alcohol *abuse* from alcohol *dependence* is not **the nature** of the problems (except for withdrawal symptoms, which indicate *physical* dependence), but the **frequency, persistence, and pervasiveness** of problems.

# Function One: Build the Relationship

## INTRODUCTION

The indignity, shame, and embarrassment associated with alcohol problems affect every physician and every patient, directly or indirectly. Almost everyone has a family member or acquaintance who is afflicted. Physicians quickly learn that intoxication not only causes mayhem and chaos in emergency rooms, but also kills and maims drivers, passengers, and countless people with cirrhosis, delirium tremens, pneumonia, and so on. People who are drunk are unkempt and messy, vomiting and bloody, disagreeable and difficult to help. Talking about alcohol is always a sensitive matter. Patients with serious problems distort facts and respond defensively, and physicians have many negative and painful experiences with such patients. The combined effects of stigma, defensiveness, and painful experience means that patients are wary of questions and physicians are skeptical and uneasy. In few other medical situations does physicians' ability to listen attentively, act compassionately, and recommend with dignity so strongly affect patients' willingness to divulge information and to participate in dialogue about possible treatment.

## CONVERSATION

For these reasons, short introductory explanations are helpful when bringing up drinking. They might sound like the following:

> *I need to ask every patient about some sensitive topics.*
>
> *Information about drinking is relevant to treatment planning for many conditions.*

Empathic, partnering, and legitimizing statements, as well as expressions of expertise, become important as interviews progress, and might sound like the following:

*I sense that this is irritating for you. Let's focus on working together on your health.*

*Many people find these questions a bit annoying.*

*I've been really pleased to see how much some of my patients have benefited from going to AA meetings.*

*Good evidence shows that no one is immune to getting hooked on alcohol; it often helps to think of it like an allergy—some people have a bad reaction whenever they eat peanuts.*

*How do my suggestions strike you so far?*

*I'm pleased that you are interested in continuing to dialogue about drinking and health.*

*Changing a pleasurable habit on physician recommendation is always a challenge, and I'll do all I can to assure your success, in both the short term and as long as necessary.*

Maintenance of an effective therapeutic relationship with patients who are abstainers, healthy drinkers, or at-risk drinkers is often straightforward. Your demonstration of good listening skills and empathic responses usually suffice to keep conversations on track. Reciprocal bonding is more difficult as physicians enter caring relationships with more seriously afflicted patients. The dynamics of shame, humiliation, discouragement, and despair in patients with alcohol abuse or dependence lead to shortened dialogues characterized by awkwardness, hostility, and challenge.

Experts in motivation, behavior change, and health care communication uniformly agree that attempts to persuade patients to cut down or quit by threatening them with serious consequences usually proves **counterproductive**.

Although many physicians feel that threatening statements may be helpful, they are **not** useful and should **not** be part of medical interventions. The following are examples of threatening statements that physicians typically make:

*I'm sure you can see that your life difficulties will continue unless you stop drinking.*

(rolling eyes, raising voice, turning away)

*You will die in a short time unless you quit.*

## Function Two: Assess and Understand the Patient's Problems

### INTRODUCTION

The biggest problem is that physicians who wish to distinguish among "healthy" drinking, "risky" drinking, and serious problems of abuse or dependence rely heavily on what patients say, and patients with the most serious problems minimize and lie effectively. The consequence is that whenever you see any level of problem, you have to assume it may be a very serious one, even though the patient seems to be drinking socially if one uses only the facts as the patient volunteers them.

Alcohol abuse is a prototypical biopsychosocial illness. The AMA declared alcoholism a disease many decades ago, and many attempts have subsequently been made to describe the pathophysiology of alcohol problems. Inevitably, the descriptions emphasize social and emotional components, and the clearly medical aspects set in later, when heavy and repetitive drinking is well established. The relationship issues mentioned above and expanded on below explain why obtaining any data from people with alcohol abuse is a process that requires careful attention to maintaining trust and understanding the strategies that have been found useful through clinical experience and associated research studies. Patients are universally reluctant to disclose amounts of alcohol they've drunk and seldom connect symptoms to alcohol intake in conversation, even when they cognitively understand the connections. Therefore adequate data collection requires that clinicians attend constantly to trust and relationship issues and use tested strategies.

## DEFINITIONS

### Intoxication

Most observers easily detect the slurred speech, lack of coorindation, and emotional lability, sometimes with changes in or loss of consciousness, that signal intoxication. Blood alcohol level (BAL) declines in a linear fashion at approximately 0.015 to 0.020 g/dl per hour. If the BAL is initially 0.225, it will not arrive at 0.08 for 7 to 9 hours (0.08 is the legal limit for driving in most states). Alcohol on the breath in clinical situations almost always signals an alcohol disorder. No person is immune to the nervous tissue effects of alcohol.

### Tolerance

Tolerance is caused by steady heavy drinking, indicates neurologic adjustment to alcohol, is inevitably toxic, and usually means *alcohol dependence*. Tolerance is present if an odor of alcohol is apparent without evidence of intoxication. A person can look and behave entirely normally with a very high alcohol level (even as high as 0.500 g/dl).

### Blackout

This term describes a state of high BAL without loss of consciousness, after which the person does not remember events of the prior few hours, and sometimes several days' prior events. A blackout means severe intoxication but like any other single problem does not by itself signal tolerance or dependence. It surely is a signal of risky drinking.

### Withdrawal syndrome

Withdrawal syndromes clinically indicate alcohol dependence and are manifest as tremor, anxiety, sweating, and stomach upset. Brain chemistry changes over weeks to months of heavy drinking, and withdrawal symptoms do not happen after simple intoxication or a short binge. People experience an intense craving, and a few trials convince them that a drink is an effective antidote. In many cases people try continuously to dampen the withdrawal sickness, drinking around the clock, barely sleeping and eating little. Individuals in this situation develop the potentially lethal complication of *delirium tremens*.

### Denial

Denial severely limits normal social interactions, triggers defensiveness and irritation in caregivers, and limits effective and compassionate care. Denial manifests as limited insight into realities that are obvious to others and springs from both neurologic and psychosocial sources—a combination of memory lapses associated with intoxication along with the emotional compartmentalization triggered by embarrassment and shame. It intensifies as continued heavy drinking produces additional cognitive deficits and more socioemotional isolation.

## ARE YOU WORRIED ABOUT THE PATIENT'S DRINKING?

In seeking to understand patients' problems, physicians usually try to make a diagnosis to signify the presence of a medical disease or a psychosocial problem. However, in any one interview or a series of interviews, denial and patients' reactivity to being questioned may severely limit data gathering. Because a physical problem such as cirrhosis, bleeding, withdrawal symptoms, another of the dozens of medical complications described in texts, or a letter from a family member or court record is often missing, you may be left with scant hard evidence and unable to ascertain whether the patient is at risk, has alcohol abuse, or has alcohol dependence. This situation is very common in many primary care situations, and too often when uncertainty is high, physicians take no action.

This section describes orderly and tested information-gathering strategies and tactics that help understand patients' problems and may result in a diagnosis. We return later to what you might recommend to a patient about whom you are concerned but for whom no diagnosis is obvious.

## PRESCREEN

First, ask every new patient a simple question about drinking:

*Do you sometimes drink alcoholic beverages?*

If the answer is no, leave this topic. The abstinent subgroup with past problems often discloses this spontaneously, although the clinician may want to explore selectively why a patient is abstinent.

## SCREENING

Follow a yes answer with a screen for at-risk drinking, abuse, and dependency.

Both a simple query about quantity and frequency and the CAGE test for alcohol dependence are feasible and reliable next steps.

If you prefer the quantity/frequency approach, ask first about heavy drinking days:

*How many times in the past year have you had five or more drinks in a day* (for men); *or four or more drinks* (for women).

(Positive screen is at least one day with five or more drinks [four for women].)

If this initial question is positive, quantify the drinking behavior. You can determine a weekly average by asking:

*On average, how many days a week do you have an alcoholic drink?* or *On a typical day, how many drinks do you have?*

Risky drinkers are those whose consumption exceeds moderate or safe amounts (more per occasion or more frequently, see the preceding). When you find an at-risk drinker, proceed next to screen for dependence with CAGE. Closed rather than open questions are helpful here. If patients answer open-ended questions vaguely, forcing you to ask clarifying questions, they feel accused of lying and become defensive.

The CAGE test (Table 29-1) is a validated screen for alcohol dependence, and for two positive responses it is 60% to 95% sensitive or 40% to 95% specific, depending on the population screened. CAGE is less accurate for women and African Americans. CAGE alone will not find

---

TABLE 29.1 ■ **CAGE Screening for Dependence Symptoms**

1. Have you ever felt that you should *cut down* on your drinking?
2. Have people *annoyed* you by criticizing your drinking?
3. Have you ever felt bad or *guilty* about your drinking?
4. Have you ever had a drink first thing in the morning to steady your nerves or get rid of a hangover? (***Eye opener***)

at-risk drinkers, but it eases conversation with more seriously afflicted patients. If CAGE is clearly negative and you did not begin by asking the quantity/frequency questions, ask them now to find risky drinkers.

Many studies of a variety of laboratory tests confirm that they are inadequate for screening.[3]

An alternative strategy is the 10-question AUDIT questionnaire (see Appendix 1), which can be self-administered in a waiting room, is sensitive throughout the spectrum of unhealthy drinking, and is the best instrument for identifying risky drinking (sensitivity 57% to 97%, specificity 78% to 96%).[3,4]

## RED FLAGS

Many times other information from the patient or other sources makes it clear that some kind of drinking problem is present. Follow up patient's spontaneous mention of partying, hangover, blackouts, or withdrawal symptoms with the CAGE test. For a positive family history, arrests for driving while intoxicated, spouses or friends who confide about problems, and prior medical records that indicate alcohol-related problems, begin with the quantity/frequency questions or the CAGE.

Interviews with family, nurses, or social workers and records from other physicians or hospitals may contain unanticipated information that establishes a diagnosis.

## CONTINUE THE CONVERSATION

A positive screening response or red flag of any kind means both that you will seek more data to fully understand the patient's problem and you will express your concern and make a recommendation (that is, conduct a brief intervention, see the following). The context, time available, and the patient's apparent levels of engagement, trust, or defensiveness shape your decision at this branch point to begin sharing information or continue seeking more information from the patient.

You can foster relationship and collaboration by weaving subsequent questions into a conversation that builds on the thread of prior exchanges with the patient.

*You mentioned feeling you should cut down. How have your attempts to do so worked out?*

Similarly, clinicians who respond to patients' irritability, defensiveness, and even suspiciousness in a respectful, dignified, and empathic way enhance the likelihood of successful intervention and treatment.[2,6] Show interest in the patient as a person with voice tone, posture, and other nonverbal gestures that convey care and concern.

# Function Three: Collaborative Management

## INITIAL STEPS

As soon as the data arouse concerns that your patient is drinking in an unsafe fashion, share your thoughts with the patient in a collaborative mode. Although only the patient can take responsibility for change and effect change, physicians can promote it by engaging and fostering patients' intrinsic motivation. Effective physicians intentionally and deliberately demonstrate empathy, listen to patients' perspectives, selectively provide information, and shore up patients' confidence about successfully making and sustaining change. Attentively listening to patients' clues about their readiness for change allows physicians to tailor their conversation and collaboratively negotiate action steps that have a higher likelihood of success. Unadjusted recommendations to "think about your drinking," "cut down to safe levels," "go to AA," or "talk with Dr. addiction specialist" seldom promote change.

## READINESS FOR CHANGE MATTERS

Studies show that more than 75% of primary care patients express some readiness for change and that higher readiness correlates positively with problem severity. These findings contradict the common belief that severe drinkers are uniformly pre-contemplative.[8]

Patients with alcohol abuse or dependence actively resist talking seriously about change (or say "yes, sir" or use other defensive strategies to avoid engagement), perhaps because they would have to leave the drinking culture in which they live or because attempts to control drinking or find contentment in life have repeatedly failed. Discouragement, depression, and despair dam up one's motivation and damn every action plan or change effort that lacks strong and persistent support from loved ones or community resources.

Asking two questions about patients' conviction and confidence steers dialogue directly toward issues of change and helps ascertain motivational readiness. A question about conviction assesses what patients believe about the *importance* of taking action, whereas a question about confidence assesses what patients believe about their *ability* to adopt or change a behavior despite obstacles or barriers. The latter is often referred to as their degree of self-efficacy.

Ask patients to help you understand where they stand by requesting that they use a numerical rating scale. Frame your questions as follows:

First:

*On a scale of 0 to 10, how convinced are you that cutting down or quitting is important?*

And then:

*Let's suppose for a moment that you were a 10, convinced that you should cut down or quit. On a 0 to 10 scale, how confident are you that you would be able to entirely abstain (or limit drinking to safe levels) for the next 4 weeks?*

Although in a given conversation the scales or answers may not be accurate, reliable, or valid, this is far less important than the fact that the conversation is focused on change. Usually, following up with this inquiry:

*I wonder why you chose X, instead of Y (a lower number)?*

encourages patients to hear themselves speak about change in positive terms (see Chapter 18 on "Change Talk"). You can then move to a conversation about next steps that is informed by having heard patients talk about motivation—its importance to them and their current evaluation of their self-efficacy. This is true even when patients protest that they do not like to use number scales.

## PROVOCATION

Physicians provoke an internal dialogue within their patients whenever they engage a topic that might require a behavior change—high cholesterol, diabetes management, smoking, or even taking a new medication are good examples. Real change is often slow, and the physician may act as provocateur of such internal dialogues over time. In the case of risky drinkers, as noted in the preceding, this time period may extend to years. Further, for patients with abuse and dependence, the physician seldom provides definitive treatment and serves as provocateur toward alcohol-specific counseling and treatment, treatment of associated or complicating mental health or substance abuse problems, and resources for community-based help, such as Alcoholics Anonymous.

In this role of provoking internal dialogue, you want patients' internal dialogue to include the fact that you are concerned, that you are a resource who has worked with similar situations, and that your continuing relationship will be trustworthy and durable. The following sections on brief intervention and Brief Action Planning elaborate further on tactics and skills that build relationships while provoking successful behavior change.

## BRIEF INTERVENTION

Brief intervention refers to 10 to 15 minutes of counseling, with feedback about drinking, personalized advice, negotiation of goals, assistance with ways to achieve goals, and follow-up contact. Brief interventions, studied in a variety of practice settings, decrease alcohol intake and decrease the prevalence of at-risk drinking by 10.5%. In long-term follow-up studies of up to 16 years, brief intervention decreased self-reported daily and binge drinking, as well as alcohol-related mortality.[5] Nonconfrontational and empathic interviewing styles aimed at enhancing patients' motivation are more effective at reducing (or stopping) drinking than confrontational counseling. Brief intervention can be effective whether patients are ready to take action to change, are thinking about change, or even seem dead set against change at the time of the interview.[6,7]

In a brief intervention, physicians provide information, listen to patients' perspectives about both the pros and the cons of possible changes, and help boost the patient's self-confidence about change. Importantly, the information you provide includes *feedback* about the patient's health and the succinct *framing* and *interpreting* of data and information about *resources* to support any action plans the patient undertakes. Finally, and of special importance, physicians demonstrate their attentiveness to this particular interaction by taking every opportunity to respond to patients' emotions, including both their verbal and nonverbal expressions of feeling (using Function One skills, see Chapter 3 and Chapter 18).

## EDUCATION

Experts agree that physicians should present information in a dialogue, check patients' understanding of the information, listen to their perspectives, and listen specifically for more clues about conviction and confidence. The steps of (e)TACCT (see Chapter 5) are useful to follow with this population: (e) refers to "elicit" baseline knowledge; "T" refers to telling the patient brief chunks of information; "C" is about caring by responding with Function One skills to emotions the patient demonstrates; the second "C" then is about counseling itself about more substantive educational messages; and the last "T" is "tell-back," that is, asking the patient to tell-back what the physician has discussed with the patient to ensure they are "on the same page." These steps are discussed in more detail below.

## (E) ELICIT BASELINE KNOWLEDGE

Ask patients what they know and are thinking before telling them what you know. Questions like the following are suitable:

> *Do you know anyone with an alcohol problem? Tell me a little about what you see.*
>
> *I'm concerned about your drinking and will share my thoughts with you. Would you tell me your view about your drinking?*
>
> *Do you know anyone who has made important changes in their drinking? How did they do that?*

## (T)(TELL) PRESENT INFORMATION IN FOCUSED AND SUCCINCT STATEMENTS

We list important baseline information here, in straightforward empathic language that you can adjust to the circumstances of any intervention. Begin by stating your concern and giving it a name.

*Our conversation causes me concern about your health. Specifically, I'm worried that your alcohol intake is … risky (or perhaps) causing serious problems for you.*

*I will give you my best advice, which is based on ideas from the experts and my experience with other patients with similar problems.*

*Most people who drink alcohol drink less than you, and about half of Americans drink less than 12 drinks in a year or abstain completely.*

*No one sets out to develop problems from drinking. Responsible drinking is a pleasure, but seeking those pleasurable effects can quickly become a habit that may go a little too far.*

*People are different from one another, and in some folks the brain's nerve cells seem to get hooked easily, almost like an allergy.*

*For better health, you should curb (or cease) your alcohol use.*

*Making a change in any habit is difficult, and we know a lot about how to help folks take successful baby steps and find the support that can produce long-lasting change.*

*The key choices are up to you, and you are the person who will decide what to do. I'd like to join with you to make plans that will work for you.*

*You are in charge, and I will stand by you even if progress is slow or intermittent.*

## (A)(ASK) CHECK UNDERSTANDING

Each time you present a bit of information, ask patients what it means to them. Examples might sound like the following:

*What do you think about my concerns?*

*Does (that statement) make sense to you?*

*I can imagine you might have another take on this. Would you share it with me?*

## (C) (CARE) RESPOND TO EMOTIONS

Wary patients who notice that their physicians are moving into the complex territory of behavior change, particularly about behaviors that are stigmatized, often have a fight-or-flight response. They try to disengage by expressing irritation or changing the topic, more or less openly. If you do not respond to their feelings, they will know you do not care about them and trust levels will predictably decrease. Rarely will helpful information, checking of readiness, or action planning reverse this situation.

Nonverbal responses of patience, or attentive, welcoming, and open gestures, or gestures of joining with the patient are helpful. Even more important is avoidance of eye rolling or turning attention away from the patient. Verbal responses that communicate respect, partnership, understanding, and support, adjusted for dialogues about drinking, include the following:

*I hear irritation in your voice as I ask you about drinking.*

*Every patient I've worked with about changing drinking finds it complicated.*

*My focus is on your health, and to see what we can do as a team if we work together.*

*I know that you have navigated troubled waters in other situations* (mention a specific if you can), *and I hope you can bring some of those strengths to bear here.*

*I have a lot of respect for the independence of spirit you show, as we discuss drinking.*

*Oftentimes in conversations about drinking, patients wonder if I can possibly understand how it fits into their full life.*

## (T) (TELL-BACK) AND INVITE QUESTIONS

Beyond checking receipt of information chunks, invite more general questions and inquire about feelings.

*Just to make sure we're on the same page, can you tell me back what we've just gone over."
And ...*

*I'm open to hearing what's on your mind as we proceed. What are your concerns or questions?*

*How are you feeling as we move along?*

*What's uppermost in your mind as we try to make plans together?*

## BRIEF ACTION PLANNING

As you move beyond data gathering, continuing to build the relationship as you proceed, your desired goals include helping patients make a behaviorally specific personal action plan for health in which they are confident they can succeed and arranging follow-up. Chapter 5 discusses this generic process in detail.

All patients with unhealthy use of alcohol will benefit from your attempt at Brief Action Planning (BAP), a core skill of Function Three, and many of these patients will make action plans for their health and start to decrease their maladaptive use of alcohol. Others may only make an action plan for health when clinicians use more advanced stepped-care action planning skills, as described in Chapter 18.

Many will not engage, and others will not follow through with what they agreed to do. Nevertheless, the process of exchanging views on need and tactics for change in a compassionate, respectful conversation has a positive impact. Changing risky drinking or recovering from abuse or dependence are complex and long-term processes. Demonstrating that you are a trusted and knowledgeable partner makes a difference. Next month, or a year, or 5 or even 10 years from now, people will be grateful, and some will remember to express that gratitude to you. Few moments in medical practice are more professionally satisfying than these, because they testify to the power of healing relationships.

## SOME SPECIFIC COMMUNICATION STRATEGIES FOR PATIENTS AT DIFFERENT LEVELS OF READINESS

Approaching patients with risky drinking or alcohol abuse/dependence is always challenging and, in addition to the suggestions described in the preceding, we provide some ideas that may be helpful if you consider strategizing according to levels of readiness for change.

Think first about a patient who expresses a desire for change at the 8 to 10 level. Even when convinced, few risky drinkers can easily imagine small steps. In fact, many make it a point to *not* track exactly how much or how often they drink. A conversation might go something like the following:

*So, we're agreed that you are drinking above safe levels, and you think cutting down is important for your health. Can you imagine a small step that you could carry out to move in that direction before we check in again?*

Patients might be very creative because they know the details of their lives and you do not, but you have some notion of the difficulties anyone faces with changing an ingrained habit, particularly one that has powerful effects on the neurochemistry of pleasure pathways in the brain and is connected with friendship and sociability (even if alcohol provides false courage for social engagement).

Patients usually imagine big steps that reflect the normal lack of awareness of the pressures from habit or from friends and social situations to overwhelm good intentions. They might suggest stopping for a week or never drinking more than two drinks. These strategies are seldom viable. Of course, if you discuss the pros and cons, and the patient is confident at more than a 7 level, give it a try. If the patient fails, reframe the situation as a learning experience and make a new plan more likely to succeed.

In the absence of viable patient suggestions, you might wonder out loud about beginning with keeping a record of time and place of drinking, or beginning to chart rough estimates of amounts, or noting effects on self or others after the usual amount of drinking. Some drinkers might agree to never drink of Wednesdays or not have more than six at the bar. If the patient's confidence level about success of a plan is less than 7, negotiate a new plan, now or at another visit, suggesting that you both will try to be creative about working out baby steps that patients think have at least a 7 chance of success. This is an iterative process, as with any important behavior change. Furthermore, major keys to success include support from the community and building trust that you will show respect and support for the patient in spite of difficulties. If trust in you or community support is lacking, sustained change is unlikely. If patients with abuse or dependence are engaged and still not succeeding, the time for consultative help is right. Few nonspecialist physicians should continue this work without specialist assistance for the patient (program, counselor, AA, etc.).

Turn now to patients with much lower readiness to change or patients with very little interest (or no interest at all) in changing. Avoid the righting reflex; that is, do not waste your time or energy trying to persuade them to change—surely they will not change, and they will resist and resent your intrusions openly or silently. Your efforts will be counterproductive. A useful conversation might sound like the following:

PHYSICIAN: *Is there anything you'd like to do about your alcohol intake before we meet again?*

PATIENT: *What do you mean? Are you trying to tell me I need to cut down on my drinking, because if that's what you're saying, you're barking up the wrong tree.*

PHYSICIAN: *I hear what you are saying. I'm expressing my own concern about connections between alcohol and health, and was just asking if there is anything about alcohol and health that you might like to discuss with me now.*

PATIENT: *I'm not interested.*

PHYSICIAN: *So it sounds like you are quite certain that alcohol hasn't led to any problems for you in any way.*

PATIENT: *That's what I've been trying to say here.*

PHYSICIAN: *Sorry to sound like I'm hassling you. I've expressed my concern, and I'm okay with leaving this topic. I'd like to follow your lead and move to the other plans we need to discuss together before we close for the day.*

For patients who do not want to change, take a long view and in future visits listen carefully for change talk; that is, anything from the patient that suggests he or she is contemplating change or has made some effort in the past, or notices what friends or some celebrity have done. Note if the risky drinker mentions any connection with any idea of planning for health that is a positive sign. Furthermore, patients who drink excessively often pursue other unhealthy habits (e.g., smoking) on which they may be able to act. The patient may be willing to develop a plan for that other behavior so long as the patient is clearly interested and convinced he or she can carry it out. Any successful lifestyle change will build self-efficacy and build trust in the relationship with you. Self-efficacy can generalize to other behaviors, like maladaptive alcohol use. You can continue data gathering over time about drinking, symptoms, and interest and commitment to change and continue to offer the patient the opportunity to develop action plans for health around alcohol use.

## SOME POSSIBLE DIALOGUES WITH PATIENTS WHO HAVE LOW READINESS FOR CHANGE

Many patients with low or very low readiness, however, are able to demonstrate some ambivalence, and clinicians may be able to starting working toward change with those patients. We suggest a few possible strategic approaches for such patients. Here is one example.

> *So, you've indicated that you are a 3 regarding your interest in making changes in your drinking. A 3 actually indicates some positive interest in making real changes. I wonder why you would say a 3 at all and not a 2, 1, or 0?[A]*

This type of comment is called a strength-based intervention and is a higher-order motivational interviewing technique, which can elicit change talk from a patient with persistent unhealthy behavior. Instead of arguing with a patient with low confidence or giving up, it aims to guide the patient to a realistic appraisal of his or her own condition. By asking the patient to state his or her own concerns, even if only at a level of 1 or 2, they are still real concerns of the patient. The idea is that when the patient starts to state the concern in his or her own words, the patient hears them in a different way (rather than as a lecture from a health professional) and they have a different meaning. In this way, they actually become "change talk," because the patient has stated the concerns him or herself, in his or her own words, and in that way with a personalized meaning to and for the patient. For example:

> *Well, you did say that if I do keep drinking like this, my liver might someday really start to fail. And my wife said she is probably going to leave me if I don't stop drinking. I'm not sure that's going to happen—but that's what she says. And I really don't drink very much anyway. But I guess I know that I am probably going to have to stop, or at least cut down some day ...*

At that point, the physician has been able to elicit some change talk and may be able to start a dialogue with the patient about change because he or she has acknowledged that he or she may have to stop someday. This conversation may lead to some small action plan for health—perhaps keeping a log about the drinking, investigating options to get help (like AA or other helping agencies), thinking about stopping, agreement to continue the discussion, and so on.

Of course, some patients will not admit to any concerns at all. The physician can say something like this:

> *So, if I understand you correctly, you are feeling absolutely fine with how you've been doing and it's okay with you for things to go on just the way they've been going so far? You don't have any concern at all.*

By reflecting the negative side (*You don't have any concern at all*), the physician uses an amplified negative reflection (see Chapter 18 on advanced skills) that may bring out the ambivalence many individuals with risky drinking experience and may be willing to admit when faced with this type of question.

> *Well, doc, I wouldn't say I have no concern at all. If you really want to know the truth, I do occasionally worry that my wife may actually leave me, or that my liver may go out on me. I really wouldn't want either of those to happen.*

Again, this type of dialogue may begin to open up a discussion that may allow some early action planning for change to begin.

## Summary

Communicating with patients about risky drinking and alcohol use is challenging and often frustrating. Physicians, however, who strategically use straightforward concepts and skills from the Three Function Model to engage, understand, and cooperatively manage patients will find significant improvement in medical outcomes as well as personal satisfaction in working with these patients who are sometimes quite difficult and challenging.

### References

1. Bondy S, et al: Low-risk drinking guidelines: the scientific evidence. *Can J Public Health* 90:264–270, 1999.
2. Bertholet N, et al: Does readiness to change predict subsequent alcohol consumption in medical inpatients with unhealthy alcohol use? *Addict Behav* 34(8):636–640, 2009.
3. Daeppen J, et al: Efficacy of brief motivational intervention in reducing binge drinking in young men: a randomized controlled trial. *Drug Alcohol Depend* 113(1):69–75, 2011. Brief Motivational Intervention Reduces Heavy Episodic Drinking in Young Men.
4. Dawson D, Pulay J, Grant B: A Comparison of two single-item screeners for hazardous drinking and alcohol use disorder. *Alcohol Clin Exp Res* 34:1–11, 2010.
5. NIAAA: *Helping patients who drink too much: a clinician's guide*, Washington, D.C., 2005, Government Printing Office, (updated, January, 2007). http://pubs.niaaa.nih.gov/publications/Practitioner/Clinicians Guide2005/clinicians_guide.htm; accessed 12/4/2012).
6. Saitz R: Unhealthy alcohol use. *N Engl J Med* 352:596–607, 2005.
7. Schermer C, et al: Trauma center brief interventions for alcohol disorders decrease subsequent driving under the influence arrests. *J Trauma* 60:29–34, 2006.
8. Williams E, et al: Readiness to change in primary care patients who screened positive for alcohol misuse. *Ann Fam Med* 4:213–220, 2006.

### Endnote

A. This approach, and most of the dialogues about change in this chapter, derive from William Miller and Stephen Rollnick and their contributions from the field of Motivational Interviewing.

# Higher Order Skills

# CHAPTER 30

# Nonverbal Communication

Cecile A. Carson

## OVERVIEW

This chapter describes how nonverbal communication affects the doctor-patient relationship. Awareness of nonverbal channels and signals as well as development of nonverbal skills can improve quality of communication and outcome of care. Nonverbal communication refers to all behavioral signals that send interpersonal messages and reflect the tenor of interactions between the physician and the patient. Attention to these signals allows the interviewer to monitor the process of an interaction—to keep a finger on the pulse of what transpires in a dynamic, moment-to-moment manner as he or she moves through the three functions of the medical interview. Most important, understanding nonverbal signals allows the interviewer to guide the physician-patient interaction in a positive direction.

*Using nonverbal communication effectively does not take extra time*, because nonverbal communication occurs in real time, simultaneously with the verbal flow of an interview. Approximately 80% of essential communication between individuals occurs nonverbally, involuntarily, and outside of conscious awareness. Verbal behavior can be deceptive and misleading; people can lie. Nonverbal behavior speaks the truth; in general, nonverbal signals cannot lie. Important information that cannot be hidden is exchanged at all times—from patient to clinician and from clinician to patient. Only 20% of essential communication is verbal and voluntary. Thus the patient and the physician have control over only a small portion of communication. A patient nonverbally signals any problems he or she has with the three functions of the interview, even if the problem is not expressed verbally. In general, the physician's problems also are expressed nonverbally outside of conscious awareness.

The four general categories of nonverbal communication are as follows:

1. *Kinesics*: facial expressions, gestures, touch, body tension, position, and angulation
2. *Proxemics*: spatial relationships and barriers
3. *Paralanguage*: voice tone, rhythm, volume, emphasis, and rate of speech
4. *Autonomic output*: flushing, blanching, sweating, tearing, piloerection, changes in breathing and pupil size, swallowing, and dry mouth

## Basic Behavior

Feeling safe is a basic human need involving self-protection and self-preservation. The patient needs to know if he or she is safe enough with the physician to expose real concerns, fears, and vulnerability.

If the patient does not feel safe, he or she will typically demonstrate behaviors such as fight, flight, or conservation-withdrawal. The alert clinician quickly reads nonverbal behavior and determines whether the patient across the nonverbal space feels safe at any one moment.

## SAFETY

Feelings of safety are reflected by body signals of engagement, relaxation, and a physically open stance. These include low general body tension and the relaxation of facial muscles, with arms and legs relaxed and uncrossed. The patient who feels safe shows more variety in both gestures and voice because a sense of safety gives rise to freer expression.

## FIGHT

The stance of the patient who demonstrates the fight response is most often a stance of engagement and of attack or retaliation as a defense against feeling unsafe. Typical nonverbal signals of a fighting feeling include a forward lean and jutting jaw, clenched fists, and a narrowing of the eyes with inner brows lowered and the mouth tense. The patient may also have a flushed face, flaring nostrils, increased voice volume, and deeper breathing.

## FLIGHT

Most of the nonverbal cues demonstrated by a patient experiencing the flight response involve disengagement and withdrawal. The patient leans away, pushes back in a chair, or turns the head down and away. The voice flees as the volume diminishes, the breath flees as it becomes shallower or is held, and facial color flees (blanching). Other typical cues include putting up physical barriers such as crossed arms and legs and averting the eyes or turning the head away.

## CONSERVATION-WITHDRAWAL

Conservation-withdrawal refers to the patient's reaction to feeling overwhelmed with excessive input and being unable to mount a defensive response. The patient reacts this way when he or she receives unacceptable news, suffers irretrievable loss, or becomes significantly depressed. The patient typically demonstrates a nonverbal pattern of disengagement and relative immobility or quiescence.[1] The patient's body appears slumped rather than relaxed. The patient has a sagging face and slack jaw and slow, shallow breathing. Usually the patient does not appear to use the arms and legs as protective barriers.

*It is important to read the overall pattern of nonverbal responses rather than to rely on any one sign. Nonverbal signals should not be oversimplified or overinterpreted.*

Patients sometimes cross their arms and legs because it is cold, because there are no arms to the chair, or as a convention of etiquette, yet their body may be quite relaxed and engaged and their voice melodious, indicating an overall sense of safety in the encounter. Although cultural differences in nonverbal behavior affect comfort levels with interpersonal distance and touch and often are expressed as a variety of gestures and eye gazes, nonverbal expressions of safety are universal. Issues of safety in the encounter show uniformly in the amount of the patient's body tension and autonomic responses and in facial expressions of anger, fear, sadness, surprise, disgust, and joy.[2] Mixed responses such as fight *and* flight are also frequent. A flushed face and loud voice combined with crossed arms or with a turn away from the physician can signal anger at the clinician or the situation and reluctance or fear of overtly expressing the anger.

# Nonverbal Skills

Helping the patient move from not feeling safe to feeling safe is crucial to creating a therapeutic milieu in which to gather high-quality information from the patient, assess readiness to change, and negotiate a treatment plan. The skilled physician can use specific nonverbal interventions to facilitate the interview process:

1. Develop nonverbal rapport.
2. Shape the space of the encounter.
3. Address mixed messages.

## DEVELOPING NONVERBAL RAPPORT

Rapport means "I am with you" and represents the *nonverbal structure of empathy*. Defined as "nonverbal synchrony between two persons," rapport behaviorally consists of two parts, *matching* and *leading*.

*Matching* is the process of moving as the other person moves in such a way as to acknowledge aspects of the other person's behavior as a reflection of his or her emotional state. The physician can use any aspect of the patient's behavior: facial expressions, voice volume and rate, body angulation, or gestures. As the physician begins to create synchrony with the patient, he or she begins to enter the patient's world. Patients unconsciously recognize this nonverbal engagement. Their *conscious* recognition is typically through a feeling of being understood by the physician, which can occur even before or without the transmission of verbal information.

The physician must be graceful, respectful, and cautious when matching. Small, gentle efforts at matching should be used; otherwise, the patient may feel manipulated and mocked rather than supported.

The beauty of enhancing rapport nonverbally is that it does not involve extra time, because it occurs simultaneously with the process of gathering verbal information from the patient. However, if rapport is ignored, the patient can feel unsupported if his or her posture and rhythms are not in synchrony with the physician's.[3] Without rapport, the interview will be inefficient and ineffective.

What might matching look like? The confident, compassionate, and skilled physician matches the patient's nonverbal behavior without conscious awareness of what he or she is actually doing. However, understanding the process of matching can increase the interviewer's efficiency and effectiveness. For example, the physician may match a withdrawn patient's posture by leaning forward, with his or her head slightly down and the shoulders drawn slightly inward (Figure 30-1). This facilitates the building of rapport and helps the patient feel understood.

A second example is that of a physician who notices rapport problems when facing a highly guarded patient whose arms and legs are crossed tightly and whose body is tense. The cautious physician begins the interaction with his or her own arms (and perhaps legs) loosely crossed, nonverbally acknowledging and accepting the patient's guardedness. The physician performs most of this matching without thinking about it. If the physician leans in too close to the patient, the patient may interpret this as an invasion of personal space and an intrusive response. Even if the physician's intent is to be inviting, the guarded patient may respond to this nonverbal intrusion by withdrawing into an even tighter presentation (Figure 30-2).

*Leading* refers to the use of the interactional synchrony that has been set up by matching. Patients who feel increased rapport are motivated to try to maintain that feeling; therefore a leading motion by one person of a pair may produce a reciprocal response by the other person. Leading invites the patient to move with the physician rather than to feel rushed or coerced into responding.

Leading can be a test of whether the interactional synchrony is present. This test consists of making a leading motion within the patient's awareness and observing to see if the patient unconsciously follows the lead. The physician's leading motion can be a behavioral shift, such as a movement, a gesture, or a change in voice or breathing. Synchrony is present if the patient follows these leading motions. The response to the lead does not have to be an exact duplication;

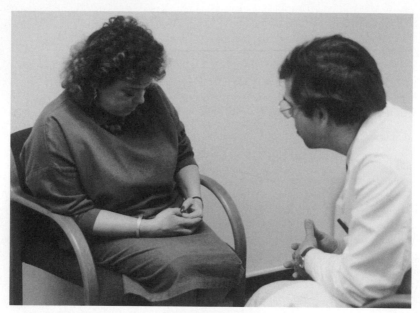

**Figure 30.1** Matching.

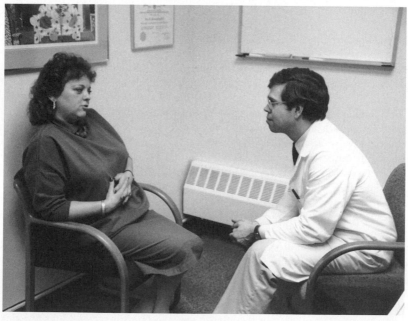

**Figure 30.2** Mismatching.

a movement or shift in the general direction of the lead is an adequate indicator. For example, the clinician may reach up and push his or her glasses higher up on the bridge of his nose; the patient may respond quite unknowingly by reaching up immediately afterward and touching his or her own chin.

If the interviewer leads the patient too fast or too dramatically, the rapport will be broken. If the interviewer becomes aware of this break, he or she can recover rapport quickly by returning to matching. Anything new or different that is introduced into the interaction can also be considered leading, either by the provider or the patient. For example, screening questions about social and sexual history and recommendations such as medication, procedures, and referrals all create something new in the interaction.

## SHAPING SPACE

Intentionally shaping the physical space of an encounter sets the form for reflective listening and the quality of the relationship. How the clinician arranges the spatial relationships in the room frequently parallels how he or she views the interpersonal relationship with the patient. Specific components of the space include the following:

1. The amount of interpersonal distance between people
2. The vertical height differences (such as lying, sitting, and standing)
3. The presence of physical barriers (such as a desk, chair sizes, charts, and bed rails)
4. The angles of facing each other (full face, shoulder-to-shoulder, or angles in between)

*Interpersonal distance* relates to territoriality. If the clinician is too close during an interview, the patient will feel that his or her space has been encroached on and may try to restore the proper distance (e.g., by looking away, crossing arms or legs to provide a "frontal barrier," flushing, or changing the topic to a less personal one) (Figure 30-3). If the clinician is too far away, true engagement with the patient may be discouraged and a sense of disinterest will be conveyed.

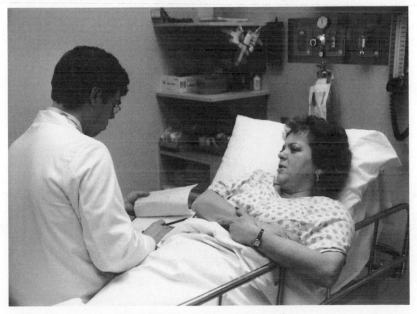

**Figure 30.3** Physician too close to patient.

*Vertical height differences* relate to power. At the start of an encounter, many patients already feel vulnerable and at a disadvantage relative to the clinician. The clinician can help minimize this feeling in the patient by being sensitive to vertical height differences that may exaggerate the patient's disadvantaged position and by being willing to shift his or her position to be at the same level as or below the patient (Figures 30-4 to 30-6).

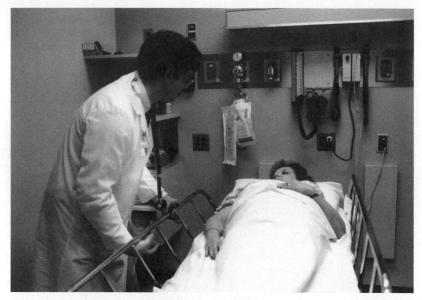

**Figure 30.4** Physician too high.

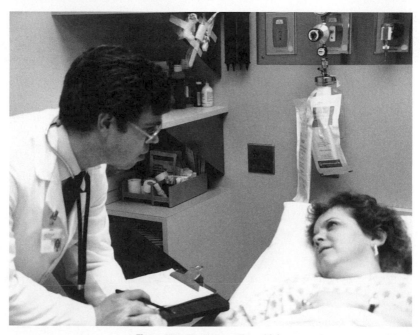

**Figure 30.5** Physician still too high.

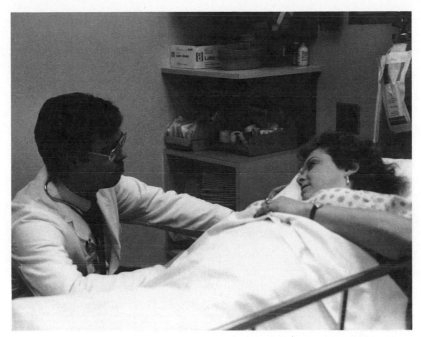

**Figure 30.6** Vertical height equal.

*Physical barriers* send the nonverbal message of protection or *keep your distance*, whether this message is intended or not. When the clinician recognizes barriers, he or she can go around them (such as with an office desk), move them out of the way (such as with charts or crossed arms and legs), or comment on them to soften their effect if they are fixed barriers in the space. It is also important to do *none* of these if it is clear that the barrier is offering the patient or the clinician a sense of protection or safety that is needed at the moment.

*Angles of facing* are an important component of the interview space. When the clinician and the patient disagree and are sitting directly opposite each other, their physical position can cause them to experience their differences as more of a confrontation than is actually intended. Once the clinician is aware that such a situation exists, he or she can defuse the confrontational aspects by shifting position to change the angle at which he or she is facing the patient. Just a slight angulation off a directly opposite position will begin to ease the tension. If the clinician moves even further into a side-by-side position with the patient, the configuration will more clearly support a collaborative effort between them, in spite of the disagreement (Figure 30-7).

## ADDRESSING MIXED MESSAGES

When there is incongruence between verbal and nonverbal modes in the patient's communication, the nonverbal message more truly reflects the patient's actual feelings and better predicts his or her behavior in response to the issue at hand. A mixed message means that the patient is not safe enough to tell the clinician how he or she feels. The patient may send a mixed message for a number of reasons: He or she may feel that disagreeing with or questioning the provider may threaten care, feelings may be too unacceptable to acknowledge, or the patient may feel overwhelmed or out of control.

A nonverbal "no" from the patient is signaled by a furrowed brow, slight shaking of the head, strained voice, breath holding, slightly increased pallor of the face, or tensing of the muscles. The

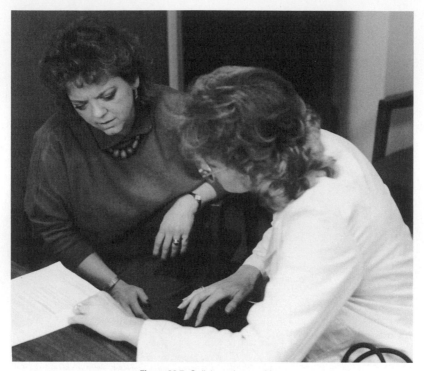

**Figure 30.7** Collaborative position.

clinician should understand that this "no," even if inconsistent with the patient's verbal response, indicates that the job is not finished. The incongruence must be addressed; if it is not, the patient will not comply with what he or she has agreed to do or will have difficulty or be frustrated in attempting to do it. The physician can also send mixed messages to the patient. If these messages are not acknowledged and discussed, they may send a powerful message about the physician not being trustworthy and will make the encounter feel less safe to the patient.

When dealing with a mixed message from a patient, the physician should try converting an incongruent "no" into a congruent "no" to make it accessible for discussion or to create enough safety for expressing the unexpressed feeling. The two major strategies for doing this are *direct acknowledgment* and *using the language of the third person.*

*Direct acknowledgment* openly reflects that the physician is receiving two messages from the patient:

> **PHYSICIAN:** *You know, even though you say you'll take the medication, I sense that you have some hesitation about it. If you have some concerns, let's talk about them.*

If the patient relaxes or nods in agreement, the physician has succeeded in transforming the incongruent "no" into a congruent "no" about which the patient can safely talk. If the patient withdraws or blanches further, the next strategy may be more useful.

*Using the language of the third person* avoids direct reflection to the patient. Instead of reflection, this method raises potential questions or fears through linguistic distancing to increase the feeling of safety. The physician can say something such as the following:

> **PHYSICIAN:** *I once worked with a patient in a situation similar to yours who was concerned about starting a new drug.*

While saying this, the physician would look carefully at the patient for the nonverbal parameters of agreement such as head nodding, deeper breathing, the return of facial color, or muscular relaxation. If the patient nonverbally agrees and remains silent, the physician can pursue potential concerns further by saying the following:

> **PHYSICIAN:** *This patient had several concerns. One was about possible side effects* (watching for nonverbal signs of agreement or disagreement), *and another one was the cost* (again looking for signs).

By this time, the patient usually feels a clear invitation to explore any of these concerns or offer additional ones.

# Application to the Three Function Approach

Each of the nonverbal skills allows the physician to monitor the process of the interaction with the patient in all three functions of the interview. The key is to track the patient's nonverbal output throughout, noticing whether the patient is feeling safe. The following are common strategies for applying the nonverbal skills as the interview progresses.

## FUNCTION ONE: BUILD THE RELATIONSHIP

The nonverbal skills set the form for beginning the relationship with the patient. Well before any words are exchanged, the patient feels the effect of how the interview space is set up. Is the clinician close or distant? Does the physician meet the patient eye-to-eye? Is the desk or chart between them, or is it shared as they work from a side-by-side position?

As the interview begins, the physician should begin matching the patient to join him or her nonverbally in the patient's world. Easy behaviors to match are body lean (left, right, or forward) and volume and rate of speech. If the patient is loud or speaking fast, it is enough for the physician to shift his or her own voice in the direction of more volume and rate without having to match the patient's voice exactly. (Remember, the patient should not be aware of the matching.)

Patients need to know if their provider can tolerate the full expression of their difficulties and suffering. If the physician detects incongruence in the affect the patient is showing versus whether the patient is verbally acknowledging the affect, the physician can use reflection or the language of the third person to help the patient express it more congruently. For example, the physician might say something such as the following:

> **PHYSICIAN:** *Mrs. Jones, you say everything is fine at home with your family, but you seem sad as you speak about them. Is there something else?*

## FUNCTION TWO: ASSESS AND UNDERSTAND THE PATIENT'S PROBLEMS

The patient who feels safe may give better information. Continuing to monitor nonverbal rapport and nonverbal output of whether the patient feels safe says "I care" in a way that allows the patient to offer spontaneously all the information and associations important to the reason he or she is seeking help. This also makes it easier for the patient to report potentially embarrassing information.

The physician is usually under time pressure and needs to organize the interview to stay on time. Often the physician needs to shift topics, bring closure to a part of the interview, or interrupt a patient who has become tangential in responding to a question. Being in rapport with the patient allows the physician to use the interruption more like a lead and makes it easier for the patient to experience the redirection without closing down on spontaneity or feeling cut off by the physician.

When the physician asks, "Is there anything else?" when developing the agenda at the beginning of the interview and at the end of history taking, he or she should ask this question without delivering a mixed message. Too often the physician accompanies this question by shaking his or her head "no" or pulling away and looking at the chart.

## FUNCTION THREE: COLLABORATE FOR MANAGEMENT

The third function of the interview represents a great opportunity for the use of nonverbal skills as the physician works to educate and motivate the patient and develop a treatment plan with him or her. Tension is frequently high between the physician and the patient when they deal with their differences about what is wrong with the patient and what would be helpful to his or her health. Too often the physician feels that the doctor's job is done after the straightforward delivery of diagnostic and treatment information. This simplistic approach can increase the suffering of many patients. Some patients may not understand what the diagnosis means, and others may face major obstacles (e.g., beliefs, emotions, limited financial and personal support, and family commitments) to complying with the physician's recommendations.

Using the nonverbal skills can be extremely important when the physician and patient are working through their differences. Any objection the patient has to the diagnosis or the treatment recommended by the physician may be signaled through the nonverbal channel.

The physician should be in nonverbal rapport with the patient when any diagnosis or treatment is offered. This state of "I am with you" allows the patient to take in the new information more readily and give it due consideration.

An astute physician can monitor the effect each utterance has on the patient by looking for safe or not-safe responses (many will be subtle). For instance, when the physician offers an explanation of the diagnosis and observes that the patient's body tension has gone up and the patient is holding his or her breath, the physician should stop and ask what significance (meaning) the explanation seems to have for the patient. The same would apply for any recommendations the physician makes regarding treatment, procedures, or referrals.

Asking whether the patient feels that he or she will be able to adhere to the treatment recommendations is an important part of the interview. If the patient says, "Sure, doc, whatever you say," while turning away and shaking his or her head "no" or if the patient flushes, the physician should know that more work is needed. The physician could move to reflection or to language of the third person to help bring the patient's objection openly to the negotiating table, to figure out a form or plan that might fit better with the patient's concerns and needs, or to offer more information and education.

## Conclusion

Combining both nonverbal and verbal modes of interaction when working with patients can be tremendously satisfying because it requires the physician to be more "real" in the professional role in which he or she is encountering patients. Many physicians fear that acknowledging the patient's affect and taking the time to work through the differences in a treatment plan will lead to burnout. The opposite is actually true. The level of honesty and support that is possible when the physician joins the patient more fully in the healing process makes time constraints and the lack of a cure for some presenting problems much easier to bear.

Beginning the nonverbal work slowly and in small segments is useful. The physician should spend time observing nonverbal behavior inside and outside the clinical arena. The physician should focus on one aspect at a time (e.g., shifts in voice tone, flushing or blanching of the face, and which members of a crowd stand in nonverbal synchrony and which do not). It is usually instructive for the physician to notice when he or she moves away or closer to the patient. The physician who takes the time and effort to practice observing nonverbal behaviors will notice that sensory acuity increases steadily and that a new world of discourse and communication opens up.

Additional references are available for further study on each of the aspects of nonverbal behavior.[4-7]

## References

1. Engel G, Schmale A: Conservation-withdrawal: a primary regulatory process for organismic homeostasis. In *Physiology, emotion & psychosomatic illness*, Amsterdam, 1972, Elsevier-Excerpta Medica.
2. Eckman P, Friesen W: *Unmasking the face*, New Jersey, 1975, Prentice-Hall.
3. Maurer RE, Tindall JH: Effect of postural congruence on client's perception of counselor empathy. *J Counsel Psychol* 30:158–163, 1983.
4. Carson C: Nonverbal communication in clinical encounters. *Cortland Forum* 129–134, 1990.
5. Milmoe S, et al: The doctor's voice: postdictor of successful referral of alcoholic patients. *J Abnormal Psychol* 72:78–84, 1967.
6. Harrigan JA, Rosenthal R: Nonverbal aspects of empathy and rapport in physician-patient interaction. In Blanck PD, et al: *Nonverbal communication in the clinical context*, University Park, Pa, 1986, Penn State University Press.
7. Carson C, Shorey J: "Nonverbal Communication," ABIM Self-Evaluation Module in Nonverbal Communication and Related Skills (CD ROM), 2002, 2010.

# CHAPTER 31

# Use of the Self in Medical Care

Dennis H. Novack

## OVERVIEW

This chapter discusses the importance of physician self-awareness, growth, and self-care to communication and the doctor-patient relationship as well as to the quality of life of the physician. Examples of problems and resolutions are presented and pathways to growth are described.

Students and practicing physicians who master the communication skills presented in this text will be more effective clinicians. Yet medicine is also an art. Physicians uniquely combine their knowledge, skills, attitudes, beliefs, and emotional responses to patients in the service of healing. Healing—making patients "whole" again—involves more than curing disease and is promoted by the human connections between physicians and patients. Much of the art of medicine involves physicians using their intuition and personal reactions to patients for their patients' benefit. Self-aware practitioners can be more "skillful artists" in applying their therapeutic interventions.[1]

Personal reactions to patients affect care in many ways. Patients will remind physicians of parents and friends; physicians may like or dislike certain patients based on these impressions. For a variety of reasons they may not fully understand, physicians feel attracted to some patients and repelled by others. Physicians balk at asking certain sensitive questions of any patients. The feelings patients evoke in physicians sometimes aid in understanding a patient's experience in illness and sometimes get in the way. Physicians communicate empathy to some and judge others, nonverbally expressing negative attitudes. They joke freely with some patients and are stiff and formal with others. Physicians may undermine their care of some patients by being too friendly and trying to do too much, or of other patients by expressing anger with the patients' behavior.

Physicians' personality characteristics, such as obsessiveness, perfectionism, impatience, idealism (or disorganization, patience, and many others), play major roles in their styles of interviewing, the quality and quantity of information they collect, and their abilities in relating to and healing their patients. Because physicians' personal qualities always affect their behaviors, how can they use self-knowledge in the service of patient care? The answers to this question are related to the physicians' activities in three domains: personal awareness, personal growth, and self-care. This chapter discusses these concepts and illustrates certain points with vignettes from my experiences or from those related by my colleagues in physician support groups.

## Physician Personal Awareness

Personal awareness is an essential foundation of practicing the art of medicine. By paying attention to the use of self in patient care, and by discussing a variety of issues with colleagues and friends in formal and informal sessions, students and physicians can continuously enhance their self-awareness. They can make it a practice to notice their feelings in relationship to patients and ask themselves how these feelings are affecting communication. If they hesitate to ask patients certain sensitive questions, they can ask themselves why. If these questions are important to their understanding of a patient's illness, they can find a way to ask such questions in spite of the difficulty (or ask their peers or teachers how they approach these questions). If physicians know that they need to perform a complete examination but want to cut corners, or if they find that they are avoiding interacting with certain patients, they can spend a few minutes reflecting on these feelings and analyzing their origins. For example, trainees in the clinical rotations often indefinitely "defer" breast and genital examinations because of embarrassment and therefore may miss critical findings. Many students feel uncomfortable sitting and talking, or simply listening, to patients who are dying, and they unwittingly cut short their time with these patients or avoid them entirely. This behavior can increase these patients' isolation and pain and rob the students of meaningful interactions.[2] Students can ask themselves what they need to do to overcome feelings and behaviors that may prevent them from offering patients optimal care. The following physician's experience demonstrates how this may be accomplished:

> *Early in my training, I had great difficulty relating to patients around issues of sexuality. I would not ask patients questions about their sex lives or sexual orientation, and I would not examine the breasts of young women patients. I thought it could be sexually stimulating to do so. Confused and ashamed of my feelings, I simply avoided the issues. One day, I admitted a 28-year-old woman with advanced breast cancer to my service. I was horrified to learn that she had a physical examination the year before by a physician who had not done a breast exam.*

> *Similarly, I avoided spending time with my dying patients. I was afraid of their pain. I was afraid they would ask me questions I could not answer. I hated feeling helpless and incompetent. I remember one patient who was dying of pancreatic cancer. As he grew more and more jaundiced, I spent less and less time with him, only staying to discuss the most pressing medical issues. One day, I passed his room on rounds and simply waved to him.*

> *I realized that my avoidance of these difficult and sensitive issues was compromising my medical care. I resolved to overcome my feelings, change my behaviors, talk to trusted colleagues about these issues, and attend conferences and courses that could help me improve my care of patients in these domains.*

Students and physicians can also increase self-awareness by reflecting on and discussing with others a variety of topics related to the effects of physicians' personal issues on medical care.[3] It is best for physicians to have these discussions with peers with whom they can be honest and who will be honest in their feedback. Although a full understanding of these issues may develop only over many years, it is worthwhile to begin addressing certain topics from the beginning of medical education. These topics include core beliefs, the effects of family of origin, gender, and culture on one's care of patients, attitudes toward vulnerability and death, love, attraction, and anger in patient care, and medical mistakes.

Students' core beliefs about themselves as future physicians will affect their patient care. If they believe that medicine is a calling, rather than just a job, they are more likely to be tolerant of the stresses of training and to feel more satisfaction with patient care. If they believe that their roles as physicians encompass attention to psychologic and social aspects of illness, they are more likely to explore these issues with their patients. If they have certain "dysfunctional beliefs,"[4] they are likely to experience more stress in training. These dysfunctional beliefs include strong convictions that any limitation in knowledge is a personal failing, that responsibility is to be borne alone by physicians, that altruistic devotion to work and denial of self is desirable, that keeping one's uncertainties and emotions to oneself is professional, and that perfection is an achievable goal.

A student's attitudes, feelings, and behaviors concerning such issues as intimacy, anger, and conflict resolution are often influenced by patterns in the student's family of origin. The student learns first from his or her family about the nature, benefits, and pitfalls of caring, the roles of the caregiver, the balance of giving and receiving, the communicative aspects of illness, and how to respond to distress. These dynamics are fundamentally important to the physician-patient relationship. Patients may remind physicians of family members with similar problems or behavioral patterns. An unrecognized identification of patients with family members can elicit feelings, including fears of harming the patient, inadequacy, loss of control, and addressing certain difficult topics.[5]

Attitudes about gender roles influence communication with those of the opposite sex. These attitudes, shaped by family and societal norms, can affect patient care and physicians' ability to accept feedback from colleagues of the opposite sex. Similarly, sociocultural norms influence physicians' attitudes toward acceptable illness behaviors, obesity, sexual behaviors, geriatric patients, "family values," the importance of work, and many other emotionally charged issues. Moreover, medical training probably constitutes a distinct culture that facilitates socialization into the profession. The culture of medical training and the culture of the individual hospital can affect physicians' medical care in many ways, and self-awareness can mitigate some of the negative effects. The following personal experience illustrates one way this can happen:

> *The stresses of training and shared misery bound our resident group together, but also fostered an "us against them" mentality toward our patients. We called patients "crocks" and "gomers," and every new admission was a "hit." We spent much more time talking about surgical service "dumps" and the intellectual challenges of certain difficult diagnoses than the suffering and humanity of our patients. One day, a senior resident told me with dismay that she had seen the obituary of one of our "dirtbag" alcoholic patients who had died a few days before. She was shocked to learn that he had been a man of great accomplishment and a real contributor to his community until alcoholism had brought him so low in his last years. She had the sudden realization that our name calling had been a way to avoid connecting certain patients' anxiety and despair with our own. She said to me, with emotion, "My God—something like this could happen to me someday." She vowed to never call a patient a "dirtbag" again.*

Physicians' love and caring for patients contribute to patients' experience of physician empathy and can be healing. However, this love and caring are beneficial only if framed within clear, mutually understood boundaries. Sometimes, perhaps because of unmet personal needs, physicians send unintended messages or become too emotionally invested in certain patients. For physicians in small towns, whose neighbors and friends become patients, and for physicians whose family members fall ill, setting clear boundaries may be especially difficult. Because physician-patient relationships often engender a special intimacy, there is the potential for powerful feelings of attraction to be aroused in both the caregiver and the patient. By understanding their emotional reactions to patients, physicians can set appropriate affective boundaries that allow them to be objective yet connect with patients.[6] The following personal report provides an example:

> *When I was an intern, I remember spending a great deal of time with a young woman diabetic patient who had taken an insulin overdose after an argument with her boyfriend. I offered her empathy and understanding, talked to her about the importance of getting counseling, and explored ways that she could improve her social situation and respond more appropriately to stress. The Sunday after her discharge, she paged me and asked if she could see me in the hospital lobby. Though I was having a busy on-call day, I met with her, listened to her latest problems with her boyfriend, and held her hand as she cried. She asked if we could have lunch the next day. I agreed.*
>
> *I realized that meeting her for lunch was inappropriate, but had felt that doctors needed to be available for their patients and should be able to "go the extra mile" to help them. I had been flattered that she found me so helpful and enjoyed feeling competent in my counseling skills, at a time when my feelings of competence were being otherwise challenged by the sick and dying patients on my service. I probably was also attracted to her, and enjoyed the intimacy of our conversations. I realized, though, that responding to my own needs was undermining my*

*ability to help her. At lunch the next day, I told her of my discomfort and discussed the need for setting appropriate professional boundaries if I were to continue caring for her in the outpatient clinic.*

Understanding your attitudes about anger can be helpful in patient care, because illness, suffering, and death often engender angry feelings for patients and their families. Reacting to patients' or their families' anger with anger can be destructive. For physicians to be effective in responding to anger, they need to know the kinds of patients that elicit an angry reaction in them, their own usual responses to their own anger and the anger of others (e.g., do they overreact, placate, blame others, suppress feelings, or become superreasonable?), and their underlying feelings when they become angry (e.g., feeling rejected, humiliated, or unworthy). Such self-awareness is the starting point for physicians learning to react to anger in a way that contributes to conflict resolution and communicates empathy.

Perhaps no other aspect of medical care demands more attention to self-awareness than the issue of medical mistakes. (See Chapter 28.) Being human, all physicians make mistakes. Sometimes these mistakes lead to patient morbidity and death. Physicians who use denial and blame others are not likely to learn from their mistakes. Those who accept responsibility for a mistake and discuss it are more likely to make constructive changes in their practices.[7] To learn from mistakes, physicians must examine the attitudes, feelings, and behaviors that led to the mistake, as demonstrated in the example of the following young attendings' experience:

*Preparing for my first rotation as an attending on the inpatient wards, I asked the most popular attending in the hospital if he had any advice. He said, "Well, I'll tell you my secret. Every evening, I go to the pharmacy and look up the orders on all patients admitted to my service. I find out the diagnoses and look up anything I don't know. The next morning, when the team presents the new patients to me, I'm never wrong. They think I'm brilliant!" I was appalled. Students and residents were having a hard enough time struggling to know enough without this attending presenting a false ideal of the all-knowing physician.*

*Still, the pressures of inpatient medicine can be intense, and most students and house staff had had the experience of feeling embarrassed on rounds that they did not know some piece of information. As an attending, I soon learned the device of turning questions back to the team when asked a question I could not answer. Usually someone on the team knew the answer, and I could add information that I did know about the subject. It seemed a benign form of deception, but I was caught one day, nevertheless.*

*I was attending on an inpatient service when my resident asked me about a patient we had admitted several days before. This middle-aged man had come to the hospital with a cellulitis and fever and was now improving on IV antibiotics. He had a benign medical history and otherwise normal examination results. The resident told me that one of the patient's blood cultures had come back with a positive result for* Enterobacter, *and he asked me if we should alter our antibiotic therapy. I was not sure of the answer, so I hedged. I asked him if the bacteria could have been a contaminant. He replied, "Well, I drew the blood from his groin, so it was a dirty stick. It was the only one of four cultures that was positive, so I guess it could have been." This was an excellent resident who in many respects had more up-to-date knowledge of inpatient medicine than I did, so I assumed he was right. In any case, the patient was improving by all measures, so we agreed that we would keep him on his current regimen. I did not know that* Enterobacter *was rarely a contaminant. Apparently the resident did not know it either but allowed that it was a possibility based on his assumption of my greater experience. Unfortunately, the patient developed a septic condition and died within a week.*

*In the end, it turned out that my guess had been correct—subsequent cultures confirmed that his sepsis was due to* Escherichia coli, *and the* Enterobacter *had actually been a contaminant. However, it would have been appropriate to start him on broadened antibiotic coverage, which would have been active against* E. coli *as well. The story of his final illness was complicated, and other factors played a role in the outcome. I'll never know if starting a new antibiotic would have saved him. Still, I was left with the knowledge and sadness that my need to be seen as a bright attending physician could have contributed to his death. I now freely admit my ignorance when asked questions that stump me, and I will not let misplaced feelings of pride affect my medical therapy.*

## Personal Growth

Attention to personal awareness is essential for personal growth. Attention to activities that promote personal awareness and growth can help physicians develop the maturity and sense of well-being that allow them to focus on patients' problems. Scholars have delineated the components of well-being:

1. *Self-acceptance*: respect and acceptance of one's past life and present identity
2. *Positive relations with others*: includes the ability to have warm, trusting, and intimate relationships
3. *Autonomy*: the ability to act from a stable sense of self and values without needing the approval of others to do what is right
4. *Environmental mastery*: the ability to advance in the world and change it creatively
5. *Sense of purpose in life*: gives one a sense of direction and meaning in work and personal life[8]

A *commitment to personal growth*, that one will continue to develop one's potential, grow and expand as a person, and grow in self-knowledge, helps physicians to develop the sense of well-being essential for optimal patient care.

Medical school can be a challenge to developing a sense of well-being. The press of work tempts students to ignore their relationships with lovers, family, and friends. Some superiors are abusive and some ask students to behave unethically. At times the rigors of clinical work lead students and trainees to feel overwhelmed, anxious, and demoralized. Students must create a context in their medical training for discussions with peers about the stresses of training, personal reactions to patient care, and personal development. Many medical schools have programs to enhance student well-being and personal growth. There are a wide variety of activities, including support, Balint, and literature in medicine discussion groups, that have proved valuable, as well as inclusion of personal reflection activities in behavioral science and clinical skills curricula.[3,9] If a school does not offer such programs, class representatives can work with deans to inaugurate them. Students who begin a pattern of attending to personal awareness, growth, and self-care during their first year of medical school can "immunize" themselves against, or at least prepare for, the stresses to come. Personal awareness and growth can be difficult and sometimes painful for students and physicians, but their rewards often are increased personal freedom and personal and professional satisfaction.

## Self-Care

Trainees and physicians cannot be maximally effective in their patient care unless they attend to self-care. Physicians who are unhappy and distracted by personal problems are less available emotionally for their patients and may take a pessimistic view of patients with similar problems. Some students and physicians who are unhappy in their personal relationships use patient care as a way of escape. Patients may be more appreciative than significant others. Patient care has unending potential for commitment, and an adage among house staff is "the longer you stay in the hospital, the longer you stay." Students and physicians who use patient care as an escape often find that their personal conflicts grow worse and that they are putting themselves at risk for burnout and other emotional problems.[10]

Physicians who are very good at prioritizing the tasks in a busy practice typically spend little time prioritizing the tasks needed to have a satisfying personal life. The ability to connect with patients often depends upon physicians' abilities to care for and respect themselves. This process involves active attention to balancing school or work and personal lives, building a support network, joining groups that meet regularly for mutual support, nourishing relationships with significant others, setting aside time for exercise, and actively maintaining some social life and outside interests. Self-care also involves heeding the warning signs of dysfunction. Mental health counselors can often be helpful when relationship problems begin interfering with work. Moreover, physicians have high rates of alcoholism, drug addiction, and depression, all of which can be effectively treated. Physicians who recognize these illnesses early and seek help for them can prevent serious future problems.

## Summary

Physicians are most effective when they can use their personal reactions to patients for their patients' benefit. Physicians are better able to experience and communicate the empathy that is crucial to patient care when they attend to and develop their abilities to use themselves as instruments of diagnosis and therapy. By focusing on personal awareness, growth, and self-care, they promote their development into physicians who are capable not only of curing disease, but of healing illness as well.

### References

1. Novack DH: Therapeutic aspects of the clinical encounter. *J Gen Intern Med* 2(5):346–355, 1987.
2. Novack DH: Adrienne. *Ann Intern Med* 119(5):424–425, 1993.
3. Novack DH, et al: Calibrating the physician: physician personal awareness and effective patient care. *JAMA* 278:502–509, 1997.
4. Martin AR: Stress in residency: a challenge to personal growth. *J Gen Intern Med* 1(4):252–257, 1986.
5. Marshall AA, Smith RC: Physicians' emotional reactions to patients: recognizing and managing countertransference. *Am J Gastroenterol* 90(1):4–8, 1995.
6. Farber ND, Novack DH, O'Brien M: Love, boundaries and the patient-physician relationship. *Arch Intern Med* 157:2291–2294, 1997.
7. Wu AW, et al: Do house officers learn from their mistakes? *JAMA* 265(16):2089–2094, 1991.
8. Ryff CD, Singer B: Psychological well-being: meaning, measurement, and implications for psychotherapy research. *Psychother Psychosom* 65:14–23, 1996.
9. Novack DH, et al: Personal awareness and professional growth: a proposed curriculum. *Med Encounter* 13(3):2–8, 1997.
10. Vaillant GE, Sobowale NC, McArthur C: Some psychologic vulnerabilities of physicians. *N Engl J Med* 287(8):372–375, 1972.

# CHAPTER 32

# Using Psychological Principles in the Medical Interview

## OVERVIEW

This chapter discusses core psychodynamic and cognitive-behavioral principles that can be usefully applied to communication and care in the general medical setting. Psychodynamic principles relevant to general medical practice include psychic conflict, mechanisms of defense, resistance, transference, countertransference, support, and interpretation. Cognitive-behavioral principles discussed of relevance to medical care are the primacy of cognition, arbitrary inference, and operant conditioning.

When and if patient encounters become difficult or problematic, this text recommends that the interviewer use higher-order interviewing skills to increase the efficiency and effectiveness of the interaction. This chapter focuses on examining the patient's psychology and behavior to provide patient-specific information that will guide the clinician toward more effective higher-order interventions. Numerous psychological theories and therapies have been applied to the medical setting, many with useful insights. Given the plethora of "schools" of psychology, however, this chapter focuses on the two most influential psychological models for pragmatic suggestions to improve troubled physician-patient relationships: (1) the psychodynamic model and (2) the cognitive-behavioral model. The interested reader is referred to other sources for information about other psychological approaches.[1]

The chapter first presents some basic principles of each of the models and then discusses a typical case to which these psychological principles can be applied.

## The Psychodynamic Model: Basic Concepts

### PSYCHIC CONFLICT

One of the key contributions of Freud and subsequent psychodynamic thinkers has been the elaboration of the concept of psychic conflict. This concept asserts that the mind is subjected to internal, generally unconscious conflicts between drives, feelings, or strivings (e.g., aggression, sex, independence, and dependence) and learned fears of the environmental or intrapsychic consequences of these feelings. The particular pattern and expression of basic feelings versus learned fears is infinitely variable from individual to individual.[2,3]

An example of psychic conflict is a great fear of anger. This fear may be innate or may be developed in the superego from the internalization of parental values. A fear of aggression also may be learned because of childhood experiences of being punished for anger. Furthermore, this fear may be conscious or entirely unconscious. To elaborate on this example, consider a patient who has to wait for 2 hours to see the doctor. He is probably angry. When the doctor finally arrives, the doctor might say something like this:

> **PHYSICIAN:** *I'm sorry to have kept you waiting so long. I'm sure this must be very frustrating for you.*

Some patients might be willing to express their irritation:

**PATIENT:** *It sure is! Your secretary promised me that you wouldn't be running behind today. I've already missed some important appointments. You know other people also have schedules. (Clearly irritated)*

Patients who are able to acknowledge their irritation (or anger) in this way do not demonstrate evidence of a conflict or fear of anger. However, another patient may become tense and monosyllabic and say, perhaps with a slightly sarcastic tone, something like the following:

**PATIENT:** *No, Doctor. I know you are very busy. I don't mind waiting. I'm not angry. What good would it do anyway to get angry?*

This patient's response demonstrates psychic conflict. Conflict can be conscious to the patient; that is, the patient may be aware of feeling uncomfortable about the admission of angry feelings. He may be aware that he is angry but may be afraid to admit this, thinking the doctor might not take good care of him if he admits he is angry.

Another patient, also consciously aware of angry feelings, may experience conflict because he thinks something like "anger is bad" or "nice people don't get angry." Therefore when asked about anger, the patient may be aware that he is angry, but because he thinks anger is a "bad" thing to feel, he may deny the feeling when asked about it by the doctor.

On the other hand, conflict can be unconscious; that is, the patient may not even be aware that he is "feeling" angry. Theoretically, the patient's superego or mechanisms of defense operate unconsciously to "protect" the patient from the conscious experience of anger, which would cause the patient to feel uncomfortable or anxious. Thus, when a patient tells the doctor that he is not angry, he may in fact be telling the truth as he believes it. However, the doctor may be aware of the other side of the patient's feelings because of other, perhaps more subtle cues, for example, incongruity between the patient's verbal statements and nonverbal rigidity or profuse or excessive denial.[4] This patient even changed the intensity of the word that the doctor assumed the patient might be feeling from "frustrated" to "angry." That is the patient didn't just deny that he was "frustrated." He actually denied that he was "angry." This increase in intensity probably indicates the strength of the feeling that is being denied.

Understanding the basic principles of psychic conflict can contribute to excellence in patient management. Many experienced physicians intuitively understand psychic conflict, but more sophisticated understanding can help physicians manage many complex and problematic situations.

## MECHANISMS OF DEFENSE

An understanding of the mechanisms of defense follows logically from an appreciation of psychic conflict. Mechanisms of defense are psychological maneuvers that operate to protect an individual from anxiety resulting from the expression or conscious awareness of inner drives, needs, or strivings.

In the example described previously, if the individual was unaware of his own anger, it was because of the mechanism of "denial" that operated to protect him from awareness of the anger that would have created internal anxiety.

There are many other mechanisms of defense in addition to denial. Some other defenses are *projection, reaction formation, isolation of affect, conversion,* and *sublimation.*[5] These other defense mechanisms can be illustrated by considering the patient described previously, who has been waiting for 2 hours. *Projection* refers to the mechanism through which the patient's own forbidden feeling or impulse is attributed (or "projected") onto others. For example:

**PHYSICIAN:** *I'm sorry to have kept you waiting so long.*

PATIENT: *I'm not angry, Doctor, but your nurse and I had a disagreement about my blood pressure, and I think she put my file at the bottom of your folders.*

*Reaction formation* refers to the reversal of the forbidden feeling into its opposite. Without ever reaching the level of conscious awareness, the patient may turn his anger into its opposite:

PHYSICIAN: *I'm sorry to have kept you waiting so long.*

PATIENT: *That's okay. I'm just grateful you have time for me at all.*

*Isolation of affect* does not deny the presence of the feeling itself, but instead enables the patient to dissociate himself from the emotions associated with the usual expression of the feeling. For example:

PHYSICIAN: *I'm sorry to have kept you waiting so long.*

PATIENT: *It's okay, I guess, but I've gotten very nervous waiting so long.* (Patient demonstrates no visible or verbal signs of affective arousal.)

*Conversion* refers to the displacement of the feeling onto a physical or body part. For example:

PHYSICIAN: *I'm sorry to have kept you waiting so long.*

PATIENT: *That's okay, but my stomach pain has been getting worse and worse. I thought you would never come.*

*Sublimation* is a higher-level, more "mature" defense because it effectively turns the energy from conflictual feelings into productive activity. For example:

PHYSICIAN: *I'm sorry I kept you waiting so long.*

PATIENT: *It was a long time, but I was able to get some work done.*

Physicians who understand the principles of defense mechanisms and can recognize common patterns are able to provide more psychologically informed care to their patients. Reading can help physicians learn these patterns, but in general the physician needs a specialized learning environment with clinical supervision to master the principles and integrate them into active practice.[6]

Individualized long-term supervision by an expert clinician of the care for specific patients is one way to learn how defense mechanisms operate in longitudinal patient relationships. Balint groups, named after the psychiatrist Michael Balint, is another mechanism for the development of such skills. In Balint groups, a group of practicing physicians meets regularly (e.g., every week or every month) with an expert to review the care for complex patients.[7] Finally, clinicians can attend brief (1-day), more extensive (weekly), or more longitudinal training programs (one half day every week) to attain additional skills.

## RESISTANCE AND MANAGEMENT OF RESISTANCE

Resistance refers to the tenacity with which patients tend to cling to their defenses. Defenses usually operate unconsciously to protect patients from anxiety. Thus, when a defense is challenged, the patient usually resists the uncovering of a defense.

For example, a patient has been kept waiting and has already denied that he is angry. The physician may continue to insist that the patient appears angry. If confronted directly, the patient may become even more insistent that he is not angry and say something like the following:

PHYSICIAN: *I'm sorry to have kept you waiting so long.*

PATIENT: *I'm not angry, Doctor, but your nurse and I had a disagreement about my blood pressure, and I think she put my file at the bottom of your folders.*

PHYSICIAN: *Well, if you think my nurse has interfered with your care, I can certainly understand why you might feel angry about that.*

PATIENT: *I told you I am* not *angry!*

In general, physicians need to respect a patient's resistance and not challenge it unless the mechanism of defense leads the patient to maladaptive behavior. To give an example: The patient who has denied his anger may be so tense, irritable, and uncooperative that the physician finds working with him difficult.

The management of resistance usually involves some attempt to draw attention to the resistance to facilitate the expression of the underlying feeling. The technical words used to describe these interventions are *confrontation* and *interpretation*. Some physicians intuitively use confrontation and interpretation quite effectively, but attaining a high degree of skill in the management of resistance usually requires dedicated and systematic study with clinical supervision.

*Confrontation* is an unfortunate choice of words because it implies some degree of conflict between the caregiver and the patient. In fact, the skillful use of confrontation describes the attempt to bring an emotional issue to the awareness of the patient in such a way as to cause as little embarrassment as possible and in a manner that can maximize the chances of the patient being able to accept the awareness of the emotion. Acceptance, gentleness, thoughtfulness, and the willingness to be wrong are all characteristics that can help a physician confront a patient with maladaptive resistance. In the case described previously, the physician might comment as follows:

**PHYSICIAN:** *Okay. I guess I was wrong about saying you might be angry. All I meant to say was that I could understand how you might feel a little bothered if you think my nurse had manipulated my files to keep you waiting so long.*

**PATIENT:** *Well, of course I feel bothered. Wouldn't you be?*

**PHYSICIAN:** *I can't be exactly sure how I would feel, but the important thing now is how I can be of help to you.*

*Interpretation* refers to the uncovering of the basic conflict itself. For example, the physician who knows this patient well might try to help him understand and "work through" this conflict about anger. This is the core process in psychodynamic psychotherapy[8] and is generally not a part of the practice of most general physicians. Nevertheless, many physicians are successful in offering patients intuitive interpretations that help them attain genuine insight or growth. However, interpretation in the service of insight and subsequent working through of psychic conflicts are generally best left to formal psychotherapy or only attempted with close supervision.

## SUPPORT

At first glance the concept of support appears simple. Examined more deeply, however, being supportive to patients can become quite complex. Trying to be nice, sensitive, or warm is part of good medical care and as such is straightforward.

When patients demonstrate resistance, however, or act in any maladaptive manner, the question of support becomes more problematic. In the patient who manifests a clear defense against anxiety or resistance, a supportive intervention becomes one that, technically, supports the patient's defense. For example, if the patient insists that he is not angry, the doctor supports this defense by making a comment such as:

**PHYSICIAN:** *Okay. I guess I was wrong about what I thought was anger on your part.*

Werman[9] has written an important book describing the complexity of supportive interventions. According to Werman, support may be difficult because the physician can be most supportive only when he or she understands the prominent defenses of the patient. Thus it is not always in the patient's best interest for the physician to support defenses. For example, the patient who denies serious illness may not take medications regularly. Similarly, the patient with hypertension may say, "I feel too healthy to have a stroke." The physician who supports such a patient will make the patient feel less anxious in the short run, but at the cost of life-threatening and maladaptive behavior on the patient's part. Confrontation or interpretation, on the other hand, increases patient anxiety in the short run but may lead to more adaptive behavior in the long run.

Thus the decision to emphasize support, which may decrease anxiety in the short run, or emphasize confrontation and interpretation, which generally increases anxiety, can be difficult. Inappropriate support may at times be dangerous or reinforce maladaptive behavior. On the other hand, the effort to confront patients' defenses generally produces anxiety for the patient and usually for the physician as well. Therefore clearheaded understanding of the difference between support and uncovering can help physicians learn to appreciate these important differences and make better decisions about intervention.

## TRANSFERENCE

The concept of *transference* refers to the tendency of patients to displace onto the physician feelings that appropriately belong to other important people.[10] This is a phenomenon that occurs in all relationships but becomes pronounced in physician-patient relationships because the physician often becomes such an important person with accompanying symbolic power to the patient.

For purposes of illustration, consider again the patient who has been kept waiting for 2 hours to see the doctor. Perhaps this is a patient who feels slighted by many of the important people in his life. His father always kept him waiting and his wife does the same. It is quite likely that the patient will be especially hurt and angry at the physician who keeps him waiting because he "transfers" the anger and hurt from his personal life to the physician who acts in similar ways or who acts in ways to provoke these painful memories. The physician may be the unwitting victim of these "surplus" emotions.

At times, physicians may be told directly about transference feelings. A patient might say something like this:

> PATIENT: *You're just like everyone else. Everything else is more important than I am. My father always kept me waiting. My wife does the same. I'm used to it, doctor. Don't worry.*

More commonly, the patient is unaware of transference feelings. The patient assumes these feelings are entirely normal (they are what he or she is used to), and the patient is unaware that the feelings gain a special charge because of his or her emotional history. However, the physician who understands transference will appreciate these problems when noticing the presence of the patient's surplus feelings that do not seem appropriate to the clinical situation.

Just being aware of the phenomenon of transference can help physicians cope with difficult situations. However, using this understanding in work with patients can be complex, and physicians interested in making these skills a part of their routine practice generally find the need to obtain further training.

## COUNTERTRANSFERENCE

Countertransference refers to the feelings caregivers develop in response to patients. These feelings emanate from the caregiver's personal life experiences. Just as patients have transference feelings to doctors, physicians experience countertransference to patients. At times, patients remind physicians of important people in their own lives. For example, an irritable geriatric patient may remind a physician of his or her own troubled relationship with a parent, or a nonadherent adolescent may provoke feelings similar to the feelings a physician has toward his or her own child.

The physician's care of patients may become compromised or unreasonably emotional because of these countertransference feelings. This happens frequently in the routine practice of medicine.

It is unavoidable. However, the physician who is aware of the principles of countertransference may realize the inappropriateness of his or her feelings and gain better emotional control for the benefit of the physician and the patient as well.[11]

Physicians may have feelings toward patients that are not just countertransference. Dying patients may provoke sympathy, sadness, or fear, and angry patients may induce anger or frustration, among other feelings. Personal awareness and acceptance of feelings toward patients help the physician cope with the patient and with his or her own attitudes toward practicing medicine (see Chapter 31).

## Cognitive-Behavioral Model: Basic Concepts

### PRIMACY OF COGNITION

The cognitive-behavioral model of psychological functioning emphasizes the profound impact of cognitive processes on subsequent behavior and feelings. According to this theory, what we think about something (even though we may not be aware of the thought at the time) determines what we feel about it and what we do. Developed by Aaron Beck and others,[12] this approach examines the effect of deeply ingrained maladaptive or dysfunctional thought processes on a patient's overall functioning. With this approach in mind, cognitive-behavioral interventions focus on interrupting and changing these dysfunctional thought patterns.

According to cognitive models (as is the case with psychodynamic models), our early experiences are powerful in shaping our future reactions. The cognitive view is that in our early years we acquire a set of core assumptions or schemas about the meaning of experiences, and that these assumptions shape the way we think about events for the rest of our lives. These core assumptions influence our initial thought when an event occurs and in turn influence our feelings and behaviors. The first thought is often rapid, automatic, and transient and may at first be difficult to identify. Beck and others have identified several common categories of dysfunctional automatic thoughts that can lead to inappropriate feelings and behaviors. Arbitrary inference (described in the following) is one such category that has the potential to lead to significant subsequent dysfunction.

### ARBITRARY INFERENCE

Arbitrary inference refers to patterns of automatic, but mistaken, conclusions patients make based on certain types of environmental input.

To exemplify the process of arbitrary inference, consider again the patient whom the doctor kept waiting for 2 hours. Imagine more background information on this patient. He was the oldest of a family of five and felt (bitterly) that his parents devoted most of their time and attention to his younger siblings. This left him automatically thinking, "I am less important than the others," whenever someone in authority paid less attention to him than he thought he deserved. In response to the physician's apology for being late, this patient might say resentfully:

> PATIENT: *That's okay, doctor. I'm used to waiting for others.*

The physician who recognizes this maladaptive pattern of thinking may be able help the patient reality test by pointing out something such as the following:

> PHYSICIAN: *I realize the fact that I kept you waiting may feel like I have done something personal to you. Please be reassured that the unexpected emergency I had to attend to was unavoidable, and that everyone else in the office has also been kept waiting. You now have my undivided attention.*

## OPERANT CONDITIONING

The contribution of behavioral principles to cognitive-behavioral psychology lies in understanding the importance of stimuli from the environment in shaping subsequent behavior. Operant conditioning theory focuses on understanding the origins of behavior (and feelings) through understanding the contingencies (reinforcement and punishment) that follow predictably from certain behaviors.[13,14] According to this view, behavior and related affects can be changed by consistently changing these contingencies. Reinforcement of desired behaviors is considerably more effective in producing lasting behavior change than punishment of undesirable behaviors.

Consider the angry patient who has been kept waiting. Perhaps he has been physically punished in early life for expressing any anger. Thus he has learned never to express anger. In response to the physician's statement about being late, the patient might respond in a sullen manner, with a remark such as the following:

PATIENT: *That's okay, doctor. I know you are very busy.*

The physician who can recognize this unexpressed anger can often facilitate rapport by changing the contingency—accepting, and not punishing, the expression of irritation.

PHYSICIAN: *I appreciate your understanding. However, many people do feel irritated when their doctors keep them waiting. So, again, I am sorry to have kept you waiting and will now listen carefully to your problems.*

## George: A Case Study Integrating Psychodynamic and Cognitive-Behavioral Interventions

Can the primary care physician attain sufficient understanding of psychodynamic and cognitive-behavioral approaches to apply them usefully in clinical practice? Although these approaches represent complex theoretical systems that require years of focused study and practice to master, the central principles elaborated above can be used by physicians interested in applying these concepts to routine care. Of course, physicians interested in developing more proficient skills in this domain must dedicate time and effort to study and practice, and receive feedback from peers and experts.

The common problem of lower back pain, described in the following example, illustrates ways in which the busy physician may begin to apply both psychodynamic and cognitive-behavioral insights to improve the quality and outcome of the clinical encounter.

The medical history is presented from the patient's point of view.

*I am a 52-year-old, highly skilled automobile mechanic. I have been a good husband, father, and provider for my wife and children for 30 years. I am seeing Dr. Smith about lower back pain. It started several years ago from lifting at work and now is much worse. I haven't been able to work for several weeks and haven't been much use at home either. I don't like being useless and dependent on my wife.*

*I was very pleased with Dr. Smith at first. He diagnosed my problem as "back strain" and said I would get better soon. He put me on analgesics and bed rest and told me to lose 30 pounds.*

*Unfortunately, my pain grew progressively worse and I was less and less pleased with Dr. Smith and each appointment that followed. The CT scan did not show "anything" to explain the pain, and I insisted on an MRI. Dr. Smith reluctantly agreed to the MRI and seemed to say, "I told you so" when the MRI failed to show any other significant problem.*

*I started to get the impression that the whole thing was being blamed on me and my weight. Each time the back got worse I had to push for an urgent appointment for stronger pain medication. I got the impression that Dr. Smith wasn't happy about all this and was starting to see me as a burden and a failure. I was already pretty fed up about the back trouble, and his attitude made me feel worse.*

*Then Dr. Smith started asking questions about my personal life and my sleep pattern and whether I was depressed. I said that I was no more depressed than anyone else would be in the circumstances. He finally said that I was suffering from "clinical depression."*

*Now it was clear to me that he saw me as a mental case and thought my back pain was all in my head. I didn't like what he said, but I didn't get angry. I just said that I wanted to see a back expert because I no longer trusted his opinion. I walked out and never returned.*

So what went wrong? There are no bad guys in this common story. George's physician was probably polite, conscientious, and sensible, as well as aware of relevant psychiatric and physical diagnoses. George himself represents a common type of patient. As the patient continued to suffer, the relationship deteriorated into an unsatisfactory one for patient and physician. The core psychodynamic and cognitive-behavioral principles delineated in the preceding section can provide guidance regarding the use of higher-order but pragmatic interventions for general medical practice.

## PSYCHODYNAMIC UNDERSTANDING AND INTERVENTIONS

Psychodynamic principles suggest that conflicts about anger and dependency led to significant psychic anxiety. Regardless of the extent of objective findings to explain his back pain, George's subjective pain and dysfunction understandably led to psychic conflict and the use of defense mechanisms and resistance to deal with the conflicts.

Being out of work and dependent led to feelings of anxiety and low self-esteem. George was angry about his situation and the physician's inability to help. Rather than express his anger or gracefully accept his dependency, George felt more anxiety, which probably exacerbated his back pain. He used the defense of denial ("I didn't get angry. I just walked out.") to help him deal with the anxiety. George also probably had some element of conversion (somatization) to help him cope with the stress of back pain, dependency, anger, and whatever other stresses were going on in his life.

George's comments about the physician's view of him as a burden and a failure probably reflected some elements of transference to previously important authority figures in his life (perhaps his father?) who disapproved of him if he did not perform "adequately." Furthermore, if Dr. Smith was indeed annoyed, Dr. Smith, himself, may have had some countertransference feelings about dependent individuals reaping undeserved benefits (of unemployment or analgesics).

What could the psychodynamically informed physician do to improve the problem encounter? From a dynamic point of view, interventions that technically were considered supportive were not working with this patient. Interventions that recognized, accepted, and supported the pain led to increased pain, increased analgesic use, and increased dependency.

Psychodynamically, the most important first principle here is to address the emotional distress and empathize with the patient's predicament. Direct questions from the patient about the underlying cause, the pain, and further medical tests should be temporarily postponed until after the physician addresses the patient's emotional turmoil.

By the time the patient starts to exit the relationship, it may be too late for psychodynamically informed interventions. However, appropriate interventions to help prevent rupture of the relationship would start with basic rapport-building skills (reflection, legitimation, partnership, support, and respect) and then address the defenses and the underlying emotional turmoil and conflicts:

PATIENT: *Doc, I'm not getting anywhere with you on this. I'm leaving. I need a specialist.*

**PHYSICIAN:** *Mr. Jones, I will be happy to work with you (partnership) regarding a referral if that is what you want. Before you walk out, I want to make sure you know that I understand how frustrating this has been for you.* (**reflection**)

*Many people would feel the same way.* (**legitimation**)

*If you want to stay a few more moments, I will do what I can to help you with this and work with you to develop a plan.* (**support and partnership**)

*I also want you to know that I am impressed by how well you are coping with a terribly difficult situation. You are in great pain, out of work, and feeling lousy—and without any real answers as yet.* (**respect**)

*I realize it must be terribly hard for you to feel so dependent on others. I am sure it also makes you angry.* (**interpretation of conflicts about dependency and anger and acceptance of patient's feelings**)

Most patients respond positively to this type of empathic intervention. Patients often then begin talking about their conflicts and feelings. If the physician can listen empathically, sufficient rapport may develop to construct a mutually acceptable management plan.

## COGNITIVE-BEHAVIORAL UNDERSTANDING AND INTERVENTIONS

Cognitive-behavioral understandings and interventions most productively coincide with and supplement psychodynamic ones. George demonstrates multiple examples of dysfunctional cognitions with faulty arbitrary inferences. He probably believes the following:

- If I don't support my family, I am not a man.
- If I am not a man, I am not worthwhile.
- Only weak people get depressed.
- If the doctor thinks I am depressed, he must think I am weak.

The physician who understands these arbitrary inferences and their effect on George can make effective interventions to strengthen the physician-patient relationship and improve George's coping mechanisms. For example:

**PHYSICIAN:** *I realize it is very upsetting to be out of work. I am sure it makes you feel bad. However, it really takes a lot of strength and courage to cope with being sick. Only the strongest of men are able to handle this kind of disability. I am sure your wife and children accept your temporary disability. I truly believe you will be back to work in a short period of time.*

*With respect to your thoughts about depression, you are quite right that most people in this situation get very distressed. It is not a sign of weakness. It is very understandable. However, if you let me treat your depression in addition to your back pain, I think I can help you return to better functioning faster.*

Cognitive-behavioral psychology also suggests using operant conditioning models to help shape behavior. The most effective contingencies for altering behavior involve rewards for desirable behavior rather than punishments for undesirable behavior. The physician should understand how to use praise from himself or herself as a source of positive reinforcement for the patient. Small, reachable goals should be established, and considerable praise should be given when these goals are met. The physician should allow the patient to set the goals. For example:

**PHYSICIAN:** *Mr. Jones, please give me an idea about how much pain medicine you are willing to stick to this week.*

or

**PHYSICIAN:** *How much exercise are you willing to commit to?*

or

    **PHYSICIAN:** *What type of diet are you willing to follow this week?*

Alternatively, this is an ideal situation in which to use skills of Brief Action Planning discussed in Chapter 5; for example:

    **PHYSICIAN:** *Is there anything you'd like to do in the next week or two that might be helpful for your back pain?* (If the patient can not think of any action plans, the physician can propose a behavioral menu of options.)

If the patient and the physician together can develop some mutually agreed-upon goals that are realistic for this patient at this time, the physician's praise for achievement of the goals will reinforce the desired behavior. Reinforcement from other sources, such as the family and the employer, is also useful in difficult situations.

## Conclusion

This chapter reviews ways for physicians to use the contributions of psychodynamic and cognitive-behavioral psychology to achieve more efficient and effective communication in difficult patient encounters. Although these concepts are complex and require considerable training and expertise to master thoroughly, elements of the core concepts can be usefully applied by interested clinicians in the routine practice of medical care.

## Summary

This chapter discusses core psychodynamic and cognitive-behavioral principles that can be usefully applied to communication and care in the general medical setting. Psychodynamic principles relevant to general medical practice include psychic conflict, mechanisms of defense, resistance, transference, countertransference, support, and interpretation. Cognitive-behavioral principles discussed of relevance to medical care are the primacy of cognition, arbitrary inference, and operant conditioning.

### References

1. Novack DH: Therapeutic aspects of the clinical encounter. *J Gen Intern Med* 2:347-354, 1987.
2. Cooper AM, Frances AJ, Sack M: The psychodynamic model. In Cavenar JO, Jr, editor: *Psychiatry, vol 1,* Philadelphia, 1989, JB Lippincott.
3. Hine FR: *Introduction to psychodynamics: a conflict-adaptational approach,* Durham, N.C., 1971, Duke University Press.
4. Hall JA: Affective and nonverbal aspects of the medical visit. In Lipkin M, Jr, Putnam S, Lazare A, editors: *The medical interview: clinical care, education, and research,* New York, 1995, Springer-Verlag.
5. Freud A: The ego and the mechanisms of defense. In Freud A, editor: *The notes of the writings of Anna Freud, vol 2,* New York, 1966, International Universities Press.
6. Levy ST: *Principles of interpretation,* New York, 1984, Jason Aronson.
7. Balint M: *The doctor, his patient, and the illness,* New York, 1976, International Universities Press.
8. Brenner C: *An elementary textbook of psychoanalysis,* New York, 1955, International Universities Press.
9. Werman D: *The practice of supportive psychotherapy,* New York, 1984, Brunner/Mazel.
10. Nemiah J: *Foundations of psychopathology,* New York, 1961, Oxford University Press.
11. Smith R: Use and management of physician's feelings during the interview. In Lipkin M Jr, Putnam S, Lazare A, editors: *The medical interview: clinical care, education, and research,* New York, 1995, Springer-Verlag.
12. Beck AT, Haaga DA: The future of cognitive therapy. *Psychotherapy* 29:34, 1992.
13. Dorsett PG: Behavioral and social learning psychology. In Stoudemire A, editor: *Human behavior: an introduction for medical students,* Philadelphia, 1998, JB Lippincott.
14. Skinner BF: *About behaviorism,* New York, 1974, Vintage Books.

# CHAPTER 33

# Integrating Structure and Function: Diagnostic Reasoning, Clinical Inference, Communication Flexibility, and Rules

Steven Cole

## OVERVIEW

This final chapter discusses several higher-order communication skills that I applied or developed and found useful in my own clinical work over almost 40 years of working with patients. Some were derived from well-known concepts in the medical literature, some arose from conversations with Julian Bird, but most of those discussed in this chapter emerged organically from the interpersonal clinical chemistry between me and my patients. They all relate to the integration of structure and function and fall within four broad concepts: diagnostic reasoning; clinical inference; communication flexibility; and "rules" of interviewing.

Six types of clinical flexibility represent higher-order skills of expert interviewers: flexibility of (1) language, (2) style, (3) control, (4) advice, (5) agenda, and (6) function. And six "rules" can help guide both beginning as well as expert communication: (1) observe your patient, (2) observe yourself, (3) when in doubt, check, (4) when the patient demonstrates an emotion, respond to it, (5) don't answer every question immediately, and (6) understand that patients are usually forgiving of mistakes in the interview.

This text focuses on the three basic functions of the medical interview with concrete, pragmatic guidelines to improve the efficiency and effectiveness of communication with patients. However, the physician-patient encounter is an extraordinarily subtle, rich, and complex phenomenon, about which even the most experienced physicians and most knowledgeable researchers continue to seek further growth. Thus, although mastery of the basic and advanced skills presented in this text yields clear competence, attainment of clinical excellence requires supplementation of these skills with a wide variety of even higher-order, subtle, as yet undefined processes and related skills.

For the purposes of this book, both basic and selected advanced skills are implemented using concrete, observable behaviors. The basic and selected advanced skills presented in this text are relatively straightforward. In fact, this book has been devoted to the presentation and illustration of operational definitions of these 30 behaviorally grounded skills.

Higher-order skills reflect more complex behaviors that do not lend themselves so readily to operational definitions. Furthermore, higher-order skills reflect behaviors emanating from complex internal processes that may be even more difficult to describe than the skills themselves.

One reason these internal processes remain so undefined is that they often operate unconsciously or only within the partial awareness of the clinician. At times it may be difficult to separate these internal processes from their corresponding outward behavior and skills.

Much of the knowledge of the higher-order skills remains tacit or personal, as described by the philosopher of science Michael Polanyi.[1] As such, they are considerably more difficult to teach and learn. On the other hand, just because these skills are tacit and difficult to teach and learn, physicians should not relegate them to the domain of the intuitive and unteachable.

The task of making the tacit more explicit and setting forth the principles of higher-order functioning is well worth the effort. When learners can understand and articulate these principles, they can begin to use them as templates to become more effective self-observers and communicators.

This concluding chapter addresses some of the more complex, subtle, and important, yet less understood, of the higher-order skills: the ability to integrate structure and function in the medical interview.

The skillful physician operates at all times within an overlapping matrix of structural and functional objectives. Regardless of whatever element of data (structure) the physician may be concerned with obtaining at any one moment of the interview, he or she simultaneously must also attend and respond appropriately to relevant input regarding the rapport (Function One), understanding (Function Two), and collaborative management (Function Three) domains of the interview process. For example, a question about cardiac history in the family may induce anxiety about a parent's heart attack (Function One) or a question about exercise (Functions Two and Three). Conversely, when offering an educational message about smoking, the physician may encounter new information concerning cardiac symptoms (Function Two) about which he or she had been unaware or new anxieties over sexuality (Function One).

This chapter describes several processes and principles that can aid physicians in accomplishing integrative goals efficiently and effectively. Understanding and using these processes and principles can help physicians achieve proficiency in integrative communication.

# Higher-Order Processes and Skills

## CLINICAL REASONING

The study of medical expertise and of the data-gathering approaches of experienced physicians indicates that expert interviews do not necessarily proceed in a completely open-ended manner of unbiased data gathering. That is, the expert medical interviewer does not act as a "blank slate," collecting neutral data for the subsequent development of diagnostic possibilities. From the first moments of meeting patients, experts generate hypotheses and explanatory models. As described by Elstein and colleagues,[2] Kassirer,[3] and Norman,[4] expert clinicians search for meaning in the patient's diverse complaints by comparing the patient's story with their own cognitive (internal) templates of known illness patterns. This search for meaning by the physician is paralleled by the patient's own search for a satisfactory explanatory model for his or her problem(s).[5]

The search for patterns leads the expert clinician to generate a limited number of explanatory hypotheses, perhaps four or five at most, very early in the interview process. This hypothesis generation reflects the highest degree of clinical expertise and has become the subject of considerable research.[6] At present, however, little is known about the exact nature of this process, and even less is known about how to teach it. After generating diagnostic hypotheses, the expert clinician pursues these possibilities by systematic questioning to test and refine hypotheses and generate new hypotheses, if necessary.

Expertise in clinical reasoning (hypothesis generation and testing) and related processes of decision analysis (to help guide physicians' choices in interviewing and investigation) are important in the efficient and effective practice of clinical medicine. Physicians' understanding and mastery of these principles will become even more important as the practice of medicine becomes increasingly complex. Nurcombe and Gallagher[7] describe a model of medical student education in clinical reasoning that could be an example for other programs.

The mastery of clinical reasoning can be added to the basic skills described in this text. Clinical reasoning enriches basic skills—it does not supplant them. Basic data-gathering skills such as open-ended questioning, facilitation, and checking remain just as important within more sophisticated models of clinical reasoning. Furthermore, the importance of the basic skills for rapport development and education and motivation does not change within a more advanced communications approach to diagnostic reasoning.

## CLINICAL INFERENCE AND FLEXIBILITY

Of all the skills addressed in this text, clinical inference and flexibility are the two most important. Clinical inference refers to the ability to observe the patient and infer what he or she is experiencing (e.g., thoughts, feelings, and concerns). There is limited information on how this clinical intuition can be learned or taught. Understanding nonverbal cues (see Chapter 30) is one element, but other factors are also important. To aid inference clinicians express empathy, moving from simple reflections of surface emotions (e.g., "I can see you feel sad") to more complex inferential reflections (e.g., "It sounds to me like you're also feeling a bit guilty about the impact the drinking is having on your family life.") Once clinicians start making inferences (hunches) about patient's thoughts, feelings, and concerns, however, they also run risks of being wrong and irritating patients and impairing rapport and trust. Generally speaking, patients understand that everyone is wrong some of the time and if the inference is presented in a humble, exploratory manner (not arrogantly), patients will forgive the mistake and the error will generally help move the discussion in a direction that more closely fits the clinical reality for the patient. On the other hand, if the inference (complex reflection) is presented in an arrogant manner or a manner *perceived* as arrogant or authoritarian by the patient, rapport may be seriously damaged. Clinical experience is invaluable for developing these inferential abilities as well as the sense of appropriate timing for presentation; training and coaching programs are available to develop these higher-order skills; and modeling from observing experienced physicians at work are all extremely helpful.[6]

Flexibility, the other skill of central importance to higher-order interviewing, is related to clinical intuition. Flexibility in interviewing is the ability to observe the impact of interventions on patients and respond appropriately and flexibly. The most important rule of flexible interviewing is to use what works. Because every patient is somewhat different from every other patient, the skilled interviewer must be prepared to change and adapt interventions according to the needs and responses of patients. The better the observational and inferential abilities of the physician, the faster he or she will be able to decide how interventions are working and the more flexible he or she will be in altering behavior to meet the needs and responses of the patient. Flexibility can be considered under several headings: flexibility of language, style, agenda, control, advice, and function.

*Flexibility of language* concerns the physician's efforts and ability to adjust his or her use of language and concepts to a level of health literacy that is readily understood by the patient. Most doctors try to do this, but ever so often they either slip into professional jargon or oversimplify, which can cause patients to either get lost in a medical minefield or feel patronized. If in doubt, the physician should ask the patient directly for his or her view about the complexity of the language being used. (see Chapter 20).

*Flexibility of style* concerns the physician's efforts and ability to emphasize aspects of his or her personality to which the patient is most responsive. This differential responsiveness is related to transference. Some patients respond best to a doctor who is parental; others need a doctor who comes across more like a friend or peer; others, often but not always older patients, are more cooperative if the doctor's style reminds them of a helpful son or daughter. Skilled physicians modify their behavior in small ways to adapt themselves to these roles while not compromising their basic integrity or indulging in phony games.

*Flexibility of agenda* concerns the physician's adaptation of his or her agenda to fit with the patient's agenda. The highly skilled physician takes care to identify the underlying concerns and expectations that prompted the patient's visit. (see Chapter 4). For reasons that may be unconscious, these true concerns are often not expressed by the patient right away. If underlying concerns are not identified and responded to, the patient may be dissatisfied and subsequently uncooperative. In effect, the doctor's time will have been wasted.

*Flexibility of control* concerns the physician's willingness to allow the patient to dictate the process and content of the interaction to varying degrees and within the constraints of good medical care. Some patients have a strong need to feel in control and will be forthcoming and cooperative only if this need is met.

*Flexibility of advice* concerns the physician's efforts to modify his or her medical advice in the light of the patient's health beliefs and health habits. Textbook advice may strike some patients as unrealistic or downright bad, in which case they will be dissatisfied and difficult. The doctor again would be wasting time. (see Chapter 23).

*Flexibility of function* indicates the willingness and ability of the physician to shift among the three functions of the interview, depending on the patient's needs at the moment. While the physician gathers data, the patient's emotional state may demand attention, or similar emotional needs may emerge when the physician discusses a treatment plan. Skillful interviewing requires movement from one function to another as appropriate based on the *patient's* needs.

Most of the higher-order processes and skills described in this chapter can be recognized in the expert clinician more easily than they can be described or taught. Michael Polanyi's argument that much knowledge remains "tacit," that is "we know more than we can say" seems applicable to this aspect of higher order communication in the medical setting.[8] In general, complex skills can be most easily attained through clinical experience, observation of experts, self-reflection, and supervision.

# Six Rules of Integrative, Higher-Order Functioning

## 1. OBSERVE YOUR PATIENT

Observe your patient is the cardinal rule of higher-order interviewing. The skilled observer can discriminate significant and often key diagnostic and management information concerning physical as well as emotional functioning from simple observation of such things as posture, gait, position of the eyes, head, tremor, and clammy skin. (see Chapter 30). Close observation also allows the interviewer to gauge the impact of his or her questions and comments on the patient and correct any interventions that have had unintended or negative effects on the patient.

Unfortunately, "Observe your patient" is one of the most commonly violated rules. Without observing the patient closely, nonverbal signals of great importance can easily go unnoticed. Physicians who read the chart while they talk to patients often miss important clues, which can be time saving and crucial for effective diagnosis. To give one example, a very experienced and caring neurologist with whom I worked closely once interviewed a man with Parkinson's disease who started crying when the physician asked a question about his spouse. Although I was able to observe this, the physician missed this dramatic moment entirely because he was reviewing the chart at that moment.

## 2. OBSERVE YOURSELF

The skilled interviewer also pays attention to his or her own emotional reactions. (see Chapter 31). For example, a feeling of frustration, anger, sadness, anxiety, boredom, or the like should be viewed as an opportunity to enrich understanding of the patient and the current physician-patient relationship. This enriched understanding of the relationship should be viewed as a vehicle for improved efficiency and effectiveness in the encounter rather than as an obstacle to care.

Just as diagnostic hypotheses are continually generated by the data from the patients' narrative history, physicians should produce relationship hypotheses as they become aware of their own feelings in the interview. For example, physicians who notice that they feel irritated should ask themselves questions about the origin of this frustration:

1. "Why am I irritated now?"
2. "Is it just that I am tired and busy?"
3. "Is there something else about this patient that bothers me?"
4. "Is the patient responding to me like someone else I know who irritates me?" (**counter-transference**)
5. "Do I remind the patient of someone important in the patient's life that can account for this tension in the relationship?" (**transference**)

Answers, or hypotheses about answers, lead the skilled interviewer to an altered line of interventions (assessment, management, or rapport development) that results in more efficient and effective interviewing. Interviews that become more efficient and effective because of increased physician self-awareness become less problematic for the physician. (see Chapter 31).

## 3. WHEN IN DOUBT, CHECK

Checking has already been described as one of the most important basic skills of assessment (of data) (see Chapter 4). It also has special importance as a higher-order, integrative skill. When a physician notices that something is not flowing smoothly in the interview process but does not fully understand the source of the difficulty, the physician should turn to the patient for help in understanding the problem and seeking the resolution. For example:

> **PHYSICIAN:** *It seems to me, Mrs. Jones, that we're getting a little stuck on this issue of the diabetes medication. We seem to be going around in a bit of a circle. Let me repeat to you what I have heard you say so far, and then you can correct any misunderstandings or fill in any gaps.*

By reviewing the circumstances of the conversation, the physician allows the patient the opportunity to clarify the source of the problem. Furthermore, while reviewing the interaction sequence, the physician gains the time and perspective to increase his or her understanding of the difficulty and develop new strategies for interventions.

## 4. WHEN THE PATIENT DEMONSTRATES AN EMOTION, RESPOND TO IT

Although a skillful interviewer begins all interviews by building rapport, the patient, especially one with acute or chronic illness, usually experiences emotions throughout the interview. If the patient shows anxiety, anger, or sadness, for example, it is almost always best to respond to this emotion immediately. Many interviewers are afraid that they will lose time in the interview or open Pandora's box if they attend to the patient's emotions every time these feelings emerge.

> *Immediate attention to the emotional domain saves time, certainly in the long run and almost always in the short term. Emotions that are not addressed will be suppressed, only to reemerge in more distressing form later.*

This rule of good interviewing is discussed earlier in the book (see Chapter 3), regarding rapport development as a basic skill. It is repeated here because of its importance as a higher-order, integrative skill as well. Most of the difficulty that interviewers encounter with their patients can be addressed by improved attention to the emotional domain of the interview.

Focusing attention on the physician-patient relationship during the interview is a higher-order, integrative skill because it often necessitates (especially for problem patients) the flexible use of the three functions simultaneously or in rapid succession. For example, if the physician notes that the patient seems angry about a recommendation to lose weight, the physician should respond to the anger with a comment like, "It seems that my recommendations to lose weight have made you short tempered with me." The patient's response to the physician's empathic (Function One, reflection) comment will contain important information (Function Two, assessment and understanding), which the physician will need to evaluate to continue with Function Three (collaborative management) effectively.

## 5. DON'T ANSWER EVERY QUESTION IMMEDIATELY

Answering questions too quickly is a common mistake that physicians, even experienced and skillful ones, make in their everyday practices. Many questions that patients ask their physicians convey significant emotional distress. If the associated emotional distress is not addressed, the answer may not satisfy the patient, not because the answer is incorrect, but because the answer did not deal with the underlying emotional concern. For example, the patient who has been waiting too long might ask the question (with an irritated tone):

> **PATIENT:** *Doctor, I guess you've been pretty busy today?*

The doctor who answers the question without addressing the emotional concern (or loss of rapport) might say something like:

> **PHYSICIAN:** *Yes, I had some unexpected emergencies to deal with.*

This reply misses the point of the patient's frustration.

When patients ask questions that emanate from emotional distress, it is usually better to address the emotional distress first or include the response to the emotion in the answer. A better response to the patient's question about the physician's schedule might acknowledge the patient's frustration and offer an appropriate apology. For example:

> **PHYSICIAN:** *I understand your impatience and frustration. I am very sorry. I had several unexpected emergencies about which I had no choice. You now have my undivided attention.*

As another example, consider a patient with unexplained abdominal pain who asks the physician (in an anxious tone), "Doctor, what do you think is wrong with me?" The physician might be tempted to answer the question by saying something like, "Well, it could be a number of things, like irritable colon, diverticulitis, a virus, (and so on)." If the patient is afraid that he might have a cancer like his father, these answers might not be reassuring. A better response would be one that addresses the observed anxiety, for example:

> **PHYSICIAN:** *You seem quite concerned about what might be causing this problem. Can you tell me what diagnosis most worries you?*

Alternatively, rapport-building interventions such as support and partnership are often effective first responses to questions containing emotional distress. Another response to the question about abdominal discomfort might be the following:

> **PHYSICIAN:** *I will answer your question in a moment. However, before I review the diagnostic possibilities with you, I want to make it clear that I see that you are worried. I*

*want you to know that I do not see any specific possibility of anything serious that should worry you.*

Of course, this statement can be made truthfully only if the physician believes there is no serious problem.

In the event that the physician is indeed worried about a potentially serious problem, the physician should still respond to the emotion with support and partnership, as part of (or even before) answering the question. For example:

> **PHYSICIAN:** *I can see that you are worried about the possible meaning of these symptoms. I want you to know that I am going to get an answer for us just as soon as possible and that whatever we find, I will work with you to develop an appropriate management plan. These are the possibilities as I see them ...*

## 6. UNDERSTAND THAT PATIENTS ARE USUALLY FORGIVING OF MISTAKES IN THE INTERVIEW

What about physicians who violate rules of basic or higher-order interviewing? What effect does this have on their patients?

Physicians often interrupt their patients, overlook key diagnostic cues, miss important emotional messages, and deliver ambiguous management suggestions. Fortunately, for many reasons, patients are generally quite forgiving of their physicians and these mistakes.

Understanding the forgiving tendency of patients can be helpful to beginning as well as experienced clinicians who are developing or using higher-order, integrative skills. If physicians actually care about their patients and try to help, as most physicians do, this caring comes through to their patients, who generally tolerate most interviewing mistakes. The skilled physician who continually observes the patient and himself or herself will have multiple opportunities to rectify these errors. For example, consider the physician who fails to notice or respond to a patient's fear of cancer. The verbal or nonverbal expression of the fear will appear again, giving the physician a second or third chance to respond appropriately.

The tendency of unacknowledged emotions to recur underscores the importance of addressing emotional or rapport problems as soon as they appear. Despite the fear of opening the gates to a flood of emotions, early attention to emotional distress saves time. Patients are far less forgiving of the physicians whom they feel are too busy to care. These are the physicians, in fact, who get sued. Not caring is the reason most patients give for starting lawsuits against physicians.[9] It does not take a long time to demonstrate caring to most patients. Most physicians do care about their patients and demonstrate this caring intuitively without conscious recourse to basic or higher-order interviewing skills. In problematic situations, the basic skills of Function Three (Chapter Three) are almost always sufficient to facilitate physician's expression of empathic caring.

## Conclusion

This text focuses on the three core functions of the medical interview and the skills that can be used to achieve the objectives of the functions most efficiently and effectively. Although the differentiation of functions, objectives, structures, and skills is somewhat arbitrary and overlapping, the ability to delineate separate tasks, understand them, and practice them contributes to achieving a higher degree of excellence in the patient encounter. This final chapter presents an integrative overview, describing several higher-order processes and principles to guide the learner and advanced practitioner in navigating the complex pathways towards the smooth integration of structure and function in the interview.

# Summary

This final chapter discusses several higher-order communication skills that all relate to the integration of structure and function and fall within four broad concepts of diagnostic reasoning, clinical inference, communication flexibility, and "rules" of interviewing.

Six types of clinical flexibility represent higher-order skills of expert interviewers: flexibility of (1) language, (2) style, (3) control, (4) advice, (5) agenda, and (6) function. And six "rules" help guide both beginning as well as expert communication: (1) observe your patient, (2) observe yourself, (3) when in doubt, check, (4) when the patient demonstrates an emotion, respond to it, (5) don't answer every question immediately, and (6) understand that patients are usually forgiving of mistakes in the interview.

### References

1. Polanyi M: *Personal knowledge: towards a post-critical philosophy*, New York, 1968, Harper.
2. Elstein A, Shilman L, Sprafka S: *Medical problem solving: an analysis of clinical reasoning*, Cambridge, Mass, 1978, Cambridge University Press.
3. Kassirer JP: Teaching clinical reasoning: case-based and coached. *Acad Med* 85(7):1118–1124, 2010.
4. Norman G, Young M, Brooks L, Non-Analytical Models of Clinical Reasoning: The Role of Experience. *Med Educ* 41(12):1140-1145, 2007.
5. Johnson TM, Hardt ES, Kleinman A: Cultural factors in the medical interview. In Lipkin M, Jr, Putnam S, Lazare A, editors: *The medical interview: clinical care, education, and research*, New York, 1995, Springer-Verlag.
6. Elstein AS: Psychological research on diagnostic reasoning. In Lipkin M, Jr, Putnam S, Lazare A, editors: *The medical interview: clinical care, education, and research*, New York, 1995, Springer-Verlag.
7. Nurcombe B, Gallagher RM: *The clinical process in psychiatry: diagnosis and management planning*, Cambridge, Mass, 1986, Cambridge University Press.
8. Polanyi M: *The Tacit Dimension*, Chicago, 1966, University of Chicago Press.
9. Levinson W, et al: Physician-patient communication: the relationship with malpractice claims among primary care physicians and surgeons. *JAMA* 277(7):553–559, 1997.8.

## The Medical Interview: The Three Function Approach Table of Skills

| Function One: Build the Relationship | Skills | Examples |
|---|---|---|
| | Non-verbal Behavior | Attentive listening (eye-contact, forward lean, appropriate pause and silence, avoid interruptions). |
| | Reflection | *"I can see this is very difficult for you." "You seem very sad." "I know you're really irritated by what's been going on."* |
| | Legitimation | *"I can understand why you feel this way." "I think most people would feel the same way."* |
| | Support | *"I want to do whatever I can to help." "I care about what happens to you."* |
| | Partnership | *"We're in this together." "Let's work on this together."* |
| | Respect (Affirmation) | *"I'm impressed with how well you're coping under the circumstances." "I think you're doing a great job managing your illness and keeping up with everything else at the same time."* |

*P(E)ARLS: Partnership, (Empathy expressed through reflection and legitimation), Affirmation, Reflection, Legitimation, Support

| Function Two: Assess and Understand | Skills | Examples |
|---|---|---|
| | Questioning Style (Open-to-Closed Cone) | *"How can I help you today? (Open-ended question)* *"What brought you to the hospital?" (Open-ended question)* |
| | Direction/ Clarification | Can you tell me more about the back pain?" *(Directed question)* *"Does the pain go down your leg?" (Closed question)* |
| | Facilitation | *"Tell me more about ... "* *"Uh-huh"* (pause, head nod) *"Okay" (attentive silence)* |
| | Checking/ Summarizing | *"Let me review what you've been saying to make sure I've gotten it right ... "* |
| | Survey Problems | *"What else concerns you?"* *"Are there any other ways I can be of help?"* *"Is there anything else on your mind?"* |
| | Negotiate Agenda | *"There are several issues you have brought up. Which ones would you like to talk about first?"* |
| | Develop Narrative of the Problem | *"Okay, you said the back pain started about three months ago. Why don't we start from that point ... what happened next?"* |
| | Explore Patient Perspective (ICE: Ideas, Concerns, Expectations) | I: *"What ideas have you had about what might be causing your problems?"* C: *"What concerns you most about these problems?"* E: *"What are your expectations for this visit?"* |
| | Impact of Illness | *"I'd like to know how these problems have affected you day-to-day—your home life, your work, how you feel in general ... "* |

**The Medical Interview: The Three-Function Approach Table of Skills** (Continued)

| Function Three: Collaborative Management | Skills | Examples |
|---|---|---|
| | Educate (Use eTACCT) | elicit patient's baseline understanding of the problem<br>Tell patient first chunk of information (adjust for culture and literacy)<br>Ask about understanding and concerns regarding first chunk<br>Care by using relationship skills (Function One) as emotions appear<br>Counsel patient regarding information needed<br>Tell back—ask patient to review his or her understanding of information |
| | Support Self-Management (Using Brief Action Planning) | Brief Action Planning (three core questions and five associated skills)<br>1. *"Is there anything you'd like to do about your health in the next week or two?"*<br>a. SMART Behavioral Planning—specific, measurable, achievable, relevant, time-specific *(what, where, when, how often?)*<br>b. Elicit the commitment statement *"Would you mind repeating back what you just decided to do?"*<br>c. For patients needing or wanting information or ideas, offer a behavioral menu<br>2. *"About how confident do you feel that you can carry out your plan, on a 0 to 10 scale, where 0 means you are not at all confident and 10 means you are very confident?"*<br>d. If confidence is less than 7, problem solve ways to overcome barriers<br>3. *"When would you like to come back to review how you've been doing with your plan?"*<br>e. Follow-up *"So, how did it go with your plan?"* |
| | Motivational Interviewing | Two Advanced Motivational Interviewing Skills<br>1. Elicit and resolve ambivalence<br>2. Develop the discrepancy |

## The Brief Action Planning Guide
16 Jul 2013
### A Self-Management Support Tool for Chronic Conditions, Health and Wellness

*Brief Action Planning is structured around 3 core questions, below. Depending on the response, other follow-up questions may be asked. If at any point in the interview, it looks like it may not be possible to create an action plan, offer to return to it in a future interaction. Follow-up is addressed on page 297. Question #1 of Brief Action Planning is introduced in clinical interactions after rapport has been established.*

1.  Ask Question #1 to elicit ideas for change.
    *"Is there anything you would like to do for your health in the next week or two?"*

    a.  If an idea is shared and permission received, specify details as they apply to the plan. (Help the person make the plan SMART - Specific, Measurable, Achievable, Relevant and Timed).

    *"Many people find it useful to get very specific about their plan. Would that work for you?"*
    With permission, proceed.
    *"What?"* (type of activity)
    *"When?"* (time of day, day of week)
    *"Where?"*
    *"How often/long/much?"* (often: once, three times, five times; long: minutes, days; much: servings, meals)
    *"When would you like to start?"*

    b.  For individuals who want or need suggestions, offer a behavioral menu.

    i.  First ask permission to share ideas.
    *"Would you like me to share some ideas that others I've worked with have tried?"*

    ii.  Then share two to three ideas ALL AT ONCE. The ideas are not too specific, relevant to their goal and varied.
    *"Some people I have worked with have _____, others have had success with _____ or _____."*

    iii.  The last idea is always one of their own. Then ask what they want to do.
    *"Do any of these ideas work for you, or is there an idea of your own that you would like to try?"*

    iv.  If an idea is chosen, specify the details in order to make the plan SMART (above).

    c.  After the individual has made a specific plan, elicit a commitment statement.
    *"Just to make sure we both understand the details of your plan, would you mind putting it together and saying it out loud?"*

2.  Ask Question #2 to evaluate confidence. The word "sure" is a synonym for the word "confident".

    *"I wonder how sure you feel about carrying out your plan. Considering a scale of 0 to 10, where '0' means you are not at all sure and '10' means you are very confident or very sure, how sure are you about completing your plan?"*

    a.  If confidence level ≥7, go to Question #3 below. *"That's great. It sounds like a good plan for you."*

    b.  If confidence level <7, problem solve to overcome barriers or adjust plan.
    *"5 is great. That's a lot higher than 0, and shows a lot of interest and commitment. We know that when confidence is a 7 or more, people are more likely to complete their plan. Do you have any ideas about what might raise your confidence to a 7 or more?"*

    c.  If they do not have any ideas to modify the plan, ask if they would like suggestions.
    *"Would you like to hear some ideas from other people I've worked with?"*

    d.  If the response is "yes," provide two or three ideas (behavioral menu). Often the following menu applies:
    *"Sometimes people cut back on their plan, change their plan, make a new plan or decide not to make a plan. Do you think any of these work for you or is there an idea of your own?"*

    e.  If the plan is altered, repeat step 1c and Question #2 as needed to evaluate confidence with the new plan.

3.  Ask Question #3 to arrange follow-up or accountability.
    *"Sounds like a plan that's going to work for you. Most people find it helpful to check in on how it is going with their plan. Would that work for you?"*
    If they want to check in, make the follow-up plan specific as to day, time and method (phone, email, in person, etc.)

www.centreCMI.ca
1

Follow-up for Brief Action Planning

1. First ask, *"How did it go with your plan?"*

    a.  If successful recognize (affirm) their success.

    b.  If partially successful, recognize (affirm) partial success.

    c.  If little or no success, say, *"This is something that is quite common when people try something new."*

2. Then ask, *"What would you like to do next?"*

    a.  If the person wants to make a new plan, follow the steps on page 296. Use problem solving and a behavioral menu when needed.

    b.  They may want to talk about what they learned from their action plan. Reinforce learning and adapting the plan.

    c.  If the person does not want to make another action plan at this time, offer to return to action planning in the future.

---

### The Spirit of Motivational Interviewing

The Spirit of Motivational Interviewing underlies Brief Action Planning.

1. Compassion: Actively promote the other's welfare.
2. Acceptance: Respect autonomy and the right to change or not change.
3. Partnership: Work in collaboration.
4. Evocation: Ideas come from the person, not the clinician or helper.

---

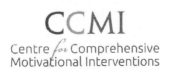

CCMI
Centre *for* Comprehensive
Motivational Interventions

*This tool was developed by Steven Cole, Damara Gutnick, Kathy Reims and Connie Davis.*

www.centreCMI.ca

2

# Learning How to Interview

There are many ways to learn better interviewing skills. A great deal depends on the level of interest, experience, and motivation of the learner and the resources and organization of the learning program.

Most of the readers of this text will be medical students or teachers of medical students. This Appendix discusses some of the educational approaches that have been used in learning about interviewing. Each of several modalities is presented with suggestions about how to use the techniques most effectively.

## Readings

Assigned reading, sometimes followed by class or group discussion, can be an invaluable source of knowledge about interviewing. Interested learners can benefit from an examination of many of the references cited throughout this text. Reading can provide a conceptual framework around which skills can be practiced and developed. However there is a clear disjunction between knowledge and the skills needed to apply this knowledge. Interviewing proficiency is a skill that can be aided by knowledge, but high degrees of knowledge do not guarantee any level of skill. Skills are most appropriately developed through the other techniques described here.

Besides providing knowledge, reading about interviewing skills can help change attitudes and dispositions to behave in certain ways. Research supporting the importance of interviewing skills in patient management and advocacy by medical leaders for interview training can help develop the attitudes that are desirable to learn for future practice.

## Lectures

The strengths and weaknesses of lectures are similar to those of reading material. Knowledge can be transmitted and attitudes can be influenced through lectures, but lectures do little toward the development of psychomotor proficiencies (i.e., skills).

## Demonstration

Demonstration plays a powerful role in influencing learner skills. The imitation model is one of the most natural and basic learning mechanisms in all animals. Whether the skill or desired behavior is interviewing, pottery, music, dancing, or almost anything else, demonstration provides an invaluable first step to learning. It is much easier for students to imitate what they actually see than to produce de novo what they are instructed to do through readings or lectures. However imitation should not be taken too literally. Direct imitation may be appropriate for learning some basic skills, but learners should also feel free to adapt what they have seen to suit their own styles. This freedom is particularly important for learning higher-order skills. Complex and higher-order skills are much subtler and cannot be easily imitated. They therefore depend a great deal more on the characteristics and style of the particular doctor.

Demonstration can be accomplished in several different ways. Learners can watch videotapes of effective interviewing or observe live demonstrations by an instructor with real patients.

Interviewing skills can also be effectively demonstrated by using role-play or standardized patient techniques.[1,2]

The most important part of effective demonstration is observing a model in discrete, digestible chunks. When the modeled behavior extends over a long time (more than 3 to 4 minutes) or contains an assortment of unclear behaviors, the model can serve more to confuse or dazzle than to aid the learner. A demonstration must be short enough for learners to remember what they saw, and it also must be structured to allow learners to analyze it in categories of behavior that are understandable and digestible.

## Practice

There is no substitute for practice. This holds true for any skill. Playing tennis, playing the piano, and performing surgery all require practice. Interviewing is the same. Interviewing can be practiced in role-play, with simulated patients, or with real patients.

Although necessary for proficiency, practice is certainly not sufficient. Just as the tennis player can develop bad habits that interfere with proficiency, so can physicians develop bad habits that interfere with their communication skills. To be maximally useful to learners, practice must be coupled with observation and feedback.

## Observation and Feedback

Learners need the opportunity to obtain feedback on their performance.[3] There are numerous ways to obtain this feedback. Most commonly, teachers offer feedback on students' performance. Motivated self-learners can audiotape or videotape their interactions with patients, review these, and become their own self-critics. Alternatively, learners can solicit feedback from colleagues. In addition, learners can request feedback from actual patients. Obtaining honest feedback from patients can be difficult, but this is possible if the learner convinces the patient that he or she is sincere in the effort to obtain both positive and negative feedback.

Feedback should be obtained immediately after the designated behavior. The longer the interval between actual performance and feedback, the lower the potential for learning. Learners should be given both positive and negative (constructive) feedback. Feedback is much more useful if it is concrete and specific. Moreover, it is usually better to give positive feedback first. Learners and teachers are too quick to focus only on the negative behaviors. To help develop skills in self-observation, learners will find it useful to give their own positive and negative feedback to themselves first and then to seek feedback from other observers.

## Re-Practice

Once a learner has obtained feedback on performance, he or she must use this feedback in repeated efforts, or re-practice. Feedback often is given in learning situations without learners having the opportunity to practice the skill again and attain a more successful outcome. An opportunity for significant learning is missed if feedback is obtained without the opportunity for repetitive practice. Repeated practice under the observation of an instructor also allows the opportunity for the learner to test whether he or she has actually mastered the problem at hand. If the learner does not succeed at this repeated attempt, he or she can be given yet another opportunity to attempt to meet the challenge at hand.

When using live patients and videotaped material, it may be difficult to obtain opportunities for immediate repetitive practice. After a review of live or videotaped patient interviews, spontaneous role-play techniques can be especially useful in crafting simulations that allow learners the opportunity for re-practice of skills that are difficult to learn.[1]

# Videotape

Videotape is an invaluable method for learners to observe their behavior with patients. Videotapes can be stopped at any point to allow for a discussion and review of specific behaviors. In addition, there is no better vehicle to discuss nonverbal communication. Both the patient's nonverbal behavior and the interviewer's nonverbal signals can be scrutinized.

Using videotape to learn interviewing has a few drawbacks. Some learners, especially those who are not skilled or confident, may be distressed by videotape-based feedback, particularly if it is given in front of their peers. Such a situation can impede learning. Videotape should be used only with some sensitivity to this issue and with some freedom of choice for the learner.

Sometimes the technology of videotape interferes with efficiency in the educational process. Ensuring that the machines are working properly, finding desired tape sections for review, and dealing with other logistical issues can take a great deal of time, time that is lost for education. When the time available for learning is limited, technology-intensive methods that take time away from actual learning should be avoided. This time might better be spent with demonstration, actual interviewing practice, role-play practice, and other "live" methods of education.

Another drawback to the use of videotape is that feedback is often delayed for a long period. The educational utility of immediate feedback may be lost when learners wait for a long time to obtain their feedback. The learner's memories of the actual event may be forgotten by the time feedback is received. Furthermore, videotape feedback is often received without providing the learner with an immediate opportunity for repeated practice.

When videotaping is used for learning interviewing, the following guidelines are suggested:

1. Sensitively negotiate the ways videotape will be used and feedback will be obtained.
2. Make sure that the equipment is working well and that valuable time is not lost with mechanical fumbling.
3. Arrange for feedback immediately or shortly after videotaping.
4. Plan for learners to use the opportunity for repetitive practice (perhaps by using role-play techniques) immediately after feedback, preferably under observation again.

# Standardized Patients

*Standardized patients* are nonpatients, often but not necessarily professional actors, who are trained to assume patient roles. Such actors and actresses can also be trained to provide students with feedback on the students' interviewing performance. Stillman and others[2,4] have used such simulated patients with great success for the teaching of interviewing and physical examination skills to medical students, house officers, and other interested learners. These simulated patients have also been used to evaluate medical students and other physicians.

When such simulators are well trained, they can repeatedly present learners with the types of patients that instructors believe to be the best training for their students. Simulated patients can be so well trained that they bear very close resemblance to actual patients. In fact, some actors actually play the roles so well that when students or house officers are "blind" to when they will interview real patients or simulated patients they may not be able to tell one from the other. However, caution is needed when standardized patients are used as teaching aids because they may not have received adequate training. When they are allowed to give independent feedback (in the absence of other instructors) to learners, their feedback may be idiosyncratic, incorrect, or even harmful to learners.

# Role-Play

Standardized patients represent a special case of the more generic use of role-play techniques.[1] Role-play, however, merits a separate section in this text because in most learning situations, it has come to mean a less formalized, less structured approach to the simulation of patient roles for communication skills training.

Role-play is a versatile technique that allows instructors to focus on particular aspects of interviewing for the benefit of demonstration, practice, or feedback. Through role-play, learners can be invited to play the role of a patient, instructors can demonstrate techniques, and learners can practice basic or advanced interviewing skills.

Like videotapes, role-play exercises can be stopped frequently for feedback. Unlike videotape, a role-play exercise can be designed for immediate feedback and repetitive practice to consolidate skills. Role-play can also be used in large groups. A small role-play exercise can be constructed for demonstration in front of a large audience. The audience can then be broken into groups of two or three to practice basic skills.

The basic drawback to role-play is that learners are sometimes anxious about participating in these exercises. Instructors who have not used the techniques before may remain unconvinced of their utility and may themselves be anxious, and therefore unconvincing and ineffective. These obstacles are easily overcome. A guide for using role-play is available,[1] and interested learners and instructors can effectively use these techniques, given some modest motivation and effort. When necessary, consultation or supervision by someone who has had role-play experience can be invaluable.

## Modified Live Patient Interviews

There is no substitute for practicing with real patients to learn good interviewing skills. Every patient is different, and the complexities of interviewing cannot be demonstrated by using only simulated patients or role-play scenarios. Practice with live patients lends a richness and credibility to training that cannot be duplicated by other techniques.

Live patient interviewing can be modified in educationally useful ways that add to the powerful effects of the method. When observed in his or her interviews with real patients, the learner has the opportunity to benefit from immediate feedback on a variety of communication techniques.

After an interview is completed, patients can be asked to provide their feedback on the learner's performance. They can tell the learner what techniques seemed to work well and what parts did not. Learners who are curious about whether patients feel that their privacy is being invaded by quality-of-life questions can ask patients about this issue directly. Patients' responses to these kinds of inquiries are often instructive and meaningful to learners.

The rotating live patient interview is a modification of live patient interviewing that has proved useful for learners. With this technique a patient is asked to allow a group of learners to interview him or her one at a time. For example, one learner might talk to the patient for about 5 minutes. He or she can pause for feedback, with or without the patient present. Then the interview can be restarted with another learner.

Live patient interviews allow students to use repetitive practice to master techniques that require more work. For example, if one learner has talked with a patient for a few minutes and the group has stopped for feedback, the patient might be willing to repeat the same interview for purposes of learning. Patients often are pleased to help in this effort to train students to become better doctors.

## Small Groups

Interviewing is best learned in groups of four to six learners. A few lectures may be useful to cover basic concepts, and some role-play may be accomplished in large groups, but close instructor feedback is invaluable for mastering key interviewing skills. A small student-to-teacher ratio allows the instructor to observe each learner and understand individual strengths and weaknesses. This effort is certainly faculty intensive, but no way has been found around this problem. Standardized patients have been used to give individualized feedback, but their usefulness is limited to the particular cases on which they have been trained. When standardized patients are allowed to give more generalized feedback, they may overstep the situations for which they have been trained. Effective learning, then, requires at least some close supervision by medical faculty.

## Learner-Centered Methods

Current educational research indicates that students may learn more effectively when they are allowed to guide their own educational efforts. This has also been called the discovery method or problem-oriented approach to education. Many exciting developments in medical education are occurring along these lines.

An educational program in communication skills lends itself well to the discovery and learner-centered process. Basic skills, however, are addressed most effectively through a creative and flexible integration of learner-centered with more traditional instructor-oriented approaches. For example, Suzuki violin, a learner-centered method for teaching basic music skills, relies greatly on independent student discovery and problem solving, but an instructor demonstrates proper finger, head, and arm positioning from the beginning. Montessori primary education, to give another learner-centered model, encourages grade school students to work independently and address topics of their own choosing at their own pace of learning. However, while encouraging this freedom, Montessori also structures the learning of basic math skills within a highly operationalized, rigid framework of materials and methods.

By analogy to the Suzuki and Montessori methods, Mack Lipkin, Jr., Craig Kaplan, and other leaders of the **American Academy on Communication in Healthcare** have pioneered approaches to learning basic interviewing skills through a flexible integration of learner- and instructor-oriented methods.[7] For example, students can and should become colleagues with their teachers at an early stage of interviewing skills training. Learners can be invited to contribute their own ideas to the goals and techniques of effective communication. A learner-centered approach repeatedly invites students to assess their level of skills and learning objectives. Furthermore, this approach suggests that learners play a role in determining with the instructor the best instructional methods for attaining their goals. Because no instructional program in interviewing can hope to attain all the objectives listed in even a basic text such as this one, instructors are encouraged to invite their students to help in determining the appropriate focus and emphasis in each instructional session, as well as the teaching methods used (e.g., live patients and role-play). The interested reader can consult relevant sources for a more detailed discussion of these topics.[5-7]

A focus on learner-centered methods should not be seen as an abdication of the instructor's responsibility to demonstrate basic techniques (such as open-ended questioning, facilitation, and reflection). Some specific interviewing techniques have been shown through research and accumulated clinical experience to be effective, and learners usually benefit from clear instruction and modeling of techniques. An analogy can be made with athletics. Consider the swing of a tennis player, usually taught through demonstration and careful imitation. However, as a tennis player advances, he or she may feel free to experiment with subtle variations of basic techniques. Similarly, basic communication skills may be modified and expanded as learners and teachers together consider the mechanism, timing, and application of their use. For all these reasons, particularly for the development of higher-order skills, learner-centered approaches can play a critical role in the development of competency in communication.

The teacher-learner relationship clearly parallels the doctor-patient relationship in several ways. In the doctor-patient relationship, there is no clearly right and wrong pattern of authority and control that is suitable for every condition and for every patient. Rather, some accept and adapt to their illness better when they are given relatively more autonomy to make decisions and to play a greater role in their overall health care. Similarly, some learners may be able to assume earlier autonomy as clinicians when they are given earlier responsibility to make decisions for their own education.

Clearly the desire or ability of patients or learners to assume more responsibility for their learning or health depends a great deal on their initial knowledge, attitudes, and skills. One common problem with encouraging patients and learners to develop confidence in their own problem-solving skills is that many are at first unwilling or unable to exercise a genuine role of autonomous decision making, with all the risks and uncertainties that this involves. In some clinical and learning situations this problem can be overcome by beginning with more structured teacher- or physician-oriented approaches. However, if the final goal is to help learners and patients achieve confidence to tackle unpredictable future problems on their own, a common educational task for both may be to move beyond early teacher- or physician-centered modes and toward patient- or learner-centered methods as the relationships unfold.

## References

1. Cohen-Cole SA: On teaching with role play.* In Lipkin M, Jr, Putnam S, Lazare A, editors: *The medical interview: clinical care, education, and research*, New York, 1995, Springer-Verlag.
2. Stillman P, et al: Results of a survey on the use of standardized patients to teach and evaluate clinical skills. *Academic Med* 65:288–292, 1990.
3. Maguire P, et al: The value of feedback in teaching interviewing skills to medical students. *Psychol Med* 8:695–704, 1978.
4. Stillman P, et al: An assessment of the clinical skills of fourth year students at four New England medical schools. *Academic Med* 65:320–326, 1990.
5. Knowles M: *The modern practice of adult education*, New York, 1980, Adult Education.
6. Burrows HS, Tamblyn RM: *Problem-based learning: an approach to medical education*, New York, 1980, Springer-Verlag.
7. Lipkin M, Jr, Kaplan C, Clark W, Novack DH: Teaching medical interviewing: the Lipkin model. In Lipkin M, Jr, Putnam S, Lazare A, editors: *The medical interview: clinical care, education, and research*, New York, 1995, Springer-Verlag.

---

*This chapter is available for download at Student Consult web site.